Stemming the Superbug Tide

JUST A FEW DOLLARS MORE

OECD
BETTER POLICIES FOR BETTER LIVES

Please cite this publication as:
OECD (2018), *Stemming the Superbug Tide: Just A Few Dollars More*, OECD Publishing, Paris.
https://doi.org/10.1787/9789264307599-en

ISBN 978-92-64-30758-2 (print)
ISBN 978-92-64-30759-9 (PDF)

The statistical data for Israel are supplied by and under the responsibility of the relevant Israeli authorities. The use of such data by the OECD is without prejudice to the status of the Golan Heights, East Jerusalem and Israeli settlements in the West Bank under the terms of international law.

Photo credits:
Cover © Jezper/Shutterstock.com

Corrigenda to OECD publications may be found on line at: *www.oecd.org/about/publishing/corrigenda.htm*.

Foreword

Antimicrobial resistance (AMR) jeopardises the effectiveness of many of the most valuable medical and public health advances achieved in the twentieth century. It occurs when the microbes that cause disease evolve so that the medicines which used to kill them no longer work. In 2016, the high-level meeting of United Nation's General Assembly acknowledged AMR as a fundamental threat to the health of populations, the global economy and society as a whole. It also highlighted the need for countries to urgently put in place policies to tackle AMR and prevent its disastrous consequences.

The Organisation for Economic Co-operation and Development (OECD) has been asked by its Member countries to assess which actions should be taken to prevent the emergence and spread of AMR, and to help governments to implement them. This report responds to that mandate and to a call from the European Commission – as part of its global strategy to tackle AMR – to conduct a health economic evaluation of AMR, determine its current and long-term public health and economics consequences, and assess the effectiveness and cost-effectiveness of public policies to contain it. The findings presented in this publication identify 'best buys' – i.e. affordable, feasible and highly cost-effective interventions – among control policy options for AMR in the human health sector.

This publication presents a series of novel analyses to guide countries in their policy-making process. The OECD has used advanced analytical approaches – including microsimulation and ensemble modelling techniques – to provide a precise assessment of the potential impact of public policy options to address AMR. The country-specific results reported, represent the most comprehensive and detailed assessment of AMR health and economic effects that have yet been undertaken in different national contexts. For the first time, empirical evidence is presented showing that AMR can be reduced significantly and its burden on population health and healthcare expenditure drastically reduced.

The work presented in this report was conducted by the OECD in close collaboration with the European Centre for Disease Prevention and Control, who provided expertise and valuable epidemiological data on AMR. It also benefited greatly from inputs and comments from member countries and various stakeholders. The Health Committee and one of its subsidiary bodies, the Expert Group on the Economics of Public Health, oversaw the preparation of the report. It is published under the responsibility of the Secretary General of the OECD, and does not necessarily reflect the views of individual member states.

Acknowledgements

The Organisation for Economic Co-operation and Development (OECD) work on antimicrobial resistance (AMR) was conducted on behalf of its Health Committee, between 2016 and 2018. Michele Cecchini oversaw the project and coordinated the production of the final report. He also led Chapters 1 and 5. Chapter 2 was led by Michael Padget. Chapter 3 was led by Tiago Cravo Oliveira. Driss Ait Ouakrim contributed to Chapter 1, and led Chapters 4 and 6. Mario Jendrossek, Stella Danek and Jennifer Deberardinis supported the main authors and contributed to different sections of the report. Invaluable editorial assistance was provided by Lucy Hulett and Suzanne Parandian.

However, many more people deserve credit for the work presented in this book than those listed as its authors. The production of this report benefited greatly from the inputs and comments received from other OECD colleagues, national experts, member states representatives and other stakeholders.

Among OECD colleagues, the authors would like to thank Chris James and Yevgeniy Goryakin for their advice on methodological issues as well as Sabine Vuik and Victoria Simpkin for their help in data preparation. Thank you also to Thierry Pellegrini, Aliénor Lerouge and Arnaud Atoch for their support on IT, software and programming issues – their contribution was critical to the various analyses and allowed us to speed up processing time and effectively manage very large quantities of data. Lukasz Lech and Guillaume Haquin did their best to minimise authors' time on administrative issues letting them work on the content. Paul Gallagher and Spencer Wilson were of great help in sharpening the key messages from this work. Stefano Scarpetta, Mark Pearson and Francesca Colombo provided senior leadership and advice throughout the project. Michael Ryan, from the Directorate of Trade and Agriculture, provided inputs and comments on issues related to use of antimicrobials in the livestock sector and 'One-Health' matters.

A special thank goes to our colleagues at the European Centre for Disease Prevention and Control (ECDC), namely Alessandro Cassini, Diamantis Plachouras, Liselotte Diaz Högberg and Dominique Monnet. Outputs presented in this book are an outstanding example of how open and constructive collaboration between intergovernmental organisations can provide added value for member countries and beyond. A significant share of the input data used to feed the OECD modelling work and to replicate AMR dynamics in European Countries was provided by ECDC and by national experts part of ECDC networks. In particular, the authors acknowledge the work performed by the staff of the participating clinical microbiology laboratories and of the national healthcare services that provided data to EARS-Net. The authors would also like to thank all the hospitals participating in the PPS 2011-2012 and in particular, the hospital staff that collected, validated and entered the data during the survey, and the national teams that coordinated the survey in each participating country.

Special thanks go to Charles Price (European Commission) and Jurgita Kaminskaite (Consumers, Health, Agriculture and Food Executive Agency of the European Commission) that followed the development of the project since its conceptualisation and provided inputs throughout on their respective areas of expertise.

The OECD maintains a close partnership with the World Health Organization (WHO) in its work on public health and authors would like to thank Elizabeth Tayler (World Health Organization), Saskia Andrea Nahrgang and Danilo Lo Fo Wong (WHO-Europe) for their inputs and comments on the different drafts of the report.

Many thanks also to the various experts who provided data and guidance on national AMR maters. In particular, Prof. Kathy Meleady and Prof. John Turnidge for Australia, experts from the Canadian Antimicrobial Resistance Alliance, Dr. Eili Klein from the Center for Disease Dynamics, Economics & Policy (CDDEP), Anna Dean from WHO, Dr. Melanie Colomb-Cotinat from France for their inputs in the calculation of AMR rates in a number of countries. Sonja Pierzchalski, Marisol Escudero Martinez, Dr. Michelle Alfa, Dr. Stephanie J. Dancer, Catherine Passaretti, Trish M Perl and Dr. Geraldine Conlon-Bingham provided inputs to the preparation of Chapter 5 and made available additional data, based on their own work.

Preliminary versions of the chapters of this book were presented and discussed at two meetings of the OECD Expert Group on the Economics of Public Health (EGEPH) chaired by Cristina Gutierrez Delgado and Brian Ferguson and by country delegates participating to the OECD Health Committee chaired by Bjorn-Inge Larsen and Olivia Wingzell. Country experts and delegates are too many to name individually, but authors would like to thank in particular delegates from Australia, Canada, Costa Rica, France, Germany, Ireland, Luxembourg, Italy, Japan, Switzerland and the European Commission for their constructive comments throughout the process. In addition, authors would like to acknowledge useful comments from the Business and Industry Advisory Committee to the OECD (BIAC) and the Trade Union Advisory Committee to the OECD (TUAC).

The work was funded through regular contributions from OECD member countries and received partial support from grants from the Health Programme of the European Union, from the Department of Health of Australia and from the Federal Ministry of Health of Germany.

Disclaimers

The contents of this book do not necessarily reflect the views of individual OECD member countries, or those of the European Commission.

This publication has been produced with the financial and substantive assistance of the European Union. The contents of this report are the sole responsibility of the OECD and can in no way be taken to reflect the views of the European Union.

The views and opinions of the authors expressed herein do not necessarily state or reflect those of ECDC. The accuracy of the authors' statistical analysis and the findings they report are not the responsibility of ECDC. ECDC is not responsible for conclusions or opinions drawn from the data provided. ECDC is not responsible for the correctness of the data and for data management, data merging and data collation after provision of the data. ECDC shall not be held liable for improper or incorrect use of the data.

Table of contents

Tables

Figures

Boxes

Acronyms and abbreviations

3GCREC	Third-generation cephalosporin-resistant *Escherichia coli*
3GCRKP	Third-generation cephalosporin-resistant *Klebsiella pneumoniae*
AMR	Antimicrobial resistance
AUD	Australian Dollar
BAPCOC	Belgian Antimicrobial Policy Coordination Committee
BC	British Columbia
CAD	Canadian Dollar
CEASAR	Central Asian and Eastern European Surveillance of Antimicrobial Resistance
CDC	Centers for Disease Control and Prevention
CDDEP	Center for Disease Dynamics, Economics & Policy
CRE	Carbapenem-resistant *Enterobacteriaceae*
CRKP	Carbapenem-resistant *Klebsiella pneumoniae*
CRP	C-reactive protein
CRPA	Carbapenem-resistant *Pseudomonas aeruginosa*
DALY	Disability Adjusted Life Year
DDD	Defined daily dose
DNA	Deoxyribonucleic acid
EARS-Net	European Antimicrobial Resistance Surveillance Network
ECDC	European Centre for Disease Prevention and Control
EEA	European Economic Area
EFSA	European Food Safety Authority
EHD	Extra Hospital Days
EMA	European Medicines Agency
ESAC-Net	European Surveillance of Antimicrobial Consumption Network
ESBL	Extended spectrum beta-lactamases
ESVAC	European Surveillance of Veterinary Antimicrobial Consumption
EU	European Union
EUR	Euro
FAO	Food and Agriculture Organization of the United Nations
FDA	US Food and Drug Administration
FREC	Fluoroquinolone-resistant *Escherichia coli*
G20	Group of 20
GBP	Great British Pounds
GDP	Gross domestic product
GLASS	Global Antimicrobial Resistance Surveillance System

Hib	*Haemophilus influenzae* type b
ICER	Incremental Cost-Effectiveness Ratio
IFPMA	International Federation of Pharmaceutical Manufacturers & Associations
INTERPOL	The International Criminal Police Organization
ISIC	International Standard Industrial Classification
LMIC	low and middle-income country
MRSA	Methicillin-resistant *Staphylococcus aureus*
NICE	National Institute for Health and Care Excellence
OECD	Organization for Economic Co-operation and Development
OIE	World Organization for Animal Health
PCV	Pneumococcal conjugate vaccine
PPP	Purchasing Power Parity
PRSP	Penicillin-resistant *Streptococcus pneumoniae*
R&D	Research and development
RDT	Rapid Diagnostic Test
SDGs	Sustainable Development Goals
SPHeP-AMR	Strategic Public Health Planning for Antimicrobial Resistance
TB	Tuberculosis
TRNC	Turkish Republic of Northern Cyprus
UK	United Kingdom
UN WPP	United Nations World Population Prospects
US	United States
USD	US Dollar
USD PPP	US Dollar purchasing power parity
UV	Ultraviolet
VRE	Vancomycin-resistant *Enterococcus faecalis* and *Enterococcus faecium*
WHO	World Health Organization

Executive summary

Around 2.4 million people could die in Europe, North America and Australia between 2015-2050 due to superbug infections unless more is done to stem antibiotic resistance. However, three out of four deaths from superbug infections could be averted by spending just USD 2 per person a year on measures as simple as handwashing and more prudent prescription of antibiotics. A short-term investment to stem the superbug tide would save lives and money in the long-run.

A five-pronged assault on antimicrobial resistance -- by promoting better hygiene, ending over-prescription of antibiotics, rapid testing for patients to determine whether they have viral or bacterial infections, delays in prescribing antibiotics and mass media campaigns – – could counter one of the biggest threats to modern medicine. A package of policies to promote hospital hygiene and policies to reduce over-prescription of antibiotics, including stewardship programmes, mass media campaigns and use of tests in general practice to detect whether an infection is bacterial or viral could save up to 1.6 million lives by 2050 across the 33 countries included in the OECD analysis. The investment in these policies would pay for itself within a year, and end up by saving 4.8 billions of dollars per year.

The challenge of growing resistance

Rising rates of Antimicrobial resistance (AMR) – the ability of bacteria to resist antimicrobials – will become a growing concern across the OECD and EU28 countries[1] unless governments embrace a more robust response to the threat, with babies and the elderly most at risk. Even small cuts in the kitchen, minor surgery or diseases like pneumonia could become life threatening.

AMR is primarily driven by inappropriate use of antimicrobials, including antibiotics, in human health, agriculture and livestock production and by contamination of the environment. The main focus of this report is tackling AMR in the human health sector. However, actions to promote prudent use of antimicrobials and to prevent the spread of existing infections in humans should be combined with similar actions in other sectors, in a truly "One Health" framework.

Dealing with AMR complications could cost up to USD 3.5 billion a year on average across the 33 countries included in the analysis, unless countries step up their fight against superbugs.

Of the 2.4 million people who could die in Europe, North America and Australia between 2015 and 2050, according to calculations from the new OECD model, if AMR rates follow the projected trend, southern Europe will be particularly affected. Italy, Greece and Portugal are forecast to top the list of OECD countries with the highest mortality rates from AMR while the United States, Italy and France would have the highest absolute death rates with almost 30 000 AMR deaths a year forecast in the United States alone.

In low and middle-income countries, resistance is already high and AMR is projected to grow more rapidly than in OECD countries. For example, in Indonesia, Brazil and the Russian Federation, between 40% and 60% of infections are already resistant, compared to an average of 17% in OECD countries. In the same countries, growth of AMR rates is forecast to be 4 to 7 times faster than growth in OECD countries between now and 2030. Such high resistance rates in health care systems, which are already weakened by constrained budgets, will create the conditions for an enormous death toll that will be mainly borne by new-borns, very young children and the elderly population.

Effective antibiotics are vital to modern medicine. Patients undergoing chemotherapy or transplants, for example, rely on antibiotics to prevent infections and complications. But growing antimicrobial resistance after half a century of over-prescription of antibiotics is raising concern that hospitals will run out of options to save lives, particularly with resistance to all three lines of antibiotics set to increase.

Bacteria resistant to specific antibiotics cause almost one in five infections in OECD and EU28 countries. Resistance will grow further unless action is taken.

While resistance proportions for eight high-priority antibiotic-bacterium combinations[2] increased from 14% in 2005 to 17% in 2015 across OECD countries, there were pronounced differences between countries:

- The average resistance proportions in Turkey, Korea and Greece (about 35%) were seven times higher than in Iceland, Netherlands and Norway, the countries with the lowest proportions (about 5%).
- For some antibiotic-bacterium combinations, as little as one in every four infections was caused by bacteria susceptible (i.e. not resistant) to drug treatment in certain OECD countries.
- Outside OECD countries, resistance proportions in 2015 were nearly double, 29%, across the same eight antibiotic-bacterium combinations, but could be above 42% in India, the People's Republic of China and the Russian Federation.

The projections produced by the OECD suggest that resistance proportions for eight antibiotic-bacterium combinations could increase from 17% in 2015 to 18% in 2030 across OECD countries.

Despite projected reductions in average resistance in Canada, Japan and Mexico, no single country is projected to reduce resistance for all eight antibiotic-bacterium combinations. Rather, some countries including Denmark, Iceland, Luxembourg and Slovenia, could see resistance increase in all eight antibiotic-bacterium combinations.

Average resistance growth seems to be slowing down, but there are serious causes for concern. Across the OECD, resistance to second and third-line antibiotics – which present the final line of defence to prevent infections – is expected to be 70% higher in 2030, compared to AMR rates in 2005. Across EU28 countries, resistance to third-line treatments will double in the same period. Resistance to second-line treatments, such as third-generation cephalosporins and fluoroquinolones, is expected to increase in a majority of countries, leading to greater consumption of carbapenems, and potentially promoting carbapenem resistance. In some countries, resistance to the last line of treatment – polymyxins – is already emerging with potentially catastrophic consequences. Growth in resistance among difficult-to-treat microorganisms, like Enterococci and Pseudomonas aeruginosa, is also worrisome.

AMR will have an enormous impact on population health and healthcare budgets

While more than two million lives would be at risk due to AMR in Europe, North America and Australia by 2050, superbugs could also have significant impact on the quality of people's lives.

The impact on quality of life, measured through disability-adjusted life years (DALYs), will be even larger. Southern Europe (Italy, Greece and Portugal in particular) would be the most affected. In the case of Italy, for example, up to one person in every 205 would lose one year of life in good health due to AMR.

Children and the elderly are most vulnerable. The probability of developing a resistant infection is significantly higher for children up to 12 months of age and among adults aged 70 and above. Men are also more likely to develop resistant infections than women.

The unchecked rise of superbugs would also significantly dent healthcare budgets.

Every year between 2015 and 2050, up to USD 3.5 billion (adjusted for differences in prices across countries, expressed as purchasing power parities or PPPs) is expected to be spent on average between 2015 and 2050 on AMR-related complications across 33 OECD and EU28 countries, according to calculations from the OECD model.

That corresponds to 10% of health care costs caused by communicable diseases, or to about USD PPP 2.4 per capita per year on average, with about USD PPP 6.2-6.6 per capita in Italy and the United States.

Policy solutions exist

The growing resistance to the second and third line of treatment is an extremely worrying scenario, as it means that, de facto, we are exhausting our antibiotics armoury.

However, governments could counter the problem with five main types of affordable solutions as part of a coherent package. The OECD model was used to identify "best buys" to tackle AMR in 33 OECD and EU28 countries. The set of policies assessed were aligned with the World Health Organization's (WHO) global action plan on AMR. Offering value for money, these "best buys" could significantly diminish the personal and economic cost of AMR.

- The first intervention would be to improve hygiene in healthcare facilities, including promotion of handwashing and better hospital hygiene.
- The second would be stewardship programmes promoting more prudent use of antibiotics to end decades of over-prescription.
- The third would be the use of rapid diagnostic tests to detect whether an infection is bacterial or viral.
- The fourth solution would be delayed prescription.
- The fifth would be public awareness campaigns.

Investment in these measures could pay for themselves within just one year and produce savings of about USD 1.5 for every dollar invested thereafter.

Simple measures, such as promoting hand washing and better hygiene in healthcare facilities more than halve the risk of death and decrease the health burden of AMR –

measured in DALYs – by about 40%, compared to a scenario in which no policy is in place in the 33 countries included in the study.

Promoting more prudent use of antibiotics through stewardship programmes is also particularly effective, producing similar results to hygiene improvements. Other interventions designed to tackle AMR outside hospitals such as delayed prescriptions, the use of rapid diagnostic tests to stop guessing if an infection is viral and bacterial and mass media campaigns would have a more limited impact on health but remain important polices to address a multifaceted and complex phenomenon.

All these interventions are affordable for OECD countries and, in some cases, for countries at lower level of income.

- Mass media campaigns, delayed prescriptions and improved hand hygiene cost from as little as USD PPP 0.3 up to USD PPP 2.7 per capita in many OECD countries.
- Interventions that are not particularly expensive, such as improved hand hygiene and mass media campaigns are also affordable in countries at lower level of income.
- More resource-intense interventions can cost up to a few hundred USD PPP per hospitalised patient, as in the case of actions to improve hygiene in health facilities.

Delayed prescriptions, improved hand hygiene and most stewardship programmes generate health care savings that are higher than the implementation cost of the intervention, according to the OECD model. They are therefore all cost-effective 'best buy' investments to tackle AMR. What is more, if they are implemented together, by combining policies into a coherent strategy, produce an even bigger impact.

The OECD analysis considered three main packages of interventions.

- The first, for hospitals (including improved hand hygiene, stewardship programmes and enhanced environmental hygiene in health care settings).
- The second one consisting of community actions (including delayed prescriptions, mass media campaigns and use of rapid diagnostic tests).
- The third one consists of a mixed intervention package (including stewardship programmes, enhanced environmental hygiene, mass media campaigns, and use of rapid diagnostic tests).

These packages would reduce the burden of disease from AMR by, respectively, 85%, 23% and 73%, while producing savings of USD PPP 4.1, 0.9 and 3 per capita per year.

In practice, this would mean millions of people in these countries would avoid AMR-related complications and health problems.

Key findings

- In 2015, about 17% of infections in OECD countries were due to bacteria resistant to antibiotics. But in four countries, more than one-third were resistant to antibiotics. In some G20 countries, including China, India and the Russian Federation, more than 40% of infections are due to bacteria resistant to some antibiotics.
- Around 2.4 million individuals could die in Europe, North America and Australia between 2015 and 2050 due to AMR.

- Between 2015 and 2050, AMR would cost about USD PPP 3.5 billion per year to the healthcare services of the 33 countries included in the analysis. This would correspond to USD PPP 2.4 per capita or, roughly, about 10% of the healthcare budget devoted to communicable diseases.
- If no effective public health action is put in place, AMR rates will grow further. Resistance to second and third-line antibiotics is forecast to grow the most, with AMR rates in 2030 projected to be 70% higher than in 2005 in OECD countries. In EU28, resistance to third-line antibiotics is forecast to double in the same period.
- A five-pronged assault on antimicrobial resistance -- by promoting better hygiene, ending over-prescription of antibiotics, rapid testing for patients to determine whether they have viral or bacterial infections, delays in prescribing antibiotics and mass media campaigns – is vital to stem the superbug tide.
- Policies to promote handwashing, hospital hygiene and stewardship programmes to reduce over-prescription of antibiotics could save between 35 000 to 38 000 lives per year across the 33 countries included in the analysis.
- Mass media campaigns, delayed prescriptions and the use of rapid diagnostic tests also produce a positive health impact, albeit more limited.
- Public health actions to tackle AMR are affordable. Implementing such policies varies from as little as USD PPP 0.3 per capita for mass media campaigns to a few hundred USD PPP per hospitalised patient in the case of enhanced hygiene in healthcare.
- All the assessed interventions are "best buys" to tackle AMR in the assessed countries given their high impact on population health, affordability to implement, and excellent cost-effectiveness ratio. Savings from delayed prescriptions, improved hand hygiene and, in most cases, from stewardship programmes exceed the cost of implementation.
- A package comprising hospital interventions; one consisting of community actions and a mixed intervention package would respectively avert around 1.3 million, 0.4 million and 1.1 million DALYs and 55 000, 14 000, and 47 000 life years saved across the 33 countries included. The *hospital-based package* would result in an annual average net saving (i.e. after accounting for the implementation cost of each intervention) of USD PPP 4.1 per capita across the 33 included countries. *Community-based interventions* would also result in an average annual saving of around USD PPP 0.9 per capita across the 33 included countries. The *mixed policy approach* would cost about USD PPP 2 per capita per year leading to an average net saving of around USD PPP 3 per capita per year.

Notes

[1] The OECD and EU28 countries included in the analysis are: Australia, Austria, Belgium, Bulgaria, Canada, Croatia, Cyprus, Czech Republic, Denmark, Estonia, Finland, France, Germany, Greece, Hungary, Iceland, Ireland, Italy, Latvia, Lithuania, Luxembourg, Malta, Netherland, Norway, Poland, Portugal, Romania, Slovakia, Slovenia, Spain, Sweden, United Kingdom and the United States.

[2] The eight antibiotic-bacterium combinations included in the analysis are: third-generation cephalosporin-resistant *Escherichia coli*, fluoroquinolones-resistant *Escherichia coli*, penicillin-resistant *Streptococcus pneumoniae*, methicillin-resistant *Staphylococcus aureus*, carbapenem-resistant *Klebsiella pneumoniae*, third-generation cephalosporin-resistant *Klebsiella pneumoniae*, carbapenem-resistant *Pseudomonas aeruginosa*, and vancomycin-resistant *Enterococcus faecalis* and *Enterococcus faecium*

Chapter 1. Antimicrobial resistance: A large and growing problem

Michele Cecchini and Driss Ait Ouakrim

Antimicrobial resistance (AMR) is a large and growing problem with the potential for enormous health and economic consequences, globally. As such, AMR has become a central issue at the top of the public health agenda of OECD countries and beyond. This chapter brings together the main messages of this publication and describes the key policy implications from new OECD analyses on the health and economic burden of AMR and on innovative actions to fight this top public health issue. The chapter presents AMR trends and projections in 52 OECD, Group of Twenty (G20) and European Union (EU) countries and makes a strong economic case to upscale investments in policies to promote prudent use of antibiotics in the human health sector and in policies to prevent the spread of infections. The chapter concludes by presenting the expected effectiveness, impact on healthcare expenditure and cost-effectiveness of such policies in 33 OECD and EU countries.

Key findings

- Despite being a natural phenomenon, antimicrobial resistance (AMR) became a prominent public health issue only in recent times, when an increasing share of infections proved to be resistant to available therapeutic options and the number of new antimicrobials reaching the market dropped significantly.
- AMR may develop and spread through exposure to antimicrobials in a number of settings including the human population in a community setting or in hospital, the animal sector or in the environment. The causes of the current growth in AMR rates are largely driven by human activity.
- In 2017, around 17% of bacterial infections in OECD countries were resistant to antibiotics; but in some countries, more than one-third of infections are resistant. In some Group of Twenty (G20) countries, more than 40% of infections are resistant to some antibiotics.
- If no effective public health actions are put in place, AMR rates are forecasted to grow further. The most worrying trend is that resistance to second and third-line antibiotics is forecast to grow the most, with AMR rates in 2030 projected to be 70% higher than in 2005.
- Around 2.4 million individuals could die in Europe, North America and Australia between 2015 and 2050 due to AMR; AMR would cost about USD PPP 3.5 billion per year to the healthcare services of this group of countries.
- Countries can put in place effective and cost-effective interventions to tackle AMR. Policies to promote hand washing, to enhance hygiene in healthcare facilities and stewardship programmes in healthcare facilities could avert between 34 931 and 37 836 deaths per year across the 33 countries included in the analysis. Other interventions such as mass media campaigns, delayed prescriptions and use of rapid diagnostic tests produce a positive, but more limited, health impact.
- Implementation costs for public health actions to tackle AMR vary between as little as USD PPP 0.3 per capita for mass media campaigns to a few hundred USD PPP per individual in the case of enhanced hygiene in healthcare services. Consistently across countries, all the assessed interventions show excellent cost-effectiveness ratios. Delayed prescriptions, improved hand hygiene and, often, stewardship programmes are cost saving.
- Based on their high effectiveness on population health, affordability to implement and excellent cost-effectiveness ratio, virtually all the assessed interventions can be defined as "best buys" to tackle AMR in the assessed countries.

1.1. Antimicrobial resistance: a growing threat to modern medicine

No innovation in the 20th century was more important to medicine than the discovery of antimicrobials. These "miracle drugs" introduced as therapeutic agents in the 1940s allowed for effective management and treatment of long-feared diseases such as tuberculosis, bacterial pneumonia, and sepsis and led to greatly improved survival and patient health outcomes.

However, today these health gains are at risk due to the development and spread of antimicrobial resistance (AMR). Pathogens which develop resistance may survive the effects of antimicrobials[1] making subsequent infections difficult or even impossible to treat and dramatically increasing the risk of developing complications and dying. The current rise of AMR and these very hard to treat infections threatens to turn back the clock on infectious disease gains and lead us toward a "post-antibiotic" world where minor infections can once again lead to fatal outcomes.

Further, once a bacterial strain develops resistance to an antimicrobial, this ability to resist antibiotics spreads rapidly. Fuelled by increasing mobility and globalisation, resistant infections can travel far and very quickly (Hawkey, 2008[1]). For instance, a carbapenem-resistant strain of *Klebsiella pneumoniae* (*K. pneumoniae*) needed only five years to spread globally from the United States, where it was first identified in 2003, to Israel in 2005 and to the United Kingdom, Italy and Colombia, in 2008 (McKenna, 2013[2]).

Despite being a process hundreds of times older than the humankind, AMR became a prominent public health issue only very recently. Overuse and inappropriate use of antimicrobials in humans (Cecchini and Lee, 2017[3]) and in the agricultural sector (FAO, 2016[4]) are key drivers underlying the growth of AMR. While, in the past, new antimicrobials were continuously made available to replace those becoming ineffective, now antimicrobials are progressively becoming more difficult to develop – only 1.5% of antibiotics in preclinical development reach the market (OECD et al., 2017[5]) – and the number of therapeutic options to treat common infections is significantly decreasing. Furthermore, clinical development of promising candidates is becoming more expensive and the business case and limited return on investment lead to declining private investment in AMR-relevant research and development (R&D) activities. This has led many pharmaceutical companies to abandon this business and, consequently, the number of new antimicrobials entering the market has decreased significantly (OECD et al., 2017[5]).

By using advanced statistical techniques, the OECD has analysed patterns and historical trends for eight key antibiotic-bacterium combinations and has projected historical trends up to 2030. Findings from these analyses are presented in the reminder of Section 1.1.

1.1.1. Almost one in five infections is caused by bacteria resistant to specific antibiotics in OECD and European Union (EU) countries and resistance proportions are expected to grow further if no effective action is put in place

The umbrella term AMR includes many different types of antimicrobial resistance. In principle, the list of antibiotic-bacterium combinations can be extremely extensive, although the World Health Organization (WHO) recognises that the majority of the health burden is caused by a relatively limited number of organisms including: *Escherichia coli (E. coli)*, *Klebsiella pneumoniae (K. pneumoniae)*, *Staphylococcus aureus (S. aureus)*, *Streptococcus pneumoniae (S. pneumoniae)*, *Nontyphoidal Salmonella*, *Shigella*, *Neisseria gonorrhoeae*, *Mycobacterium tuberculosis* and *Plasmodium malariae* (WHO, 2014[6])[2]. More recently, WHO complemented this list of microorganisms with a list of 12 antibiotic-bacterium combinations for which there is an urgent need to produce new antimicrobials due to the high AMR rates and limited new therapeutic options in the R&D pipeline (WHO, 2017[7]).

Cross-country comparability of AMR data is difficult, due to the varying use of multiple drugs, standards, guidelines, methods and equipment in different parts of the world. However, the development of guidelines, as well as the establishment of international surveillance networks, such as EARS-Net (the European Antimicrobial Resistance

Surveillance Network), CEASAR (Central Asian and Eastern European Surveillance of Antimicrobial Resistance), GLASS (Global Antimicrobial Resistance Surveillance System) and ATLASS (Assessment Tool for Laboratory and Antimicrobial Surveillance Systems) have facilitated the collection and aggregation of international data on AMR.

The OECD used advanced statistical techniques to analyse and forecast data on AMR for eight high-priority antibiotic-bacterium combinations[3] for 52 countries. Results point to high resistance proportions across the globe:

- Between 2005 and 2015, estimated resistance proportions for eight high-priority antibiotic-bacterium combinations increased from 14% in 2005 to 17% in 2015 across OECD countries. The average resistance proportions in the countries with the highest resistance proportions (about 35% in Turkey, Korea and Greece) were five times higher than in countries with the lowest proportions (around 5% in Iceland, Netherlands and Norway). For some antibiotic-bacterium combinations, in certain OECD countries, only one in every four infections was caused by bacteria susceptible (i.e. not resistant) to drug treatment.
- Outside OECD countries, resistance proportions in 2015 were estimated at 29% across the same eight antibiotic-bacterium combinations, but could be in excess of 42% in India, the People's Republic of China and the Russian Federation. For some country-antibiotic-bacterium combinations, only 20% of infections were caused by bacteria susceptible to drug treatment.
- Within the EU, the average resistance proportion was 18% with countries in Eastern and Southern Europe generally showing higher resistance proportions, compared to countries in Northern and Western Europe.
- Members of the G20 averaged higher resistance proportions of 30%, while key partners of the OECD[4] had the highest estimated average resistance proportions, at 41%.

According to the OECD analyses, between 2005 and 2015, only seven countries were estimated to have achieved reductions in average resistance proportions. In Switzerland, the United Kingdom, Japan, Belgium, Germany, Iceland and Canada, resistance proportions went down by an average of 2.5 percentage points, across the eight antibiotic-bacterium combinations. However, not a single country, including those just mentioned, achieved reductions in all eight antibiotic-bacterium combinations. In contrast, in eight countries (Brazil, China, Peru, Argentina, Colombia, Saudi Arabia, Israel and the Russian Federation) resistance proportions are estimated to have increased for all eight antibiotic-bacterium pairs between 2005 and 2015. In Italy and the Slovak Republic, average resistance proportions went up by 13 percentage points.

A large majority of countries have seen both increases and reductions in drug resistance, depending on the microorganism and antimicrobial agent being considered. In France, for example, the proportion of *K. pneumoniae* resistant to third-generation cephalosporins increased by an estimated 27 percentage points (from 5% to 32%, a growth rate of 540%) while the proportion of *S. pneumoniae* resistant to penicillin went down by 13 percentage points over the same ten years (from 36% to 23%, a growth rate of -36%).

Taking resistance proportions in 2005 as the base value and averaging country-specific growth rates, resistance proportions for methicillin-resistant *S. aureus* (MRSA) went down by an estimated 17% across OECD countries, while the share of *E. coli* resistant to third-generation cephalosporins grew by an estimated 222%. On average across all eight antibiotic-bacterium combinations, growth rates varied between 140% (in Italy and the United States) and -10% (in Belgium). In non-OECD countries, the range was even bigger, indicating significant heterogeneity in the evolution of resistance proportions across countries, microorganisms and antimicrobial agents between 2005 and 2015.

1.1.2. AMR is projected to keep growing at least until 2030, with resistance to second and third-line antibiotics expected to grow the most

The projections produced with the OECD model suggest that, should antibiotic consumption, economic and population growth, and out-of-pocket health spending evolve along the trends observed in the past, and should no policy action be taken, resistance proportions for eight antibiotic-bacterium combinations are estimated to increase moderately from 17% in 2015 to 18% in 2030 across OECD countries. Despite reductions in average resistance proportions in some countries, no single country is projected to reduce resistance proportions for all eight antibiotic-bacterium combinations. On the other hand, in some countries, resistance proportions could increase in all eight antibiotic-bacterium combinations.

There will continue to be significant heterogeneity across not only countries and regions, but also antibiotic-bacterium pairs. For example, while growth in third-generation cephalosporin resistance in *K. pneumoniae* and *E. coli* will slow down significantly compared to the last decade, growth in vancomycin resistance among *Enterococci* is projected to accelerate in most OECD countries. MRSA could continue to decline in OECD countries overall while actually growing in EU countries. Growth in carbapenem-resistant *K. pneumoniae* proportions is projected for all regions but could be especially great in G20 countries.

While average growth rates seem to be slowing down, there are causes for concern. The OECD model suggests that resistance to second-line treatments, such as third-generation cephalosporins and fluoroquinolones, is expected to increase in a majority of countries, leading to greater consumption of carbapenems and potentially promoting carbapenem resistance. In some countries, resistance to the last line of treatment – polymyxins – is already emerging with potentially disastrous consequences. Growth in resistance proportions among difficult-to-treat microorganisms, like *Enterococci* and *P. aeruginosa*, is also worrisome. Overall, across OECD countries, resistance to second and third-line antibiotics is expected to be 70% higher in 2030, compared to AMR rates in 2005 for the same antibiotic-bacterium combinations. Similar trends are projected for G20 countries and for resistance to second-line treatments in EU countries. Should trends continue, resistance to the last line of treatment is expected to more than double in EU countries in the period 2005 30.

1.2. Factors underpinning the growth of AMR rates

The cause of the current exacerbation of growth in AMR rates is largely driven by human activity and is two-fold. On the pathogen level, AMR may develop and spread through exposure to antimicrobials in a number of settings including among humans in the community or healthcare setting, in the animal sector, or in the environment (e.g. waste treatment). The combination of resistance across sectors creates a global population of resistant bacteria which may be transferred within and among sectors including to and from humans. On the human level, a number of different factors may influence the probability of being infected, including hygiene and living conditions, vaccination, general health status of the population and access to healthcare services and medicines, among others. Other interactions also exist which can create a vicious circle, for example increased infection rates can lead to a higher use of antimicrobials, which in turn, may lead to more resistance.

1.2.1. Inappropriate use of antimicrobials: a leading cause of AMR

Inappropriate use of antimicrobials – including over-prescription, under-prescription, and the prescription and dispensing of unnecessary antimicrobial combinations – is widely considered as a principal factor underpinning AMR. This also includes the use of broad-spectrum antimicrobials when not needed, as well as incorrect dosage and or duration, and poor adherence to prescribed course. Overall, the proportions of inappropriate use may consist of up to 50% of all antimicrobials consumed in human health care. Primary and long-term care services are the areas of most concern, with consistently high levels of inappropriate use. Between 45% and 90% of antibiotic prescriptions in general practices do not meet guidelines (Cecchini and Lee, 2017[3]).

Inappropriate prescription of antimicrobials in humans, from the production and commercialisation of the antimicrobials to the final user, play a role in triggering inappropriate use (Paget et al., 2017[8]). While in many cases diagnostic uncertainty is reported to be the main reason for over-prescription, often inappropriate use of antimicrobials is the result of rational behaviour by one or more actors, driven by cognitive biases or some form of incentive, including economic incentives. In some cases, inappropriate antimicrobial use may be caused by illegal actions, (e.g. sale of counterfeit and poor quality products). Four main categories of actors are involved in ensuring prudent use of antimicrobials in the human sector: prescribers of antimicrobials, patients, health care organisations and producers and dispensers of antimicrobials. Different drivers may support inappropriate use of antimicrobials in each of these categories.

Too often, cognitive biases, perceived pressure and poor information may cause prescribers of antimicrobials not to follow best practices.

- While physicians usually identify the most appropriate antimicrobial therapy, they also often decide not to follow these guidelines to privilege local attitudes and usual business practices.
- The fear of a possible infection, especially in fragile patients, and even if there is no sign of an infection, has been identified as another strong factor promoting use of antimicrobials.
- Finally, physicians may decide to prescribe an antimicrobial, even if they feel it is not needed, to meet patients' expectations or requests, or to prescribe a second-line antibiotic if they feel that resistance to first-line antibiotics is high in the local environment. According to a survey among general practitioners in the United Kingdom, about 50% of practitioners admitted having prescribed antibiotics for a viral infection (Cole, 2014[9]).

Patients' inadequate knowledge of AMR and of the benefits of prudent use of antimicrobials also drives inappropriate use:

- In some OECD countries, use of self-prescribed antibiotics and self-medication with leftovers from previous therapies or with antibiotics provided by friends or pharmacies in the absence of a medical prescription occurs up to 40% of the occasions where antibiotics are used (Morgan et al., 2011[10]).

- When therapies are prescribed by a physician, patients may decide to stop the course earlier than prescribed, for example because they feel better (e.g. about 10% of patients in Spain and Sweden stop taking the medication before the end of its course (Axelsson, 2013[11]; Llor et al., 2014[12])). Patients may also decide to switch to another antibiotic or skip some doses (e.g. up to 44% of patients in the United States admit to skipping doses (Edgar, Boyd and Palamé, 2009[13])).
- Patients put some pressure on physicians to prescribe antibiotics even when they would not need one, for instance if they have a viral infection, or shop around physicians to obtain multiple prescriptions for the same diagnosis. Up to 7.5% of prescriptions in Japan were considered as duplicative prescriptions (i.e. prescription for the same condition from two or more health care providers in a month) (Takahashi et al., 2016[14]).

Ineffective organisational arrangements also lead to an imprudent use of antimicrobials.

- Antimicrobials can be used as a cheap and quick fix for lack of time or resources to carry out further diagnostic tests that could guide prescription. Lack of reimbursement from health care insurances for specific tests or diagnosis may also contribute to imprudent use.
- Poor implementation of guidelines or stewardship programmes in health care settings also supports inappropriate use of antimicrobials.
- Ineffective use of antimicrobials may also be the result of the unwanted effects of policies, such as a lack of separation between prescribing and dispensing which is still normal practice in a number of countries outside those of the OECD, particularly in Asia.
- Similarly, it was argued that different reimbursement systems for general practitioners may foster higher imprudent use of antimicrobials. For example, in systems based on a fixed budget, doctors may increase prescriptions because this practice would minimise the risk of a short-term re-examination of the patient (Kaier, Frank and Meyer, 2011[15]). Conversely, in different payment systems, patients may have incentives to shop around physicians until they find one prescribing the antimicrobial therapy they want.

Producers and vendors of antimicrobials also play a significant role in supporting prudent use.

- In the majority of European countries, sales of antibiotics without prescription were estimated to account for between 2% and 8% of total antibiotic sales (Safrany and Monnet, 2012[16]); this figure may become as high as 60% in some low and middle-income countries (Adeyi et al., 2017[17]).
- Sales of antimicrobials may be also supported by promotional efforts: in the past, antimicrobials have been among leading drug classes for promotional expenditure (Ma et al., 2003[18]).
- Finally, counterfeit antimicrobials, which are often of poor quality or have a reduced active principle, amount to about 5% of the global antimicrobial market (Delepierre, Gayot and Carpentier, 2012[19]). More than one in four counterfeit antimicrobials are sold in Europe or in the Americas (Kelesidis and Falagas, 2015[20]).

The extensive use of antimicrobials in livestock production makes agriculture a critical sector in the fight against AMR. In the United States, antimicrobial use in the livestock sector accounted for about 80% of the total annual antimicrobial sales (Spellberg et al., 2016[21]). At the global level, antimicrobial consumption in livestock production is predicted to increase by 70% by 2030 due to increases in demand for meat and changes in livestock production, particularly in low and middle-income countries (Van Boeckel et al., 2015[22]). These estimates do not take into account antimicrobial use in aquaculture where use is also high. Importantly, antimicrobials in the agriculture sector are also used for disease prevention and growth promotion, including use of low-level doses of antimicrobials in feed which presents a high risk for AMR development. Once a resistant bacterium develops, it could be passed on to humans via direct contact with animals. Also, animal faeces can spread antimicrobial-resistant bacteria to food crops and the environment.

The environment also plays a fundamental role in promoting AMR. Antimicrobials used in humans or agriculture as well as waste products from drug manufacturing can end up in the environment through sewage water. Once in the environment, the continued antimicrobial activity of these drugs affects local microbial communities and favours resistance development and spread. Poor environmental hygiene also underpins the spread of infections. The environment represents a reservoir of bacteria that can eventually contaminate individuals. The hospital environment represents a particularly important setting, given the high susceptibility of patients to infections. In the United States alone, 722 000 cases of health care-associated infections were documented in 2011 (Magill et al., 2014[23]).

AMR is a prominent "One Health" issue. Human health is interconnected with animals, agriculture and the environment. Addressing public health issues in a "One-Health" framework entails a close collaboration among different professionals including, for example, human and veterinary health experts.

1.2.2. Cross-country differences in AMR rates can be explained by key determinants but no single factor stands out for all the antibiotic-bacterium combinations

The OECD has assessed the relationship between AMR rates and some of the abovementioned dimensions that, on theoretical grounds, are believed to be key determinants of AMR. OECD analyses conclude that:

- Higher antibiotic consumption in humans is generally associated with higher resistance proportions, but this is not always the case. For example, resistance proportions in Belgium are lower than expected when considering antibiotic consumption in the human sector in the country, while the reverse is true in Mexico. While these associations could reflect the fact that the appropriateness of consumption also matters (Zilberberg et al., 2017[24]), they also suggest there are other factors at play.
- At the global level, the bulk of antimicrobials are consumed in the animal sector, mostly by food-producing animals, but there is evidence that resistance may spread to humans. For a subset of countries for which data are available, the OECD calculates that total antibiotic consumption (i.e. combined consumption in the human and animal sectors) is highly correlated with resistance in *E. coli*,

which can cause infections and sepsis in many organs (e.g. urinary tract, bloodstream, skin and soft tissues and gastro-enteric tract).

- Out-of-pocket health expenditure, which captures access to health care services including antimicrobial drugs, is positively associated with the share of *K. pneumoniae* infections that are resistant to third-generation cephalosporins.
- Per capita gross-domestic product (GDP), a proxy of the broader socio-economic environment of countries, is highly correlated with carbapenem-resistance among *P. aeruginosa*, which can cause infections and sepsis in many organs (e.g. urinary tract, respiratory tract, bloodstream, skin and soft tissues and gastro-enteric tract).
- The World Bank Worldwide Governance Indicators[5] scores, which capture governance and policy-related dimensions, are a very strong predictor for resistance proportions (Kaufmann, Kraay and Mastruzzi, 2011[25]): lower average scores, corresponding to poorer governance, are associated with higher resistance proportions.

Findings from the OECD analyses suggest that, while certain factors (e.g. governance, country income, out-of-pocket health expenditure, antimicrobial consumption in human and animal sectors) probably play a role in determining resistance proportions, particularly for specific antibiotic-bacterium combinations, there is no single major driver of drug resistance. The emergence and spread of AMR is a complex phenomenon with multiple interrelated causes and consequences and requires a multifaceted set of actions.

1.3. AMR is a significant burden on population health

Since their discovery, antimicrobials have become an essential instrument in medical therapies and surgical treatments. The introduction of antimicrobial therapies has markedly decreased the burden of infectious disease. In addition, by preventing hospital-acquired infections, antimicrobials have allowed the introduction of complex medical interventions such as organ transplantations, advanced surgery, chemotherapy and care of premature babies, just to cite a few. The number of clinical situations in which the use of an antimicrobial is essential is countless and covers the whole lifespan.

Even after accounting for methodological shortcomings, available evidence concludes that the burden of AMR in significant and infections could become a major cause of death in a "post-antibiotic" world. Previous analyses concluded that, at the current rates of resistance, about 23 000 and 25 000 deaths per year are directly attributable to AMR in the United States (CDC, 2013[26]) and Europe (ECDC and EMEA, 2009[27]), respectively.

By feeding its microsimulation model on AMR with cross-country comparable and updated evidence and by considering a more comprehensive set of infections susceptible of developing resistance, the OECD calculates that, under a business-as-usual scenario in which no new policy action is put in place:

- Around 2.4 million individuals could die in Europe, North America and Australia between 2015 and 2050. Italy, Greece and Portugal top the list with an annual mortality rate of, respectively 18.2, 14.8 and 11.3 deaths per 100 000 persons. In absolute terms, the United States has the highest number of AMR deaths with an average of almost 29 558 per year (9.0 deaths per 100 000); followed by Italy and France with around 10 778 and 5 620 deaths per year, respectively. Other populous European countries including Poland, Germany, the United Kingdom and Spain, despite substantially lower mortality rates (from 2.6 to 6.1 deaths per 100 000), would be affected by 1 800 to 2 300 AMR deaths per year.

- The impact on population health, measured in terms of quality of life, will be even larger than the impact on life expectancy. Accounting for the population size of the countries, Southern Europe (Italy, Portugal, France and Greece in particular) would be the most affected. For example, in Italy, up to one person in every 205 could lose one year of life in good health because of AMR.
- Children and the elderly are the two population groups whose health status is most affected by resistant infections, with probability of AMR several times higher in the age groups 0-1 and 70+, compared to the rest of the population. Men are more likely to develop resistant infections than women.

In the so-called "post-antibiotic" world, in which virtually no antibiotic would be effective, the burden caused by AMR could become significantly bigger as even small infections could lead to death. In OECD countries, every year, at least 47 million individuals develop an infection which has the potential to become resistant to antimicrobials[6] (IHME, 2017[28]) and many would die. In addition, in the absence of valid therapeutic alternatives or effective actions to prevent the spread of infections, the incidence rate for communicable diseases may grow further as people would be infected for a longer period and would have more opportunities to infect others.

In the same scenario, surgical operations for non-life threatening conditions, even if highly disabling, would be avoided or postponed, with a significant decrease in the quality of life of patients, as the risk of infection, and subsequently, death would be too high. For example, prophylactic use of antibiotics in hip replacement surgery reduces postoperative infection rates by up to 50% and death due to infection by 30% (Smith and Coast, 2013[29]).

In a scenario in which antibiotics would become almost completely ineffective for therapeutic and prophylactic use, the OECD calculates that the ten most common procedures carried out in hospitals in the European region in 2014, would have produced an additional 435 000 infections leading to an additional 30 000 deaths. A previous analysis, focused on the United States, concluded that the same scenario would produce an additional 400 000 infections and 21 000 deaths in 2010 (Teillant et al., 2015[30]). Such estimates roughly correspond to the yearly number of deaths due to motor vehicle accidents in the same regions.

Poor access to effective and high-quality antimicrobials is already causing a significant health burden in low and middle-income countries. In OECD countries, it is calculated that less than 450 000 individuals (i.e. about one person in every 3 000) die because of diseases such as lower respiratory infections, diarrhoea and neonatal sepsis which can be easily treated when good access to high-quality antibiotics is ensured. Conversely, more than 4.5 million people died in 2016 from this group of diseases in low and middle-income countries, accounting for about 12% of total mortality. Children would pay a particularly high toll as more than 25% of the 4.5 million deaths would be in the under-five age group (IHME, 2017[28]).

1.4. AMR is a significant source of welfare loss

AMR damages health, society and the economy of countries. Much of this is due to the incremental health care costs caused by resistant infections in the hospital setting. The additional costs caused by a resistant infection, compared to a susceptible infection, generally vary between USD 10 000 and USD 40 000 per case (Cecchini, Langer and Slawomirski, 2015[31]), depending on the type and body site of the infection, the country and the patient mix.

Such additional expenditure is caused by the use of more intensive health care procedures for the carrying out of surgical interventions or the treatment of complications. These include extra investigations or advanced laboratory tests to identify the most effective therapy; excess length of stay until the infection is eradicated; and, finally, the use of more aggressive antimicrobial therapies based on either second-line antimicrobials or combinations of different antimicrobials. More than half of the costs for all of these extra procedures are due to additional medical and nursing care while another 25% is for the payment of support services and diagnostics (Tumbarello et al., 2010[32]).

A number of previous country or region-specific studies evaluated the economic burden of AMR. Produced estimates are difficult to compare across countries as studies differ in terms of methodology, accounting approach, number of diseases included in the analyses and so on. Despite limited cross-country comparability, the impact of AMR on the budget of health care systems is estimated to be significant:

- In Europe, costs due to AMR were estimated at about EUR 940 million to treat the resistant strains of a limited set of the most common infective agents in 2007 (ECDC and EMEA, 2009[27]).
- In Canada, the total medical care costs associated with AMR are estimated at CAD 1 billion (PHAC, 2015[33]).
- In the United States, up to USD 20 billion could be spent on AMR (CDC, 2013[26]).

By using its microsimulation approach, with cross-country comparable data and an identical accounting system, the OECD calculates that, on average, every year between 2015 and 2050 up to USD PPP 3.5 billion are expected to be spent on AMR-related complications across the 33 OECD countries included in the analyses, corresponding to about USD PPP 2.4 per capita in those countries. In Italy, Malta and the United States this amount could be as high as USD PPP 6.2-6.6 per capita. In comparison, previous OECD analyses found that the average expenditure per capita for all infectious diseases in a group of 11 OECD countries was about USD PPP 20 (OECD, 2016[34]), meaning that AMR would be responsible for more than 10% of all healthcare costs caused by communicable diseases. The impact of AMR on health care expenditure (and on human health) would be even greater if, instead of considering as a comparator a scenario in which patients develop a susceptible infection (i.e. the closest alternative to a resistant infection), the analyses were based on a scenario assuming that no infection develops.

1.4.1. AMR has a greater impact on the economy of a country than its health care budget

Broader societal costs caused by AMR include time away from work, increased disability claims, loss of productivity and premature deaths. In addition, increased morbidity also affects the supply of labour if ill health requires the attention of a caregiver who would otherwise be economically productive. In the United States in the year 2000, the cost attributable to increased mortality and productivity losses due to AMR was about USD 38 000 per hospital patient, more than double the associated medical costs to treat the patients (Roberts et al., 2009[35]). Scaling up to the national level, in 2000 the

United States lost USD 35 billion (or about 0.35% of the national GDP) due to AMR. By using a different cost accounting technique and a different set of resistant infections, productivity losses due to absence from work caused by resistant infections in the European Union and the European Economic Area amounted to about EUR 600 million in 2007 (ECDC and EMEA, 2009[27]).

Societal costs caused by AMR are particularly high in low and middle-income countries. In such settings, high prevalence rates for key antibiotic-resistant infections combined with poor hygiene in health care services as well as limited protection against out-of-pocket expenditure and ineffective social safety nets significantly increases the probability that developing a resistant infection may lead to catastrophic expenditures. A non-trivial share of the 80 million individuals each year that experience impoverishment due to surgical care in low and middle-income countries (Meara et al., 2015[36]) could be already caused by AMR. Should resistance proportions keep increasing, an additional 19 million individuals in low and middle-income countries will fall into a situation of extreme poverty by 2030 due to negative repercussions on, for example, labour productivity and health care costs (Ahmed et al., 2017[37]).

Summing up the health and economic effects of AMR, the macroeconomic impact caused by resistant infections is considerable. The World Bank (Adeyi et al., 2017[17]) calculated that, at the global level, AMR could reduce GDP output by between 1.1% and 3.8%, depending on how severely the AMR epidemic develops up to 2050. Compared to a scenario without AMR, the total losses in the period 2015-50 in the worst-case scenario would add up to USD 85 trillion in GDP and USD 23 trillion in global trade. Low and middle-income countries would suffer the most, with an economic impact on GDP which would be up to 80% greater than for high-income countries. The detrimental effects caused by AMR on the labour force participation rate and productivity as well as on the size of the population would be the major drivers of this reduction in GDP. International trade and livestock production, in addition to the health care sector, would suffer the most due to reduced productivity and reduction in sales.

1.5. A strong economic rationale for taking action

Imprudent use of antimicrobials produces significant externalities imposing costs on others. The main externalities associated with imprudent use of antimicrobials include the additional costs borne by publicly-funded health care systems to treat resistant infections, the extra health burden and deaths attributed to the lack of available antimicrobial treatment borne by the population, as well as all the negative consequences on productivity and household income suffered by individuals developing a resistant infection.

Compared to other common causes of externality in public health, imprudent use of antimicrobials presents some specific characteristics. First, the consumption of an antimicrobial contributes to creating an environment supportive of AMR development, with effects deferred to a point after the direct consumption of a course of antimicrobials. The external costs associated to antibiotic consumption was calculated at about EUR 5 to EUR 12 for a single defined daily dose of common antibiotic therapies, or between EUR 101 to EUR 143 for a complete course of antibiotic therapy in hospitals (Kaier, 2012[38]). Second, both prudent and imprudent use of antimicrobials supports the development of AMR. When antimicrobials are used inappropriately, the benefits produced by the therapy tend to be zero as the antimicrobial does not produce any positive health effect, but the cost of the externalities associated with consumption increases. The deadweight loss to societal welfare attributed to inappropriate use of amoxicillin alone in the United States was estimated at USD 225 million in 1996 (Elbasha, 2003[39]).

Although outside the main focus of this report, a second strong economic rationale for governments to take action on AMR is the market failure affecting the R&D of new antimicrobials. Antimicrobials are inexpensive drugs but the cost of developing new molecules and bringing them to the market has increased over time. In addition, any newly developed product would likely be held in reserve, further discouraging private sector investments. In this context, a number of large pharmaceutical companies have decided to abandon the market and stop investments in antibiotic R&D, which has resulted in a failure in the supply of new antimicrobials that can substitute old therapies with reduced effectiveness (OECD et al., 2017[5]).

1.6. Governments need to put in place a comprehensive set of public health actions to tackle AMR

The rationale for government intervention to curb AMR is strong, with a wide range of policies potentially available. The ability of governments to design and implement wide-ranging prevention strategies, combining the strengths of different policy approaches is critical to success, including in the case of initiatives promoted in collaboration with the various stakeholders. This requires, however, drawing on objective and verified evidence. By taking as a starting point the Global Action plan on AMR, the OECD has reviewed the available evidence on the effectiveness of key public health policy options to tackle AMR and their level of implementation in OECD and G20 countries to evaluate the effectiveness and the cost-effectiveness of scaling up policy approaches at the national level. This work led to the identification of a first set of "best buys" of public health actions to tackle AMR in the human sector.

1.6.1. Global policy responses to tackle AMR is growing

Many countries have made substantial progress on policies to tackle AMR in the last few years. Following the approval of the WHO Global Action Plan on AMR in 2015 (WHO, 2015[40]), the World Health Assembly urged all Member States to develop and put in place, by 2017, national action plans on AMR. Half of the WHO Member States had a national action plan on antimicrobial resistance in place as of 2017, and another quarter had such a plan under development. According to the same survey, 84% of OECD, G20, and EU countries had developed a national action plan, with the remaining countries undertaking the development of a plan at the time of the survey (WHO, FAO and OIE, 2018[41]).

When designing action plans, countries have a broad arsenal of policy options from which to choose and the opportunity to tailor each of these policies to their unique needs. Effective policy implementation requires coordination of many different types of stakeholders, even at the local and regional levels, making antimicrobial policy making in a "One Health" (WHO, 2017[42]) perspective particularly challenging. In addition, strategies need to be tailored to specific cultures, existing practices and the resistance profile as the appropriateness of different interventions is shaped by factors such as the legal environment and how health care services are delivered in that country. Given the complex and cross-border nature of AMR, international coordination and cooperation is particularly important.

Traditional policy approaches to tackling AMR in the health care sector can be divided into two broad categories:

- interventions to promote rational use of antimicrobials which aim to prevent, or at least minimise, the emergence of new resistant microorganisms, and
- interventions to prevent the spread of existent infections by enhancing hygiene and minimising transmission.

In addition, by preventing the development of infections and by enhancing herd immunity, vaccination policies may also play a fundamental role in tackling AMR. Finally, policies in other areas, notably to promote prudent use of antimicrobials in agriculture and livestock production, also play a critical role in combatting AMR as part of a "One Health" approach.

Among the most widely deployed types of interventions in OECD countries, stewardship programmes involve the simultaneous implementation of regulations, guidelines, monitoring, education and campaigns to influence the prescribing of antimicrobials. These programmes help to determine whether a patient should be prescribed an antimicrobial, which antimicrobial should be prescribed, and for how long it should be taken. Provision of information to the public through mass media campaigns is another widely implemented intervention in OECD countries. This action aims to raise public awareness about the dangers associated with inappropriate antimicrobial prescription. Campaigns are usually delivered during the winter season as this is the period of the year during which antibiotics are more likely to be used for inappropriate purposes (e.g. to treat a cold).

Prescriber education entails a wide range of informative activities to enhance prescribers' knowledge of evidence-based medicine or to improve prescribers' communication skills as they relate to antimicrobial prescribing. While all OECD and G20 countries have in place some sort of education programme for physicians, only two countries, the United Kingdom and Norway, systematically incorporate courses on AMR in pre-service training curricula for all relevant health cadres. Use of new medical technologies, such as rapid diagnostic tests, is increasingly allowing clinicians to rapidly acquire information that can guide antimicrobial prescribing decisions.

Finally, selected countries are testing the use of delayed prescriptions, in which a patient receives a prescription that can only be filled after a certain period. For example, the National Institute for Health and Clinical Excellence, in the United Kingdom, recommends this intervention in patients with specific diseases. The use of financial incentives, usually in the form of pay-for-performance programmes, was also implemented in a few countries (e.g. in Sweden and in the United States), to tackle inappropriate prescription of antibiotics.

Interventions to enhance hygiene are formally in place in virtually every country in the world, but adherence to guidelines should be improved. Interventions such as hand hygiene and environmental hygiene in a health care setting are highly effective and, compared to interventions promoting the prudent use of antimicrobials, they produce an effect on both resistant and susceptible infections. Countries have experimented with policies to increase adherence to hand washing guidelines, which is still poor in many countries, and have tested more effective approaches to cleaning health care devices or facilities. In some countries, as for example in Hong Kong, health care services have implemented policies to systematically screen patients for infections at admittance with the objective of isolating or decontaminating infected individuals before they could spread the infection among the other patients.

Vaccination has been shown to be extremely effective in reducing the incidence of many clinical diseases, including those pathogens with high rates of resistance. For example, the introduction of the pneumococcal conjugate vaccine in children younger than two years reduced the incidence of infections (e.g. in the respiratory tract, meninges, ears, and bloodstream) by over 80% in countries at all levels of income (Kyaw et al., 2006[43]); (von Gottberg et al., 2014[44]). However, implementation of more widespread vaccination faces a number of issues, including ideological, logistical, and financial hurdles. In addition, further efforts should be invested into the R&D of new vaccines. Currently, there are no licensed vaccines for bacteria in the most critical categories of the WHO Priority Pathogens List (WHO, 2017[7]), and only 4% of R&D spending on products to prevent infections specifically related to AMR is spent on diagnostics, vaccines, or other technologies (OECD et al., 2017[5]).

1.6.2. Public health actions to tackle AMR have a positive impact on population health and are an excellent investment for OECD countries

Drawing on the available evidence, the OECD has assessed a set of policies aligned with the WHO global action plan on AMR. The OECD used its microsimulation model on AMR to examine stewardship programmes, media campaigns, actions to enhance hygiene in health care facilities, including promotion of hand-washing and enhanced environmental hygiene, delayed prescriptions and the use of diagnostic tests in 33 OECD and EU countries, and to identify "best buys" for tackling AMR.

Findings from the OECD microsimulation model on AMR show that substantial health gains may be achieved by scaling up to the national level many of the assessed policies. More specifically, results show that:

- Policies to promote hand washing and to enhance hygiene in health care facilities consistently rank as the most effective policies both in terms of reduction of mortality and burden of disease measured in disability-adjusted life years (DALYs). In the 33 countries included in the study, the implementation of these two policies could respectively avert about 37 836 and 34 931 deaths per year and increase the number of persons living in good health by about 21 000 and 17 000 per year. This means that, compared to a scenario in which no policy is in place, hand-washing promotion and hygiene enhancement would be expected to reduce the risk of death from AMR by more than half and to decrease its health burden, measured in DALYs, by about 40%. Compared to policies to promote rational use of antimicrobials, this group of policies tackle both susceptible and resistant bacteria. However, they do not tackle some of the key determinants of AMR associated with imprudent use of antimicrobials.
- Stewardship programmes are particularly effective, too, producing similar effects to hygiene-enhancing actions.
- Other interventions such as delayed prescriptions, use of rapid diagnostic tests and mass media campaigns produce more limited results, mainly because they are designed to tackle AMR in the community, which would have a more limited impact on the population health.

Implementation costs vary substantially across interventions and countries, but interventions are consistently shown to be an excellent investment, often resulting in cost savings. The cost of implementing the policy actions varies on a number of factors, including whether the intervention is targeted at the population level (e.g. mass media campaigns) or to individual patients (e.g. delayed prescriptions), with the latter generally being more costly. Other factors such as the purchasing of medical devices (e.g. rapid diagnostic tests) or the setting up of specific teams to support antibiotic prescriptions (e.g. in stewardship programmes) also have a higher implementation cost.

Interventions entailing a lower consumption of resources, including mass media campaigns, delayed prescriptions and improved hand hygiene cost from as little as USD PPP 0.3 up to USD PPP 2.7 per capita in many OECD countries. More resource-intense interventions can cost up to a few hundred USD PPP per hospitalised patient, as in the case of actions to enhance hospital environmental hygiene.

When both implementation costs and impact on health care expenditure are taken into account, the OECD model concludes that, consistently across interventions and geographical settings, all the considered policy actions are a cost-effective investment and, in a number of cases (e.g. delayed prescriptions, improved hand hygiene and, very often, stewardship programmes), the implementation cost of the intervention is lower than the corresponding savings on health care expenditure produced by the intervention. Thus, in other words, investing in public health actions to tackle AMR is a very good investment for the countries included in the analysis and the implementation cost of the public health actions completely pays for itself and produces some additional savings.

Based on the three quantitative criteria to identify the best policy options in public health (i.e. effectiveness on population health, affordability to implement the intervention, and cost-effectiveness ratio), virtually all the interventions considered in the analysis can be generally considered "best buys" to tackle AMR in the assessed countries. For some interventions, particularly those in the community (e.g. mass media campaigns and delayed prescriptions) the effectiveness is more limited but, due to their lower implementation cost, these interventions result in cost-effective investments. Extrapolation of these results beyond OECD countries is more difficult to assess as organisational arrangements and other factors may significantly influence the results of the analysis.

Combining AMR policies into a coherent prevention strategy that combines actions both to promote prudent use of antibiotics and to prevent the spread of infections in the health care sector and in the community, would help countries reach a critical mass having a greater impact on susceptible and resistant infections and their associated negative health and economic effects. The three package options considered: one for hospital measures, one for community actions and a mixed intervention package (based on a combination of selected hospital and community strategies) would each reduce the health burden of AMR by 85%, 23% and 73%, respectively. This corresponds to a total of approximately 1.3 million, 0.4 million and 1.1 million DALYs averted and 55, 15 and 47 life years saved across the 33 countries included in the study. In terms of health expenditure, the hospital-based intervention package would result into an annual average net saving (i.e. after accounting for the implementation cost of each intervention) of USD PPP 4.1 per capita (ranging from USD PPP 0.08 in Iceland to USD PPP 13.2 in Malta). The community-based intervention approach would also result in an average annual saving of around USD PPP 0.9 per capita across the 33 included countries. The mixed policy approach would result in an average net reduction in health expenditure of around USD PPP 3 per capita per year. In practical terms, this would mean that millions of people in these countries would avoid AMR-related complications and health problems, with major potential gains for themselves in terms of their health well-being, for society and economic outcomes.

Notes

[1] The term "antimicrobials" refers to a broad family of agents including any agent killing or inhibiting the growth of microbes. There are many classes of antimicrobials depending on the type of microbes targeted or the composition of the antimicrobial. Antibiotics (or antibacterials) are a sub-category of antimicrobials specifically targeting bacteria. "Antimicrobial" is used in this chapter to specifically describe those agents that exert a killing function against bacterial pathogens, or agents that work as treatment or prophylaxis against bacterial infections. In most contexts of this chapter, antimalarial, antifungal and antiviral medicines are not included under the term "antimicrobials".

[2] Throughout this chapter, the name of the infectious microorganisms, rather than the name of the most common infections caused by such microorganisms, are used as virtually all the considered microorganisms can cause infections in many different organs. So, for example, *Neisseria gonorrhoeae* is used, rather than gonorrhea (which is commonly used to refer to the infections of the reproductive organs), as the same bacterium can also cause, among the others, infections of the musculoskeletal system (e.g. septic arthritis), of the gastrointestinal tract (e.g. pharynx and rectum), of the bloodstream, and other infections.

[3] The eight antibiotic-bacterium combinations included in the analysis are: third-generation cephalosporin-resistant *Escherichia coli*, fluoroquinolones-resistant *Escherichia coli*, penicillin-resistant *Streptococcus pneumoniae*, methicillin-resistant *Staphylococcus aureus*, carbapenem-resistant *Klebsiella pneumoniae*, third-generation cephalosporin-resistant *Klebsiella pneumoniae*, carbapenem-resistant *Pseudomonas aeruginosa*, and vancomycin-resistant *Enterococcus faecalis* and *Enterococcus faecium*.

[4] OECD key partners include the following countries: Brazil, China, India, Indonesia and South Africa.

[5] The World Bank Worldwide Governance Indicators capture dimensions associated with traditions and institutions by which authority in a country is exercised, including the capacity of the government to effectively formulate and implement sound policies and the respect of citizens and the state for the governing institutions. More specifically, the indicators monitor the following six dimensions of governance: voice and accountability, political stability and absence of violence, government effectiveness, regulatory quality, rule of law, control of corruption.

[6] This number is calculated by summing up the number of cases of the following infections in OECD countries: gonococcal, chlamydial, lower respiratory, syphilis, tuberculosis, whooping cough, paratyphoid fever, typhoid fever, and meningitis. The list does not aim to be exhaustive of all the clinical conditions potentially caused by microorganisms with the ability to develop AMR.

References

Adeyi, O. et al. (2017), *Drug-resistant infections : a threat to our economic future (Vol. 2) : final report*, World Bank Group, Washington (DC), http://documents.worldbank.org/curated/en/323311493396993758/final-report (accessed on 09 May 2018). [17]

Ahmed, S. et al. (2017), "Assessing the Global Economic and Poverty Effects of Antimicrobial Resistance", *Policy Research Working Paper*, No. 8133, World Bank, Washington (DC), http://documents.worldbank.org/curated/en/190151498872848485/pdf/WPS8133.pdf (accessed on 11 May 2018). [37]

Axelsson, M. (2013), "Report on personality and adherence to antibiotic therapy: a population-based study.", *BMC psychology*, Vol. 1/1, p. 24, http://dx.doi.org/10.1186/2050-7283-1-24. [11]

CDC (2013), *Antibiotic Resistance Threats in the United States, 2013*, Centers for Disease Control and Prevention, Atlanta (GA), https://www.cdc.gov/drugresistance/threat-report-2013/pdf/ar-threats-2013-508.pdf (accessed on 11 May 2018). [26]

Cecchini, M., J. Langer and L. Slawomirski (2015), *ANTIMICROBIAL RESISTANCE IN G7 COUNTRIES AND BEYOND: Economic Issues, Policies and Options for Action*, OECD, Paris, http://www.oecd.org/els/health-systems/Antimicrobial-Resistance-in-G7-Countries-and-Beyond.pdf (accessed on 19 January 2018). [31]

Cecchini, M. and S. Lee (2017), "Low-value health care with high stakes: Promoting the rational use of antimicrobials", in *Tackling Wasteful Spending on Health*, OECD Publishing, Paris, http://dx.doi.org/10.1787/9789264266414-6-en. [3]

Cole, A. (2014), "GPs feel pressurised to prescribe unnecessary antibiotics, survey finds", *BMJ*, Vol. 349/aug19 15, pp. g5238-g5238, http://dx.doi.org/10.1136/bmj.g5238. [9]

Delepierre, A., A. Gayot and A. Carpentier (2012), "Update on counterfeit antibiotics worldwide; public health risks.", *Medecine et maladies infectieuses*, Vol. 42/6, pp. 247-55, http://dx.doi.org/10.1016/j.medmal.2012.04.007. [19]

ECDC and EMEA (2009), *The bacterial challenge: time to react*, ECDC and EMEA, Stockholm (SE), https://ecdc.europa.eu/sites/portal/files/media/en/publications/Publications/0909_TER_The_Bacterial_Challenge_Time_to_React.pdf (accessed on 10 October 2018). [27]

Edgar, T., S. Boyd and M. Palamé (2009), "Sustainability for behaviour change in the fight against antibiotic resistance: a social marketing framework.", *The Journal of antimicrobial chemotherapy*, Vol. 63/2, pp. 230-7, http://dx.doi.org/10.1093/jac/dkn508. [13]

Elbasha, E. (2003), "Deadweight loss of bacterial resistance due to overtreatment.", *Health economics*, Vol. 12/2, pp. 125-38, http://dx.doi.org/10.1002/hec.702. [39]

FAO (2016), *Drivers, Dynamics and Epidemiology of Antimicrobial Resistance in Animal Production*, FAO, Rome, http://www.fao.org/3/a-i6209e.pdf (accessed on 08 May 2018). [4]

Hawkey, P. (2008), "The growing burden of antimicrobial resistance.", *The Journal of antimicrobial chemotherapy*, Vol. 62 Suppl 1, pp. 1-9, http://dx.doi.org/10.1093/jac/dkn241. [1]

IHME (2017), *GBD Compare Data Visualization*, http://vizhub.healthdata.org/gbd-compare (accessed on 11 May 2018). [28]

Kaier, K. (2012), "Economic implications of the dynamic relationship between antibiotic use and hospital-acquired infections.", *Value in health*, Vol. 15/1, pp. 87-93, http://dx.doi.org/10.1016/j.jval.2011.09.005. [38]

Kaier, K., U. Frank and E. Meyer (2011), "Economic incentives for the (over-)prescription of broad-spectrum antimicrobials in German ambulatory care.", *The Journal of antimicrobial chemotherapy*, Vol. 66/7, pp. 1656-8, http://dx.doi.org/10.1093/jac/dkr134. [15]

Kaufmann, D., A. Kraay and M. Mastruzzi (2011), "The Worldwide Governance Indicators: Methodology and Analytical Issues", *Hague Journal on the Rule of Law*, Vol. 3/02, pp. 220-246, http://dx.doi.org/10.1017/S1876404511200046. [25]

Kelesidis, T. and M. Falagas (2015), "Substandard/counterfeit antimicrobial drugs.", *Clinical microbiology reviews*, Vol. 28/2, pp. 443-64, http://dx.doi.org/10.1128/CMR.00072-14. [20]

Kyaw, M. et al. (2006), "Effect of Introduction of the Pneumococcal Conjugate Vaccine on Drug-Resistant <i>Streptococcus pneumoniae</i>", *New England Journal of Medicine*, Vol. 354/14, pp. 1455-1463, http://dx.doi.org/10.1056/NEJMoa051642. [43]

Llor, C. et al. (2014), "Access to point-of-care tests reduces the prescription of antibiotics among antibiotic-requesting subjects with respiratory tract infections.", *Respiratory care*, Vol. 59/12, pp. 1918-23, http://dx.doi.org/10.4187/respcare.03275. [12]

Magill, S. et al. (2014), "Multistate Point-Prevalence Survey of Health Care–Associated Infections", *New England Journal of Medicine*, Vol. 370/13, pp. 1198-1208, http://dx.doi.org/10.1056/NEJMoa1306801. [23]

Ma, J. et al. (2003), "A statistical analysis of the magnitude and composition of drug promotion in the United States in 1998.", *Clinical therapeutics*, Vol. 25/5, pp. 1503-17, http://www.ncbi.nlm.nih.gov/pubmed/12867225 (accessed on 09 May 2018). [18]

McKenna, M. (2013), "Antibiotic resistance: The last resort", *Nature*, Vol. 499/7459, pp. 394-396, http://dx.doi.org/10.1038/499394a. [2]

Meara, J. et al. (2015), "Global Surgery 2030: evidence and solutions for achieving health, welfare, and economic development", *The Lancet*, Vol. 386/9993, pp. 569-624, http://dx.doi.org/10.1016/S0140-6736(15)60160-X. [36]

Morgan, D. et al. (2011), "Non-prescription antimicrobial use worldwide: a systematic review.", *The Lancet. Infectious diseases*, Vol. 11/9, pp. 692-701, http://dx.doi.org/10.1016/S1473-3099(11)70054-8. [10]

OECD (2016), *Expenditure by disease, age and gender*, OECD, Paris (FR), [34]
https://www.oecd.org/health/Expenditure-by-disease-age-and-gender-FOCUS-April2016.pdf
(accessed on 18 May 2018).

OECD et al. (2017), *Tackling Antimicrobial Resistance Ensuring Sustainable R&D*, [5]
http://www.oecd.org/els/health-systems/G20-AMR-Final-Paper-2017.pdf (accessed on
08 May 2018).

Paget, J. et al. (2017), *Antimicrobial resistance and causes of non-prudent use of antibiotics in* [8]
human medicine in the EU, European Commission, Brussels,
https://ec.europa.eu/health/amr/sites/amr/files/amr_arna_report_20170717_en.pdf (accessed
on 27 September 2018).

PHAC (2015), *Canadian Antimicrobial Resistance Surveillance System - Report 2015*, Public [33]
Health Agency of Canada, Ottawa (CA),
http://publications.gc.ca/collections/collection_2015/aspc-phac/HP37-21-2015-eng.pdf
(accessed on 11 May 2018).

Roberts, R. et al. (2009), "Hospital and societal costs of antimicrobial-resistant infections in a [35]
Chicago teaching hospital: implications for antibiotic stewardship.", *Clinical infectious*
diseases : an official publication of the Infectious Diseases Society of America, Vol. 49/8,
pp. 1175-84, http://dx.doi.org/10.1086/605630.

Safrany, N. and D. Monnet (2012), "Antibiotics obtained without a prescription in Europe", *The* [16]
Lancet Infectious Diseases, Vol. 12/3, pp. 182-183, http://dx.doi.org/10.1016/S1473-
3099(12)70017-8.

Smith, R. and J. Coast (2013), "The true cost of antimicrobial resistance", *BMJ*, [29]
http://dx.doi.org/10.1136/bmj.f1493.

Spellberg, B. et al. (2016), "Antibiotic Resistance in Humans and Animals", *Discussion paper*, [21]
National Academy of Medicine, Washington (DC), https://nam.edu/wp-
content/uploads/2016/07/Antibiotic-Resistance-in-Humans-and-Animals.pdf (accessed on
09 May 2018).

Takahashi, Y. et al. (2016), "Social network analysis of duplicative prescriptions: One-month [14]
analysis of medical facilities in Japan.", *Health policy (Amsterdam, Netherlands)*, Vol. 120/3,
pp. 334-41, http://dx.doi.org/10.1016/j.healthpol.2016.01.020.

Teillant, A. et al. (2015), "Potential burden of antibiotic resistance on surgery and cancer [30]
chemotherapy antibiotic prophylaxis in the USA: a literature review and modelling study.",
The Lancet. Infectious diseases, Vol. 15/12, pp. 1429-37, http://dx.doi.org/10.1016/S1473-
3099(15)00270-4.

Tumbarello, M. et al. (2010), "Costs of Bloodstream Infections Caused by Escherichia coli and [32]
Influence of Extended-Spectrum- -Lactamase Production and Inadequate Initial Antibiotic
Therapy", *Antimicrobial Agents and Chemotherapy*, Vol. 54/10, pp. 4085-4091,
http://dx.doi.org/10.1128/AAC.00143-10.

Van Boeckel, T. et al. (2015), "Global trends in antimicrobial use in food animals", *Proceedings of the National Academy of Sciences*, Vol. 112/18, pp. 5649-5654, http://dx.doi.org/10.1073/pnas.1503141112. [22]

von Gottberg, A. et al. (2014), "Effects of Vaccination on Invasive Pneumococcal Disease in South Africa", *New England Journal of Medicine*, Vol. 371/20, pp. 1889-1899, http://dx.doi.org/10.1056/NEJMoa1401914. [44]

WHO (2017), *Global priority list of antibiotic-resistant bacteria to guide research, discovery, and development of new antibiotics*, World Health Organization, http://www.who.int/medicines/publications/WHO-PPL-Short_Summary_25Feb-ET_NM_WHO.pdf (accessed on 10 October 2010). [7]

WHO (2017), "One Health", http://www.who.int/features/qa/one-health/en/ (accessed on 10 October 2018). [42]

WHO (2015), *Global Action Plan on Antimicrobial Resistance*, World Health Organization, http://www.wpro.who.int/entity/drug_resistance/resources/global_action_plan_eng.pdf (accessed on 10 October 2018). [40]

WHO (2014), *Antimicrobial resistance: global report on surveillance 2014*, World Health Organization, Geneva, http://www.who.int/drugresistance/documents/surveillancereport/en/ (accessed on 10 October 2018). [6]

WHO, FAO and OIE (2018), *Global Database for AMRCSAT Country Self-Assessment Test*, https://extranet.who.int/sree/Reports?op=vs&path=%2FWHO_HQ_Reports/G45/PROD/EXT/amrcsat_AnswersForPublic (accessed on 18 May 2018). [41]

Zilberberg, M. et al. (2017), "Carbapenem resistance, inappropriate empiric treatment and outcomes among patients hospitalized with Enterobacteriaceae urinary tract infection, pneumonia and sepsis", *BMC Infectious Diseases*, Vol. 17/1, p. 279, http://dx.doi.org/10.1186/s12879-017-2383-z. [24]

Chapter 2. Antimicrobial resistance: A frightening and complex public health challenge

Michael Padget

This chapter introduces the background and history of antimicrobial resistance (AMR) including its biological underpinnings. It offers a comprehensive look at the leading causes and consequences of AMR. It highlights the multi-sectorial aspects of resistance development and spread and describes antibiotic use and misuse across a range of sectors. The chapter then provides a framework for understanding how AMR develops and leads to infections and provides intervention targets aimed to disrupt this process. Finally, the chapter concludes by highlighting the need for multi-sectorial and multi-national solutions. This chapter provides the reader with the foundation for the following analytical chapters.

The statistical data for Israel are supplied by and under the responsibility of the relevant Israeli authorities. The use of such data by the OECD is without prejudice to the status of the Golan Heights, East Jerusalem and Israeli settlements in the West Bank under the terms of international law.

Key findings

- Antimicrobial resistance (AMR) is a large and growing problem with the potential for enormous health and economic consequences globally. Rising AMR threatens the achievement of several Sustainable Development Goals (SDGs) related to health and poverty reduction.
- The threat of AMR is heightened by the lack of new drugs. As resistance has grown in recent years, the antimicrobial research and development (R&D) pipeline has shrunk due to insufficient economic incentives.
- AMR arises principally through use of antimicrobials. As pathogens are exposed to drugs designed to treat them, they can develop defence mechanisms to resist their effects. High rates of inappropriate drug use may play a large role in drug exposure and AMR development.
- AMR is a multi-factorial and multi-sectorial problem necessitating multi-factorial solutions with the involvement of all the key stakeholders. The rise and spread of AMR occurs across human, animal, and environmental sectors, which must all be accounted for when developing prevention strategies.

2.1. Infectious disease in the 20th century: Rise of resistance

The 20th century was marked by tremendous improvements in life expectancy and health outcomes across Europe, North America and other developed countries. Driving these improvements were dramatic reductions in the burden of infectious disease. Contributing factors included public health advances such as water and waste management along with food regulation. This period also witnessed medical breakthroughs that lowered incidence rates and provided better treatment for infectious diseases such as tuberculosis and diarrhoea. Mortality due to infectious diseases in the United States fell from almost 600 deaths per 100 000 individuals per year in 1900 to 24 in 1980. In England and Wales deaths per 100 000 individuals dropped from approximately 550 to under 10 during the same period (see Figure 2.1).

Of all the medical discoveries in the 20th century, perhaps none was more important than that of antibiotics. These "miracle drugs" introduced as therapeutic agents in the 1940s allowed for effective management and treatment of long-feared diseases such as tuberculosis, bacterial pneumonia, and sepsis, leading to greatly improved survival and patient outcomes (Zaffiri, Gardner and Toledo-Pereyra, 2012[1]). With the help of penicillin, case fatality rates for bacterial pneumonia and bloodstream infections dropped from over 80% to under 20% between 1935 and 1952. Similar results were seen for other bacterial diseases (Austrian and Gold, 1964[2]).

The period following the Second World War was considered the golden age of antibiotic discovery and a number of important and widely used antibiotics were discovered (Davies and Davies, 2010[3]). The effectiveness of these drugs combined with their relatively few side effects and cheap costs quickly led to wide use and antibiotics became standard treatment for a number of common illnesses.

In recent years however, the potency of these drugs has started to wane with the development and spread of AMR. Pathogens that develop AMR may survive the effects of antimicrobials, including antibiotics, making subsequent infections difficult or even impossible to treat. The current rise of AMR and these hard to treat or untreatable infections threaten to turn back the clock on infectious disease gains and lead us toward a "post-antibiotic" world where minor infections can once again lead to death.

Figure 2.1. Total death rate vs. infectious disease death rate: United States, England and Wales

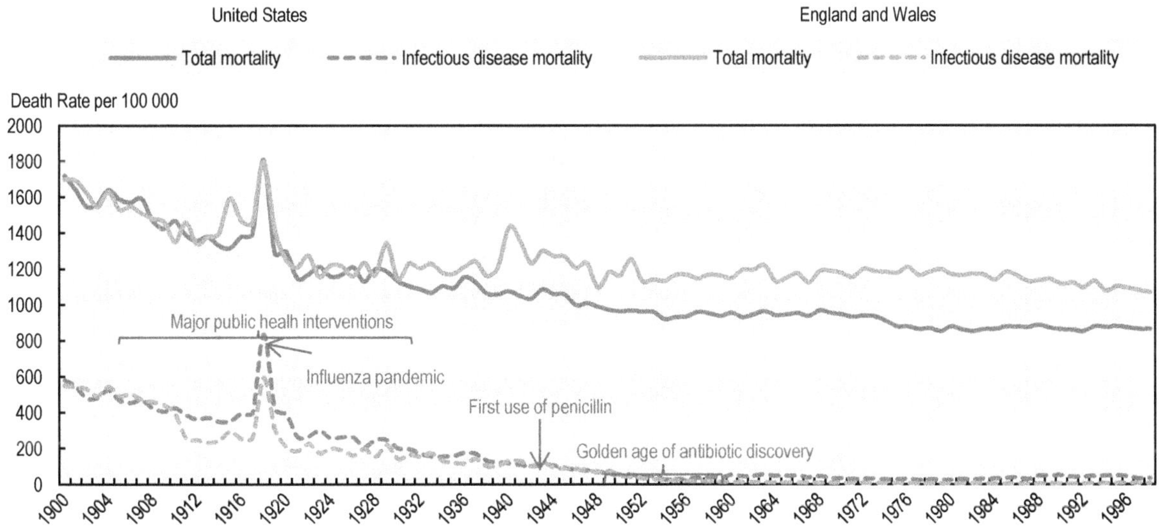

Source: CDC (2018[4]) and Office of National Statistics (2018[5]).

StatLink http://dx.doi.org/10.1787/888933854649

2.2. What is antimicrobial resistance (AMR)?

AMR evolves naturally as a result of antimicrobial use and is an example of natural selection (see Section 2.4). Because of the selection pressure exerted by antimicrobials, pathogens may develop or acquire mechanisms allowing them to survive and reproduce in environments where antibiotics are present (see Box 2.3). Increasing pathogenic exposure to antimicrobials increases the chance that they become resistant. This means that the more antimicrobials are used, the less effective they become.

AMR is also a multi-sectoral or "one health" issue. The human, animal, and environmental health sectors influence the rates of AMR and resistant infections. This then necessitates a multi-sectorial response to AMR.

Finally, AMR is a "one world" issue. Resistant pathogens do not recognise national borders and can spread easily among populations, regions, and countries. Recent studies have shown that travel and tourism can lead to greater global spread of antibiotic resistance bacteria including powerful new forms of resistance (McNulty et al., 2018[6]) (Kumarasamy et al., 2010[7]). All countries, regardless of their economic situation or strength of their health system are vulnerable to rising resistance levels and risk devastating consequences in the absence of a global solution.

2.3. Why should we be worried about AMR?

AMR poses a particular threat to public health in OECD countries and globally due to four main causes.

First, bacterial infections are highly frequent. Figure 2.2 shows the number of yearly infections by country due to bacteria susceptible to becoming resistant to antibiotics. These numbers include a wide range of infection types and are a product of both the size of the population and the infection rate in each country. The total of these infections across all countries is just over 47 million per year with nearly 60% of these infections due to lower respiratory infections. Gonococcal infections (the cause of gonorrhoea) were another leading cause of bacterial infections making up over 20% of total infections.

Figure 2.2. Infections by microbes susceptible to the development of resistance in OECD countries

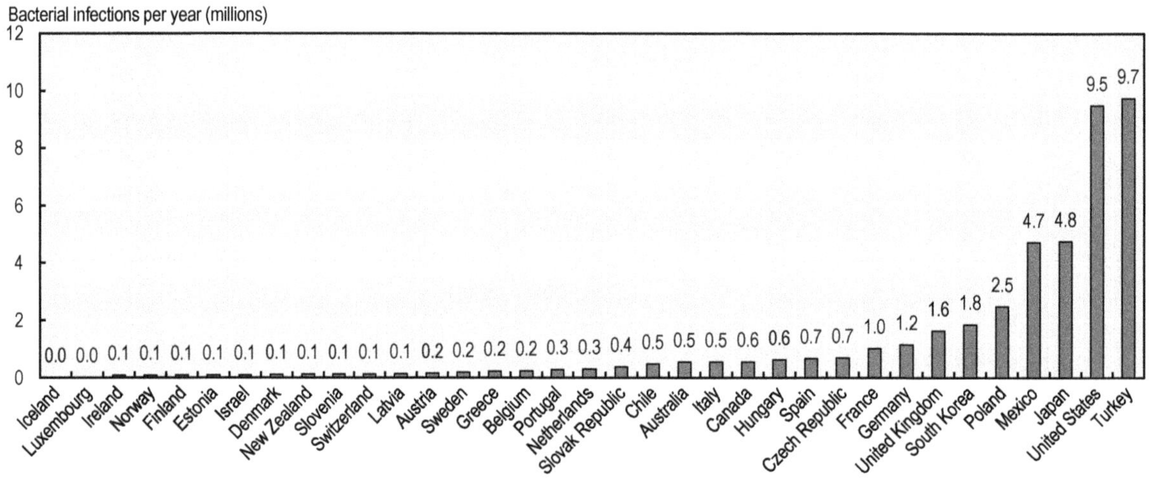

Note: The graph includes the following infections: gonococcal, chlamydial, lower respiratory, syphilis, tuberculosis, whooping cough, paratyphoid fever, typhoid fever, and meningitis.
Source: IHME (2018[8]).

StatLink http://dx.doi.org/10.1787/888933854668

Second, resistant infections lead to considerable additional morbidity and mortality and previous estimates concluded that AMR may be responsible for 23 000 deaths in the United States and 25 000 deaths across Europe each year (CDC, 2018[9]) (European Commmission, 2018[10]). Recent data from Europe highlight growing rates of AMR including bacterial infections with resistance to carbapenems, an antibiotic used as a final treatment option for already highly resistant organisms (ECDC, 2017[11]). On a larger scale, rising AMR threatens progress toward global objectives such as the Sustainable Development Goals (SDGs), in particular those targeting child health, maternal health, and mortality (WHO, 2017[12]).

Third, the economic impact of AMR may also be devastating to local and global economies in coming years. Resistant infections are significantly more expensive for health systems, resulting in longer hospital stays, more intensive treatment and more expensive second line treatments.[1] Second line treatment for tuberculosis for example may cost between 3 to 18 times more than first line treatments and on average a hospitalised patient infected with an antibiotic-resistant infection costs an additional USD 10 000 to USD 40 000 (Cecchini, Langer and Slawomirski, 2015[13]). AMR also results in lost productivity from death, longer periods of illness, and increased morbidity. In high-income countries productivity losses for resistant infections, including time away from work and informal care requirements are estimated at USD 38 000 per patient (Cecchini, Langer and Slawomirski, 2015[13]). In low and middle-income countries (LMICs) the cost of AMR may be even higher (See Box 2.1).

Box 2.1. The health and economic burden of AMR in LMICs

The burden of AMR may be much higher in LMICs than other countries given the high rates of infectious disease and the lack of access to quality medicines and care in some areas. (Gwatkin, Guillot and Heuveline, 1999[14]) (Newton et al., 2006[15]) Whereas in high-income countries the effects of resistance may include increased morbidity and economic costs, resistance in LMICs may translate directly into increased mortality (Okeke et al., 2005[16]). Mortality due to diseases such as lower respiratory infections, diarrhoea, and neonatal sepsis which could be easily managed through good health care and access to medicines accounted for an estimated 4.5 million deaths in LMICs in 2016 (IHME, 2018[8]).

LMICs are also particularly financially vulnerable to resistance. Rising resistance rates could lead to an additional 19 million individuals in LMICs falling into extreme poverty by 2030 due to the negative impacts on labour productivity and health care costs (Ahmed et al., 2017[17]). If solutions are not found, GDP losses in low-income countries due to the impacts of AMR may top 5% by 2050, 80% higher than the impact in high-income countries (World Bank, 2017[18]).

On a global scale, these costs, combined with AMR's impact on the agricultural sector and on international trade are projected to reduce the global economic output to between 1.1% and 3.8% by 2050. This will result in a large increase in extreme poverty worldwide and will threaten the achievement of the SDGs related to poverty, hunger, and inequality reduction (World Bank, 2017[18]).

Finally, the impact of rising resistance levels on health outcomes has been exacerbated in recent years by the relative lack of new antibiotics available to treat these bacteria. In the past, development of resistance was quickly met with a steady stream of new anti-infective drugs. However, the antibiotic pipeline has dried up due to a lack of financial incentives to invest in antibiotic R&D (see Box 2.2).

Box 2.2. Lack of investment in antibiotic R&D

Unlike past eras where doctors could count on continued development of new antibiotics to combat bacterial resistance, scientific challenges and insufficient market incentives have slowed research and development in this area (see Figure 2.3). This issue was examined in depth in a 2017 paper authored by the OECD, WHO, FAO and OIE (2017[19]). The following is based on the results of this analysis.

New antibiotics have become increasingly difficult to discover and typically only 1.5% of antibiotics in preclinical development reach the market. Furthermore, clinical development of promising candidate molecules is expensive. This high cost of antibiotic R&D, the low chance of success, and low reimbursement prices on market entry have led to a number of actors in the pharmaceutical industry abandoning antibiotic research. Small and medium-sized enterprises where the majority of current antibiotic R&D now occurs typically lack the funds necessary to take early stage research through to clinical development. Some initiatives have been launched to stimulate R&D although current efforts are insufficient to guarantee a robust and sustainable pipeline. To respond to this need, in 2017, G20 leaders called for the creation of a global AMR R&D Hub, (G20, 2017[20]). Launched in 2018 and open to any interested countries or invited philanthropic foundations with a commitment to investing in AMR R&D, the Hub's purpose is to increase R&D investment through facilitating information exchange between existing funding streams, promoting alignment of funding to avoid overlaps, and mobilising additional resources for R&D investment. While solutions must be found to correct R&D market incentives in the short term, longer-term solutions (e.g. greater prevention of infectious diseases and the use of alternative treatments) may also be needed to ensure these antibiotics continue to work into the future.

Figure 2.3. The decline in antibiotic R&D

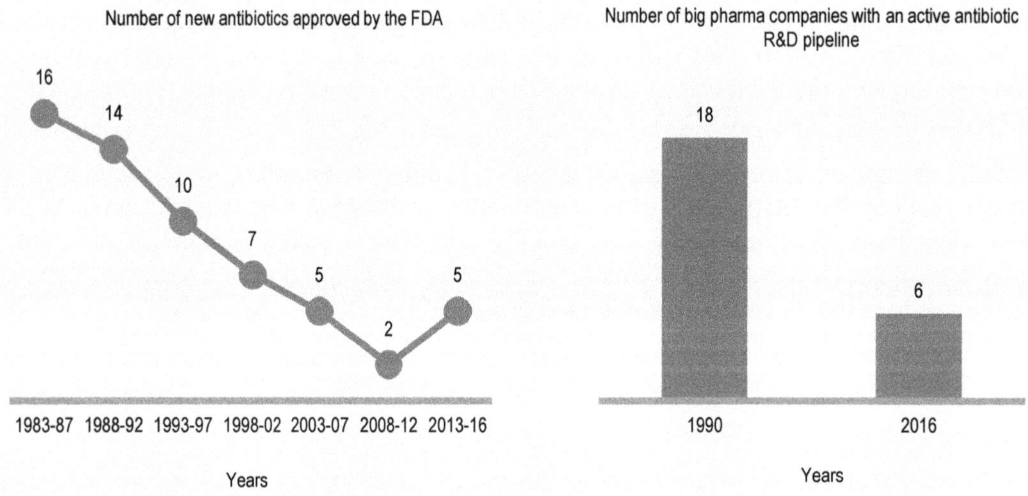

Source: OECD, WHO, FAO and OIE (2017[19]).

2.3.1. Antibiotics and the effects on the microbiota

Along with exerting selection pressure leading to resistance, antibiotics may have additional negative health consequences through the modification of the human microbiota (Langdon, Crook and Dantas, 2016[21]).

The human microbiota is the sum of all microorganisms that live in and on humans including importantly in the human gut. These naturally occurring microorganisms including bacteria are important for activities such as digestion, protection from pathogens and immune system development (Zhang et al., 2015[22]). Indeed, bacteria and humans have evolved together over centuries and humans cannot live or develop normally without the presence of bacteria (Young, 2017[23]).

Antibiotics taken regularly may disturb this delicate balance between man and bacteria. When oral antibiotics are taken to treat an infection they can disrupt naturally occurring bacterial populations and frequent use of antibiotics may lead to permanent changes in these bacterial populations (Francino, 2015[24]). Recent research has found that changes in the composition of the microbiota, particularly during young childhood, may increase the risk of development of a wide range of health problems including allergies, obesity, and even autism (Riiser, 2015[25]; Parekh, Balart and Johnson, 2015[26]; Strati et al., 2017[27]).

2.4. How did AMR originate?

Almost as soon as new antibiotics were discovered, bacteria capable of resisting their effects were identified (see Figure 2.4). Only one year after the discovery of tetracycline, a powerful broad-spectrum drug, resistant clinical isolates started to appear (Nelson and Levy, 2011[28]). Similarly, only two years after the discovery of methicillin, a drug designed to treat penicillin-resistant *Staphylococcus aureus*, were methicillin resistant strains discovered (Davies and Davies, 2010[3]). Famously, resistance to penicillin was discovered even before the introduction of this drug as a therapeutic agent (Davies and Davies, 2010[3]). The accumulation of these resistance mechanisms over the past 70 years has led to an increase in multi-drug resistant bacteria that are difficult to treat.

Figure 2.4. Timeline of antibiotic discovery and detection of antibiotic resistance

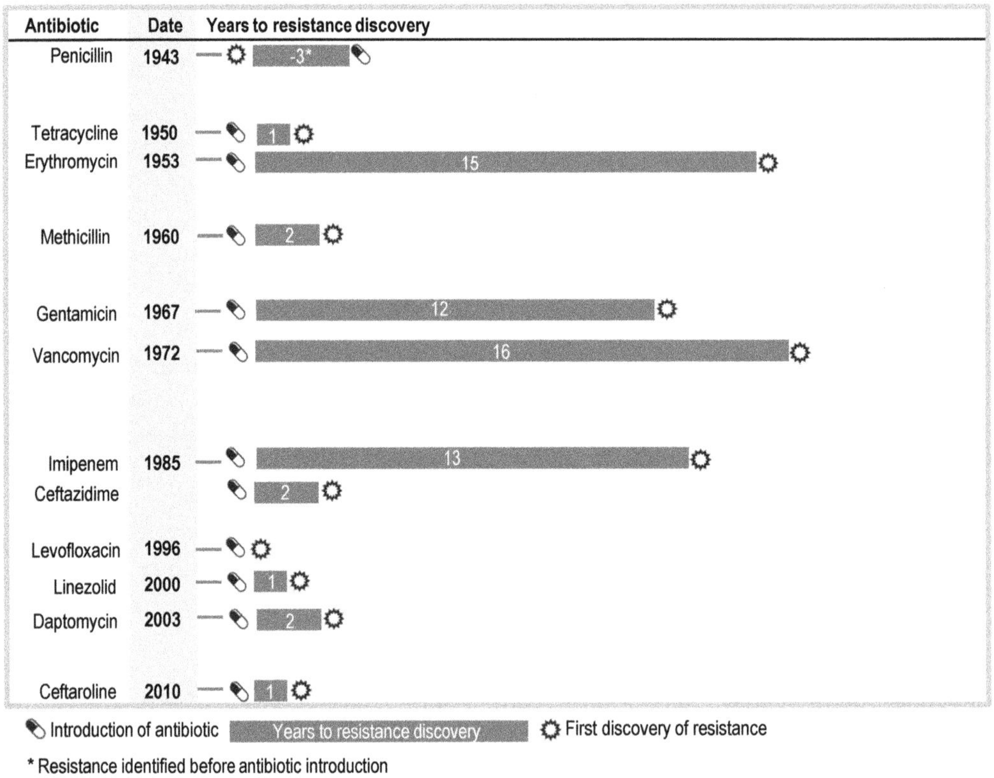

Source: Adapted from CDC (2013[29]), (Nelson and Levy, 2011[28]).

The rapid rise in resistance seen in recent years is not surprising given the fundamental and ancient role resistance plays in bacterial survival. Long before the discovery of antibiotics by humans, microorganisms have been using them to gain survival advantages over other competing organisms. Bacteria exposed to these antibiotics in nature have developed an extensive array of defense mechanisms including effective antibiotic resistance gene activation and exchange.

Bacterial antibiotic resistance is thus not a recent phenomenon and bacteria from as long ago as 30 000 years have been found to contain antibiotic resistant genes (D'Costa et al., 2011[30]) which helped them survive then as today.

Over time, this continuous struggle between microorganisms has resulted in a deep reservoir of antibiotic resistant genes known as the resistome that bacteria may access when necessary (Brown and Wright, 2016[31]).

Box 2.3. Antibiotic resistance: Acquisition and techniques

Bacteria can acquire antibiotic resistance through either spontaneous gene mutations or acquisition of resistance genes from other bacteria. This transfer of resistance genes is particularly effective in the dissemination of resistance and includes transfer of genes between different bacterial strains, species, or even genera. Mobile genetic elements shared between bacteria are capable of transmitting powerful multi-drug resistance genes such as extended spectrum beta-lactamases (ESBLs) or carbapenemases.

Antibiotic exposure increases the frequency of gene transfer increasing the likelihood of resistance spread. Even extremely low levels of antibiotics have been found to induce a stress response in bacteria provoking increased gene transfer (Andersson and Hughes, 2014[32]).

This selective pressure and gene transfer can occur in any situation where multiple bacteria are found in the presence of antibiotics. The human gut, home to an estimated 1 000 species of bacteria, is one such environment. Oral antibiotics, taken for one type of infection for example will affect all bacteria in the gut stimulating gene transfer and promoting resistance. Similar dynamics can be found in other types of environments such as water treatment plants, antibiotic contaminated soil, or any other area where large numbers of bacteria are exposed to antibiotics (Wachter, Joshi and Rimal, 1999[33]) (Xu and Gordon, 2003[34]). Limiting unnecessary exposure to antibiotics in these contexts is thus an important component in combatting rising resistance rates.

Resistance to antibiotics, whether acquired through gene mutation or gene transfer, is achieved through a number of diverse mechanisms. Some bacteria simply pump the antibiotic out of the cell wall before it reaches its target using efflux pumps. This technique can be effective against a range of antibiotics. Another resistance strategy involves modification of the antibiotic target. For example, some bacteria may alter the proteins that penicillin target rendering this antibiotic ineffective. Common antibiotic targets and resistance mechanisms can be seen in Table 2.1.

Table 2.1. Antibiotic targets and resistance mechanisms

Resistance mechanism	Action	Effective against
Efflux pumps	Pumps antibiotic out of cell before it reaches target	Fluoroquinolones Aminoglycosides Tetracyclines Beta-lactams Macrolides
Immunity and Bypass	Antibiotics or antibiotic targets bound by proteins preventing antibiotic binding	Tetracyclines Trimethroprim Sulfonamides Vancomycin
Target modification	Antibiotic targets are modified to prevent antibiotic binding	Fluoroquinolones Rifamycins Vancomycin Penicillins Macrolides Aminoglycosides
Inactivating enzymes	Destroys antibiotic through catalysation	Beta-lactams Aminoglycosides Macrolides Rifamycins

Source: Adapted from Wright (2010[35]).

2.5. What are the priority pathogens?

The umbrella term AMR includes many different types of antimicrobial resistance. In principle, the list of antibiotic-bacterium combinations can be extensive, although the World Health Organization (WHO) recognises that the majority of the health burden is caused by a relatively limited number of organisms including: *Escherichia coli* (*E. coli*), *Klebsiella pneumoniae* (*K. pneumoniae*), *Staphylococcus aureus* (*S. aureus*), *Streptococcus pneumoniae (S. pneumoniae)*, *Salmonella, Shigella, Neisseria gonorrhoeae* (*N. gonorrhoeae*), *Mycobacterium tuberculosis* (*M. tuberculosis*) and *Plasmodium malariae* (*P. malariae*) (WHO, 2014[36]).

In 2017, WHO developed a list of priority pathogens in order to help focus efforts on reducing the impact of AMR at the global level (see Box 2.4). The WHO Pathogens Priority List Working Group and a group of experts used a multi-criteria decision analysis to categorise resistant bacteria into critical, high, and medium priority categories (Tacconelli et al., 2018[37]). These categories represent the relative threat level of each pathogen to human health. Efforts to reduce AMR should focus on the highest categories. Criteria for category inclusion included: mortality, health-care burden, community burden, prevalence of resistance, 10-year trend of resistance, transmissibility, preventability in the community setting, preventability in the health-care setting, treatability, and the treatment pipeline. Inclusion in each priority category was based on the total score from these variables with higher scores going into higher priority categories. *M. tuberculosis,* the bacteria responsible for tuberculosis and for which AMR is highly problematic was not included in the list of priority pathogens as WHO consider that this bacteria is already specifically targeted by other dedicated programmes.

The bacteria on the list of priority pathogens are responsible for a wide range of infections from skin to respiratory and bloodstream infections and include both those in hospital and outside. In order to avoid the worst effects of AMR, efforts to reduce resistance and to find new treatment solutions should focus on these priority pathogens.

Box 2.4. Priority pathogens

In 2017 WHO published a list of priority pathogens (Tacconelli et al., 2018[37]) for which urgent action is needed. This list divided pathogens into critical, high, and medium priority groups according to the threat level each poses to human health. Bacteria and specific antibiotic resistances, according to priority category, are:

Critical priority pathogens:

- *Acinetobacter baumannii*, carbapenem-resistant
- *Pseudomonas aeruginosa*, carbapenem-resistant
- *Enterobacteriaceae*, carbapenem-resistant, third-generation cephalosporin-resistant

High priority pathogens:

- *Enterococcus faecium*, vancomycin-resistant
- *Staphylococcus aureus*, methicillin-resistant, vancomycin intermediate and resistant
- *Helicobacter pylori*, clarithromycin-resistant
- *Campylobacter spp.*, fluoroquinolone-resistant
- *Salmonella spp.*, fluoroquinolone-resistant
- *Neisseria gonorrhoeae*, third generation cephalosporin-resistant, fluoroquinolone-resistant

Medium priority pathogens:

- *Streptococcus pneumoniae*, penicillin-non-susceptible
- *Haemophilus influenzae*, ampicillin-resistant
- *Shigella spp.*, fluoroquinolone-resistant

The OECD analyses presented in the following chapters focus on a comprehensive set of bacteria, taking as starting point the two WHO lists mentioned above as well as other dimensions, including data availability. More specifically, the OECD analyses include:

- *Escherichia Coli*: a gram-negative commensal bacterium carried in the human gut and a common cause of infection including serious diarrhoea and urinary tract infections. *E. Coli* is also the leading cause of bloodstream infections in the community and the second leading cause of these infections in hospitals globally. Standard treatment for infection due to *E. Coli* includes third-generation cephalosporin antibiotics.
- *Klebsiella pneumoniae*, a common disease-causing pathogen also found in the human gut. *K. pneumoniae* can cause a wide range of infections from urinary tract and upper respiratory tract infections to sepsis and meningitis. It is also an important cause of hospital-acquired infections. Antibiotic treatment may depend

on the infection site and local resistance profiles but can include third-generation cephalosporins, carbapenems, aminoglycosides, and quinolones.

- *Pseudomonas aeruginosa* (*P. aeruginosa*) can be found living in a wide variety of settings including natural environments such as on human skin or built environments including hospitals or on hospital equipment. This pathogen is naturally resistant to a number of antibiotics and is a major cause of nosocomial infections and infections among people with reduced immune function. Infections may include respiratory tract, urinary tract, or bloodstream infections. Treatment of infections with *P. aeruginosa* often relies on a combination of antibiotics including certain beta-lactams, aminoglycosides, carbapenems, and quinolone antibiotics.
- *Streptococcus pneumoniae* is often carried asymptomatically in the human respiratory tract or sinuses and is a leading cause of pneumonia and meningitis. Individuals with weakened immune systems including the elderly or young are particularly vulnerable to infection with *S. pneumoniae* which can also cause a range of localised and general invasive infections. Treatment guidelines may vary with infection site but beta-lactam antibiotics such as amoxicillin or cephalosporins are often recommended for treatment.
- *Staphylococcus Aureus* is commonly found on the skin or carried asymptomatically in the nares and is a frequent cause of skin, respiratory, and bloodstream infections. *S. Aureus* is also serious problem in hospitals including notably methicillin-resistance *S. Aureus* and is responsible for a large proportion of nosocomial infections. A number of treatment recommendations exist depending on local resistance profiles and may include penicillins, cephalosporins, or clindamycin.
- *Enterococcus faecium* (*E. faecium*) and *Enterococcus faecalis* (*E. faecalis*) are both commensal bacteria of the intestinal tract and important causes of nosocomial infections including sepsis and meningitis. Ampicillin or vancomycin is commonly used to treat enterococcal infections and rising vancomycin resistance among these bacteria make these infections hard to treat.

2.6. How do AMR bacteria spread and infect humans?

Human infection with resistant pathogens is the product of two separate but related phenomena: development of resistance and infection (see Figure 2.5).

Antibiotic resistance among bacteria may develop and spread through exposure to antibiotics in a number of settings including among humans in the community or in hospital, in the animal sector, or in the natural environment. The combination of resistance across sectors creates a global population of resistant bacteria which may be transferred within and among sectors including to and from humans.

The second part of the resistance-infection equation is infection. Like resistance, a number of different factors influence infection including hygiene and living conditions, vaccination, the general health status of the population and access to medicines.

Interactions also exist between these two branches and the factors leading to resistance infections. Increased infection rates for example can lead to higher antibiotic use, which in turn may lead to more resistance and resistant infections. These resistant infections may also have variable effects on infection rates. Some studies have suggested that resistant and susceptible bacteria compete with each other and that resistant infections may replace susceptible infections (Popovich, Weinstein and Hota, 2008[38]). Others suggest that there is no competition between these bacteria and resistant infections simply add to the baseline number of susceptible infections (Mostofsky, Lipsitch and Regev-Yochay, 2011[39]).

The factors outlined in Figure 2.5 are further detailed below. Section 2.7 explains how each sector contributes to the development and spread of AMR, with a special emphasis on the misuse of antibiotics across sectors in Section 2.8. Section 2.9 discusses specific factors related to bacterial disease burden.

Figure 2.5. Factors influencing bacterial resistance, bacterial infections, and resistant infections

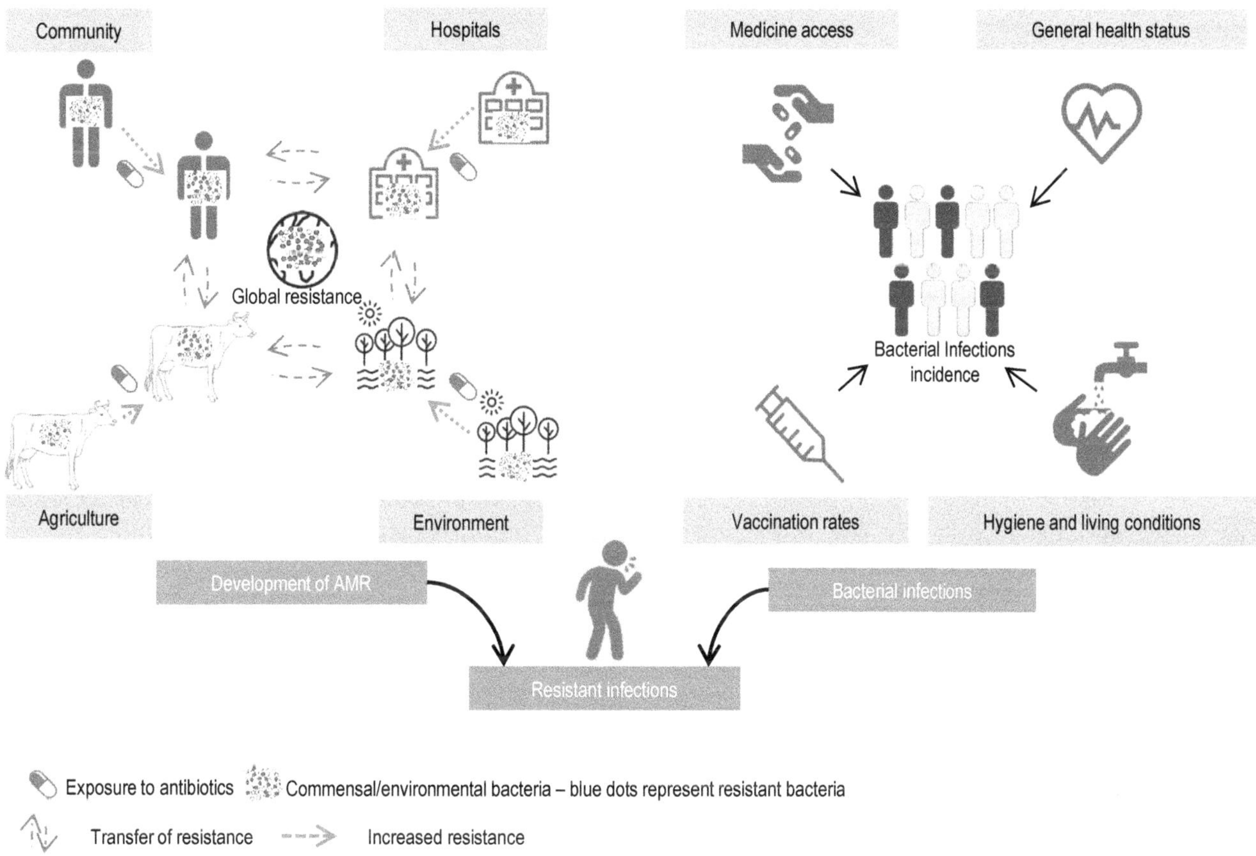

Source: Adapted from Chereau et al. (2017[40]).

2.7. How does each sector contribute to resistance development?

2.7.1. Animal sector

Use of antibiotics is particularly high among food animals and continues to grow worldwide. In the United States alone use in the animal sector represents an estimated 80% of all antibiotic use by weight (Spellberg et al., 2016[41]). Worldwide agricultural consumption is also predicted to increase by 70% by 2030 due to increases in demand for meat and changes in livestock production particularly in low and middle-income countries (Van Boeckel et al., 2015[42]). Furthermore, these estimates do not take into account antibiotic use in aquaculture where use may be high (Henriksson, Troell and Rico, 2015[43]).

Importantly, much of the antibiotic use in the agriculture sector is not for disease treatment but for disease prevention and growth promotion. This includes use of low-level doses of antibiotics in feed which presents a high risk for antibiotic resistance development (Van Boeckel et al., 2017[44]).

This high use has resulted in high rates of resistant bacteria detected in this sector including the emergence and spread of dangerous new forms of resistance such as colistin resistance or strains of methicillin-resistant *Staphylococcus aureus* (MRSA) (Price et al., 2012[45]).

2.7.2. Community

The largest source of antibiotic use and misuse in humans is in the outpatient or community sector (doctors, dentists, etc.). In the United States the majority (>60%) of antibiotic expenditure and consumption (80-90%) is associated with the outpatient setting (CDC, 2017[46]) with similar proportions reported in Europe (ECDC, 2017[11]). In 2014, there were nearly as many outpatient antibiotic prescriptions in the United States as people living in the country. In Europe, an average of 2.2 standard doses of antibiotics were consumed per 100 people per day in 2016 (ECDC, 2017[47]).

Certain sectors contribute heavily to high community antibiotic use such as long-term care where over half of nursing home residents use antibiotics each year (van Buul et al., 2012[48]). Dentistry is another important source of antibiotic consumption and can make up over 10% of community use in some countries (Marra et al., 2016[49]).

Like the animal sector, this heavy use of antibiotics in the community over recent years has led to a steady rise in the incidence of antibiotic resistance infections, including resistant tuberculosis as well as respiratory, skin, and sexually transmitted infections (CDC, 2013[29]).

2.7.3. Hospitals

Antibiotic resistance has historically been a hospital problem because these environments create a perfect storm for resistance development and infection by combining high antibiotic use with high infection rates. CDC data for 2016 showed that over half of US hospital inpatients received at least one antibiotic during their hospital stay (CDC, 2017[46]). Across Europe antibiotic use in hospitals made up nearly 10% of total human antibiotic use (ECDC, 2017[11]) despite the relatively small proportion of the population hospitalised.

Resistant infections are particularly common and problematic in hospitals due to the additional risk factors for infection among inpatients. Surgery patients or those using medical devices such as catheters, intravenous devices, or respirators are at heightened risk of infection as bacteria may infect surgical wounds or use medical devices as a vehicle for infection. Use of antibiotics is in itself a risk factor for resistant infection as it may increase the number of resistant bacteria in and around the patient while eliminating potentially protective susceptible bacteria.

Between 2008 and 2014, one in six central line-associated bloodstream infections in US hospitals were caused by dangerous resistant bacteria, as were one in seven surgical site infections. One in ten catheter-associated urinary tract infections were due to these bacteria during a similar period (CDC, 2016[50]).

2.7.4. Natural environment

While the role of human antibiotic use in resistance has been widely studied and described, the role played by the environment may be just as important. Antibiotics used in the community, hospitals, or the agricultural sector may end up in the environment through sewage water, farming activities including use of manures, or waste water from hospitals or antibiotic manufacturers (Amador et al., 2015[51]). Along with antibiotics used in terrestrial farming, those used in aquaculture may also pollute the environment and studies show a large proportion of these antibiotics end up in sediment (Henriksson, Troell and Rico, 2015[43]).

Once in the environment, the continued antimicrobial activity of these drugs may affect local microbial communities and favour resistance development and spread. Indeed, the majority of antibiotics consumed by humans or animals are excreted unmetabolised and some antibiotics such as fluoroquinolones may remain active for months in the environment (UNEP, 2017[52]).

Evidence of high rates of resistant bacteria in the environment due to antibiotic contamination has been reported and Li et al. (2015[53]) found up to three times as many antibiotic resistant genes among bacteria in natural environments affected by human activity versus those which were relatively unaffected.

2.7.5. Spread between sectors

Resistance, once developed, can easily spread to other sectors. For example, MRSA, a dangerous resistant bacteria which first developed in the hospital sector, has spread outside of that environment in recent years and is now responsible for a rising proportion of community acquired infections (Salmenlinna, Lyytikäinen and Vuopio-Varkila, 2002[54]). The animal sector is also an important development and transmission point for resistance. High levels of antimicrobial use and resistance in animals has been linked to human disease both through natural environmental contamination and direct contact with animals or animal products such as meat or meat products (Nadimpalli et al., 2018[55]). A study by Fjalstat and colleagues found that the abundance of antibiotic resistance genes in the human gut is correlated with consumption of antibiotics in animals (Fjalstad et al., 2018[56]).

2.8. Use and misuse of antibiotics

2.8.1. High antibiotic use across OECD countries

The major factor contributing to increased resistance across sectors is antibiotic use. Across OECD countries, antibiotic use among humans has increased significantly since 1980. Most of this increase occurred from 1980 to 1995 with rates remaining relatively stable in the following years (OECD, WHO, FAO, OIE, 2017[19]). Figure 2.6 shows the trends in antibiotics for systemic use in OECD countries since 2000. On average 22.15 defined daily doses (DDD) were consumed per 1 000 inhabitants in 2015 across OECD countries. A number of countries such as France and Greece showed consistently higher consumption rates while others such as Ireland have seen growing rates over this period. Notably, consumption rates show no significant reduction during this period despite rising resistance and calls to action.

Figure 2.6. Trends in antimicrobial consumption for systemic use in selected OECD countries

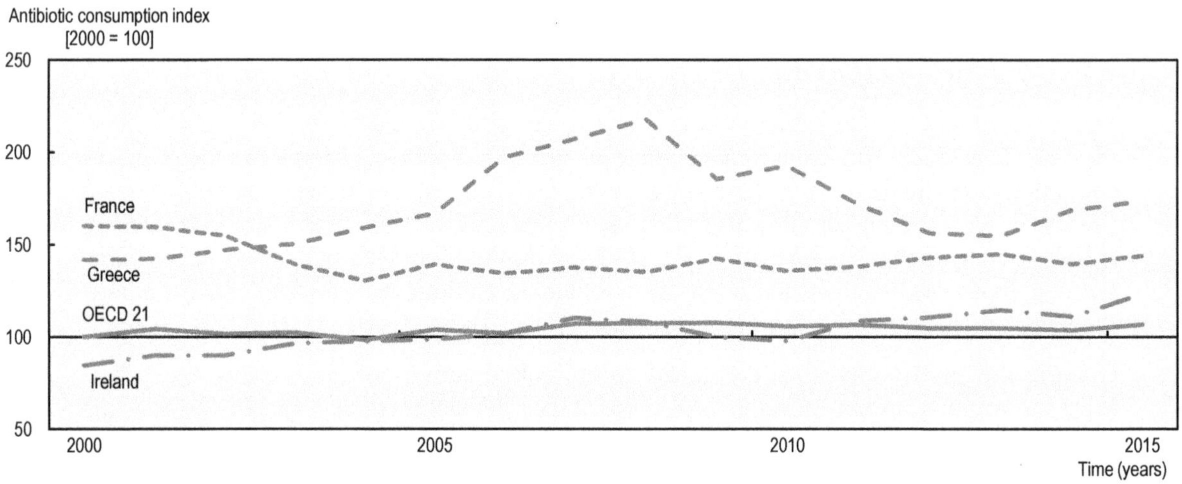

Note: Data were normalised to average antimicrobial consumption in OECD 21 in 2000 (equal to 100). Data for missing years were estimated by linear interpolation. OECD 23 includes: Australia, Belgium, the Czech Republic, Denmark, Estonia, Finland, France, Germany, Greece, Hungary, Iceland, Ireland, Luxembourg, Netherlands, Poland, Portugal, Slovak Republic, Slovenia, Spain, Sweden, and the United Kingdom

Source: Analyses of OECD Health Statistics (2018), http://dx.doi.org/10.1787/health-data-en.

StatLink http://dx.doi.org/10.1787/888933854687

2.8.2. Antibiotic misuse

Along with high use of antibiotics, there is also significant overuse and misuse in OECD countries. An estimated 50% of antibiotics prescribed by general practitioners in OECD countries are used inappropriately including situations where antibiotics were not needed or the wrong antibiotic was prescribed (OECD, 2017[57]; Paget et al., 2017[58]).

In hospitals, roughly one-third of antibiotics used may be unnecessary (CDC, 2017[46]). Hospitals also use and misuse higher proportions of last-line antibiotics which can favour the development of powerful forms of resistance including to carbapenem and polymixin antibiotics.

2.8.3. Factors related to misuse

Many factors underpin the high levels of inappropriate use of antimicrobials in the human sector including those related to doctors, patients, health care organisations, and producers and vendors of antimicrobials.

Prescriber factors

Prescribers face various pressures leading to inappropriate prescription of antimicrobials including previous practice inertia, fear of treatment failure, perceived pressure from patients and a lack of time.

Many doctors prescribe antibiotics out of habit and studies show that doctors who prescribe the most antibiotics tend to be those longest out of university or those having spent the longest time in the same practice (Mainous III, Hueston and Love, 1998[59]) (Steinke et al., 2000[60]).

Doctors may also prescribe antibiotics out of fear of treatment failure and the possibility of a secondary bacterial infection. This may be particularly likely in patients with comorbidities such as old age and chronic disease (Vazquez-Lago et al., 2012[61]).

Some antibiotic misuse results from real or perceived patient expectations. A 2015 study showed that 55% of participating general practitioners in Britain felt pressure to prescribe antimicrobials and 45% admitted to prescribing an antimicrobial, even when they knew it would be ineffective, in response to patient pressure (Cole, 2014[62]).

Issues such as time limitations, patient health coverage, and organisation actions to control AMR are also drivers of inappropriate prescribing (Cabana et al., 1999[63]) (Teixeira Rodrigues et al., 2013[64]).

Patient factors

A number of patient factors may also lead to higher misuse of antibiotics including those related to an inadequate knowledge of AMR.

Many patients use antibiotics without a prescription, often leading to unnecessary and/or incorrect use. This usage represented between 3% and 44% of antibiotic use across a sample of OECD countries in a systematic review. (Morgan et al., 2011[65]). Countries in Southern and Eastern Europe as well as Mexico showed higher rates of non-prescription use. Sources of these non-prescription antibiotics include pharmacies, unfinished courses, or friends and family. This type of consumption is particularly frequent in LMICs (See Box 2.5).

Poor adherence to antimicrobial prescriptions by patients is another cause of inappropriate use if a patient does not follow guidelines on dose or duration. Up to 44% of patients in the United States may skip antibiotic doses (Edgar, Boyd and Palame, 2008[66]). Patients may also seek additional care including antimicrobial treatment if symptoms do not disappear immediately after beginning antimicrobial treatment. A study in Japan showed that 7.5% of antimicrobial prescriptions were given for a condition for which the patient had already received a prescription from another provider (Takahashi et al., 2016[67]).

Health care organisation factors

The organisation of health care also plays a role in inappropriate antimicrobial prescribing. For example, a prescription may be an easy solution for doctors when time or diagnostic resources are lacking. Insurance that does not reimburse diagnostic testing can affect the willingness to use these services and favour inappropriate prescribing.

Reimbursement systems also influence prescribing patterns by affecting the cost/benefit of a re-examination of the same patient. Doctors working with a fixed budget may be more likely to prescribe an antimicrobial to lower the risk of seeing the same patient again within a short time (Kaier, Frank and Meyer, 2011[68]). Under some payment systems, patients are incentivised to change physicians if one doctor does not provide the antimicrobial therapy they would like.

Policies regulating the separation of drug prescription and sales can also affect inappropriate prescribing. In some countries, and particularly in LMICs, doctors may be the ones selling drugs to patients giving them an economic incentive for overprescribing.

Industry factors

Lastly, the pharmaceutical industry can contribute to inappropriate antimicrobial use. Efforts to promote drug use including antimicrobials among both patients and doctors increase the likelihood that these drugs will be prescribed regardless of need (Wazana, 2000[69]).

Drug producers and vendors also play a role. Sales of antibiotics without a prescription make up an estimated 2% to 8% of total sales among European countries (Safrany and Monnet, 2012[70]) and counterfeit antimicrobials which are often of poor quality, make up 5% of the global market (Delepierre, Gayot and Carpentier, 2012[71]).

Box 2.5. Drivers of inappropriate antibiotic use in LMICs

Antibiotic misuse may be highly prevalent in LMICs due to the high infectious disease burden, the availability of non-prescription drugs, and lack of healthcare access in some regions. The topic of non-prescription antibiotic use is particularly important as it may represent up to 100% of antibiotic use among certain populations in LMICs as is correlated with a number of factors related to inappropriate use such as unnecessary consumption, inappropriate dosage and duration, and inappropriate molecule choice. (Morgan et al., 2011[65]).

Non-prescription antibiotic use is also associated with poor quality or counterfeit drugs which are common in LMICs and an estimated 60% of antimicrobials used in Africa and Asia contain little or no active ingredients (World Bank, 2017[18]).

2.9. Other public health factors that influence infection rates and AMR

A number of factors related to infection rates among humans include vaccination coverage, hygiene, access to medicines, and general health status.

2.9.1. Vaccination coverage

Vaccination coverage is one important factor in determining infection rates and may provide an important tool in reducing antibiotic resistance. (Rappuoli, Bloom and Black, 2017[72]). Vaccines target both bacterial and viral infections and have proven to be extremely successful in preventing or even eliminating infectious diseases such as smallpox, measles, and polio. Today vaccination is no less important in preventing the re-emergence of these diseases.

Across OECD countries, vaccines are used widely to effectively prevent bacterial diseases susceptible to the development of AMR including those from *Corynebacterium diphtheriae* (diphtheria), *Haemophilus influenzae* type B, *Neisseria meningitides*, *S. pneumoniae*, *Bordetella pertussis* (whooping cough), and *M. tuberculosis* (tuberculosis). Various vaccination strategies exist across OECD countries in terms of coverage and population. A number of countries ensure vaccination coverage through mandating vaccination for school attendance. Other countries such as Australia and Israel have tied family assistance payments or child tax credits to compliance with vaccination schedules to encourage coverage.

Because vaccination prevents rather than treats disease, it could automatically reduce the number of resistant infections by reducing overall infection numbers. This reduction would reduce the need for antibiotics to treat these infections having a positive effect on AMR. A review of the impact of the conjugate pneumococcal vaccine in 2008 showed not only reductions in overall disease burden but also in antibiotic use and resistant infections among vaccinated groups (Dagan and Klugman, 2008[73]). Unlike antibiotics, and despite the absence of any vaccine for priority pathogens, the vaccine pipeline continues to produce effective and important new products. Research is ongoing for development of vaccines for a number of important bacteria such as *E. coli, K. pneumoniae, S. aureus, Salmonella, P. aeruginosa*, and *A. baumannii* (Huttner et al., 2017[74]; Lee et al., 2015[75]; Giersing et al., 2016[76]; Erova et al., 2016[77]; Yang et al., 2017[78]; Ni et al., 2017[79]).

2.9.2. Hygiene

Hygiene is another major factor in the spread of infectious disease including those with AMR. In hospitals, hygiene includes infection prevention and control practices such as hand-washing practices, sterilisation of instruments and the cleaning of rooms, corridors, and other common spaces. Poor hygiene can result in greater rates of hospital-acquired infections (McLaws, 2015[80]). Poor hygiene also favours the spread of resistant pathogens from one patient to another within the hospital resulting in hospital outbreaks (Rampling et al., 2001[81]). Hygiene campaigns in hospitals have been shown to be effective in reducing infections and a study by Kirkland et al. (2012[82]) found that a hand hygiene initiative in a US hospital reduced infection rates by over 30%.

In the community, hygiene on an individual level should include good hand washing and food handling practices, avoiding putting individuals in contact with infectious (including resistant) pathogens (Landers et al., 2012[83]). On a population level poor hygiene can be linked to a lack of sufficient public health and sanitation infrastructure such as water treatment, urban planning, and food treatment and inspection, resulting in a much greater exposure of the population to infectious pathogens (WHO, 2001[84]).

2.9.3. Access to medicines

While many countries are working to restrict antimicrobial use to avoid resistance, insufficient access to medicines including antimicrobials may be a large driver of infectious disease burden in others. Restricted access to health care in some LMICs can lead to an increased burden of infectious disease. Normally treatable infections, including lower respiratory infections, diarrhoea and neonatal sepsis, account for an estimated 12% of deaths in LMICs (IHME, 2018[8]). Ensuring timely access to antibiotics would avert an estimated 445 000 pneumonia deaths alone in children living in low and middle-income countries (Laxminarayan et al., 2016[85]). In order to maximise the benefit of life-saving antimicrobials globally counties must not only work to reduce unnecessary use but also expand access when needed.

2.9.4. General health status

The general health status of a person or an entire population can influence the susceptibility to infectious diseases. Immunocompromised, elderly, or otherwise sick individuals run a much greater risk of contracting infectious diseases (Rubin, 1993[86]). As discussed in Section 2.7.3, many of these individuals also spend time in hospital and under antibiotic treatment thus increasing the chances of developing an antibiotic resistant infection (WHO, 2017[87]).

Factors such as malnourishment, a high burden of HIV, or malaria found in some populations in LMICs, put these populations at particular risk for infectious diseases (Katona and Katona- Apte, 2008[88]). Investing in measures for greater overall population level health such as increased health care access is an important strategy in lowering the infectious disease burden.

2.10. How can promoting prudent use of antimicrobials decrease AMR?

A number of existing strategies to reduce the burden of AMR focus on reducing the use of antimicrobials. These may include public health campaigns, doctor training, or the use of delayed prescriptions. These strategies rely on both a decrease in the "upward" selection pressure toward higher resistance, and an increase in the "downward" selection pressure toward less resistance through the relative bacterial fitness of resistant and susceptible bacteria to be effective.

2.10.1. Reducing "upward" resistance selection

AMR develops through a system of natural selection where bacteria or other organisms adapt to their environment through resistance development in response to the selection pressure exerted by the presence of antimicrobials (see Section 2.2). The presence of antibiotics pushes resistance rates "upward" by killing susceptible bacteria and providing an environment available only to resistant bacteria. Antibiotics also promote gene transfer including resistant genes to increase resistance rates (see Box 2.3). Continued presence of antibiotics in an environment will put continued pressure on bacteria pushing them toward greater and greater resistance levels (Baym et al., 2016[89]). Removal or reduction of antibiotics will thus remove or reduce this upward pressure and slow or stop increasing resistance.

2.10.2. Increase "downward" selection for susceptibility

While removing antibiotics may stop resistance rates from increasing, a second mechanism is needed for rates to decrease. Removing antibiotics may also allow for a "downward" pressure on resistance through the replacement of resistant bacteria by susceptible bacteria which may be better adapted to environments where antibiotics are not present (Andersson and Hughes, 2011[90]).

This downward pressure through replacement is created by differences in bacterial "fitness", which is the ability to replicate in a given environment. Bacteria with a greater fitness thus have a survival advantage over less fit bacteria. By acquiring resistance mechanisms, some bacteria may pay a "fitness cost" which can make them less able to replicate in environments without antibiotics (Melnyk, Wong and Kassen, 2015[91]). By removing antibiotics, these less fit resistant bacteria could theoretically be replaced with the more fit non-resistant bacteria over time reducing resistance levels.

This is an attractive idea and a key to strategies aiming to reduce antibiotic resistance through reduction in antibiotic use. Indeed, a number of interventions based on reduction of antibiotic use have reported lower resistance rates which may support the effectiveness of these interventions and the theory (Guillemot et al., 2005[92]) (Baur et al., 2017[93]). However, the reality of fitness is more complicated.

Along with the wide range of resistance mechanisms is a wide range of potential fitness costs. While some resistance mechanisms come with a clear fitness cost, others seem to incur no observable cost, meaning that these resistant bacteria are just as capable of reproducing in environments with no antibiotics as susceptible bacteria. For bacteria with "cost free" resistance, simply removing antibiotics will not reduce the underlying levels of resistance (Mclnyk, Wong and Kassen, 2015[91]).

While fitness may not be able to reduce underlying resistance levels this does not mean that strategies to reduce antibiotic use should not be pursued. Regardless of the relative downward pressure induced by fitness costs, a reduction in antibiotic use will reduce the upward pressure for development of new resistance mechanisms, the transfer of resistance genes, and the growth of resistant bacteria in the absence of competing susceptible bacteria.

Note

[1] Lines of treatment correspond to the order of recommended treatment options for a given illness. First-line treatment is the first recommended treatment option. Second-line treatment is generally recommended only if a first-line treatment is insufficient.

References

Ahmed, S. et al. (2017), "Assessing the Global Economic and Poverty Effects of Antimicrobial Resistance", http://documents.worldbank.org/curated/en/190151498872848485/pdf/WPS8133.pdf (accessed on 11 July 2018). [17]

Amador, P. et al. (2015), "Antibiotic resistance in wastewater: Occurrence and fate of Enterobacteriaceae producers of Class A and Class C β-lactamases", *Journal of Environmental Science and Health, Part A*, Vol. 50/1, pp. 26-39, http://dx.doi.org/10.1080/10934529.2015.964602. [51]

Andersson, D. and D. Hughes (2014), "Microbiological effects of sublethal levels of antibiotics.", *Nature reviews. Microbiology*, Vol. 12/7, pp. 465-78, http://dx.doi.org/10.1038/nrmicro3270. [32]

Andersson, D. and D. Hughes (2011), "Persistence of antibiotic resistance in bacterial populations", *FEMS Microbiology Reviews*, Vol. 35/5, pp. 901-911, http://dx.doi.org/10.1111/j.1574-6976.2011.00289.x. [90]

Austrian, R. and J. Gold (1964), "Pneumococcal Bacteremia with Especial Reference to Bacteremic Pneumococcal Pneumonia", *Annals of internal medicine*, Vol. 60, pp. 759-76, http://www.ncbi.nlm.nih.gov/pubmed/14156606 (accessed on 27 April 2018). [2]

Baur, D. et al. (2017), "Effect of antibiotic stewardship on the incidence of infection and colonisation with antibiotic-resistant bacteria and Clostridium difficile infection: a systematic review and meta-analysis", *The Lancet Infectious Diseases*, Vol. 17/9, pp. 990-1001, https://doi.org/10.1016/S1473-3099(17)30325-0. [93]

Baym, M. et al. (2016), "Spatiotemporal microbial evolution on antibiotic landscapes", *Science*, Vol. 353/6304, pp. 1147-1151, http://dx.doi.org/10.1126/science.aag0822. [89]

Brown, E. and G. Wright (2016), "Antibacterial drug discovery in the resistance era", *Nature*, Vol. 529/7586, pp. 336-343, http://dx.doi.org/10.1038/nature17042. [31]

Cabana, M. et al. (1999), "Why don't physicians follow clinical practice guidelines? A framework for improvement.", *JAMA*, Vol. 282/15, pp. 1458-65, http://www.ncbi.nlm.nih.gov/pubmed/10535437 (accessed on 23 May 2018). [63]

CDC (2018), *Antibiotic / Antimicrobial Resistance | CDC*, https://www.cdc.gov/drugresistance/index.html (accessed on 15 May 2018). [9]

CDC (2018), *Leading Causes of Death, 1900-1998*, https://www.cdc.gov/nchs/data/dvs/lead1900_98.pdf (accessed on 13 June 2018). [4]

CDC (2017), *Antibiotic Use in the United States, 2017: Progress and Opportunities | Antibiotic Use | CDC*, https://www.cdc.gov/antibiotic-use/stewardship-report/hospital.html (accessed on 27 April 2018). [46]

CDC (2016), *Superbugs threaten hospital patients | CDC Online Newsroom | CDC*, https://www.cdc.gov/media/releases/2016/p0303-superbugs.html (accessed on 27 April 2018). [50]

CDC (2013), *Antibiotic Resistance Threats in the United States, 2013*, https://www.cdc.gov/drugresistance/pdf/ar-threats-2013-508.pdf (accessed on 27 April 2018). [29]

Cecchini, M., J. Langer and L. Slawomirski (2015), "Antimicrobial Resistance in G7 Countries and Beyond: Economic Issues, Policies and Options for Action", https://www.oecd.org/els/health-systems/Antimicrobial-Resistance-in-G7-Countries-and-Beyond.pdf (accessed on 27 April 2018). [13]

Chereau, F. et al. (2017), "Risk assessment for antibiotic resistance in South East Asia.", *BMJ (Clinical research ed.)*, Vol. 358, p. j3393, http://dx.doi.org/10.1136/BMJ.J3393. [40]

Cole, A. (2014), "GPs feel pressurised to prescribe unnecessary antibiotics, survey finds.", *BMJ (Clinical research ed.)*, Vol. 349, p. g5238, http://www.ncbi.nlm.nih.gov/pubmed/25143516 (accessed on 23 May 2018). [62]

D'Costa, V. et al. (2011), "Antibiotic resistance is ancient", *Nature*, Vol. 477/7365, pp. 457-461, http://dx.doi.org/10.1038/nature10388. [30]

Dagan, R. and K. Klugman (2008), "Impact of conjugate pneumococcal vaccines on antibiotic resistance", *The Lancet Infectious Diseases*, Vol. 8/12, pp. 785-795, https://doi.org/10.1016/S1473-3099(08)70281-0. [73]

Davies, J. and D. Davies (2010), "Origins and Evolution of Antibiotic Resistance", *Microbiology and Molecular Biology Reviews*, Vol. 74/3, pp. 417-433, http://dx.doi.org/10.1128/MMBR.00016-10. [3]

Delepierre, A., A. Gayot and A. Carpentier (2012), "Update on counterfeit antibiotics worldwide; public health risks.", *Medecine et maladies infectieuses*, Vol. 42/6, pp. 247-55, http://dx.doi.org/10.1016/j.medmal.2012.04.007. [71]

ECDC (2017), *Antimicrobial resistance surveillance in Europe 2015. Annual Report of the European Antimicrobial Resistance Surveillance Network (EARS-Net).*, https://ecdc.europa.eu/sites/portal/files/media/en/publications/Publications/antimicrobial-resistance-europe-2015.pdf. [11]

ECDC (2017), "Summary of the latest data on antibiotic consumption in the European Union", https://ecdc.europa.eu/sites/portal/files/documents/Final_2017_EAAD_ESAC-Net_Summary-edited%20-%20FINALwith%20erratum.pdf (accessed on 27 April 2018). [47]

Edgar, T., S. Boyd and M. Palame (2008), "Sustainability for behaviour change in the fight against antibiotic resistance: a social marketing framework", *Journal of Antimicrobial Chemotherapy*, Vol. 63/2, pp. 230-237, http://dx.doi.org/10.1093/jac/dkn508. [66]

Erova, T. et al. (2016), "Protective Immunity Elicited by Oral Immunization of Mice with Salmonella enterica Serovar Typhimurium Braun Lipoprotein (Lpp) and Acetyltransferase (MsbB) Mutants", *Frontiers in Cellular and Infection Microbiology*, Vol. 6, p. 148, http://dx.doi.org/10.3389/fcimb.2016.00148. [77]

European Commmission (2018), *EU Action on Antimicrobial Resistance - European Commission*, https://ec.europa.eu/health/amr/antimicrobial-resistance_en (accessed on 15 May 2018). [10]

Fjalstad, J. et al. (2018), "Antibiotic therapy in neonates and impact on gut microbiota and antibiotic resistance development: a systematic review", *Journal of Antimicrobial Chemotherapy*, Vol. 73/3, pp. 569-580, http://dx.doi.org/10.1093/jac/dkx426. [56]

Francino, M. (2015), "Antibiotics and the Human Gut Microbiome: Dysbioses and Accumulation of Resistances.", *Frontiers in microbiology*, Vol. 6, p. 1543, http://dx.doi.org/10.3389/fmicb.2015.01543. [24]

G20 (2017), *G20 Leaders' Declaration: Shaping an interconnected world*, http://www.oecd.org/els/health-systems/G20-leaders-declaration.pdf (accessed on 14 June 2018). [20]

Giersing, B. et al. (2016), "Status of vaccine research and development of vaccines for Staphylococcus aureus", *Vaccine*, Vol. 34/26, pp. 2962-2966, http://dx.doi.org/10.1016/j.vaccine.2016.03.110. [76]

Guillemot, D. et al. (2005), "Reduction of Antibiotic Use in the Community Reduces the Rate of Colonization with Penicillin G--Nonsusceptible Streptococcus pneumoniae", *Clinical Infectious Diseases*, Vol. 41/7, pp. 930-938, http://dx.doi.org/10.1086/432721. [92]

Gwatkin, D., M. Guillot and P. Heuveline (1999), "The burden of disease among the global poor", *The Lancet*, Vol. 354/9178, pp. 586-589, https://doi.org/10.1016/S0140-6736(99)02108-X. [14]

Henriksson, P., M. Troell and A. Rico (2015), "Antimicrobial use in aquaculture: Some complementing facts.", *Proceedings of the National Academy of Sciences of the United States of America*, Vol. 112/26, p. E3317, http://dx.doi.org/10.1073/pnas.1508952112. [43]

Huttner, A. et al. (2017), "Safety, immunogenicity, and preliminary clinical efficacy of a vaccine against extraintestinal pathogenic Escherichia coli in women with a history of recurrent urinary tract infection: a randomised, single-blind, placebo-controlled phase 1b trial.", *The Lancet. Infectious diseases*, Vol. 17/5, pp. 528-537, https://doi.org/10.1016/S1473-3099(17)30108-1. [74]

IHME (2018), *GBD Results Tool | GHDx*, http://ghdx.healthdata.org/gbd-results-tool (accessed on 14 June 2018). [8]

Kaier, K., U. Frank and E. Meyer (2011), "Economic incentives for the (over-)prescription of broad-spectrum antimicrobials in German ambulatory care.", *The Journal of antimicrobial chemotherapy*, Vol. 66/7, pp. 1656-8, http://dx.doi.org/10.1093/jac/dkr134. [68]

Katona, P. and J. Katona- Apte (2008), "The Interaction between Nutrition and Infection", *Clinical Infectious Diseases*, Vol. 46/10, pp. 1582-1588, http://dx.doi.org/10.1086/587658. [88]

Kirkland, K. et al. (2012), "Impact of a hospital-wide hand hygiene initiative on healthcare-associated infections: results of an interrupted time series.", *BMJ quality & safety*, Vol. 21/12, pp. 1019-26, http://dx.doi.org/10.1136/bmjqs-2012-000800. [82]

Kumarasamy, K. et al. (2010), "Emergence of a new antibiotic resistance mechanism in India, Pakistan, and the UK: a molecular, biological, and epidemiological study.", *The Lancet. Infectious diseases*, Vol. 10/9, pp. 597-602, https://doi.org/10.1016/S1473-3099(10)70143-2. [7]

Landers, T. et al. (2012), "A review of antibiotic use in food animals: perspective, policy, and potential.", *Public health reports (Washington, D.C. : 1974)*, Vol. 127/1, pp. 4-22, http://dx.doi.org/10.1177/003335491212700103. [83]

Langdon, A., N. Crook and G. Dantas (2016), "The effects of antibiotics on the microbiome throughout development and alternative approaches for therapeutic modulation.", *Genome medicine*, Vol. 8/1, p. 39, http://dx.doi.org/10.1186/s13073-016-0294-z. [21]

Laxminarayan, R. et al. (2016), "Access to effective antimicrobials: a worldwide challenge", *The Lancet*, Vol. 387/10014, pp. 168-175, https://doi.org/10.1016/S0140-6736(15)00474-2. [85]

Lee, W. et al. (2015), "Vaccination with Klebsiella pneumoniae-derived extracellular vesicles protects against bacteria-induced lethality via both humoral and cellular immunity.", *Experimental & molecular medicine*, Vol. 47/9, p. e183, http://dx.doi.org/10.1038/emm.2015.59. [75]

Li, B. et al. (2015), "Metagenomic and network analysis reveal wide distribution and co-occurrence of environmental antibiotic resistance genes", *The ISME Journal*, Vol. 9/11, pp. 2490-2502, http://dx.doi.org/10.1038/ismej.2015.59. [53]

Mainous III, A., W. Hueston and M. Love (1998), "Antibiotics for Colds in Children", *Archives of Pediatrics & Adolescent Medicine*, Vol. 152/4, pp. 349-352, http://dx.doi.org/10.1001/archpedi.152.4.349. [59]

Marra, F. et al. (2016), "Antibiotic prescribing by dentists has increased: Why?", *The Journal of the American Dental Association*, Vol. 147/5, pp. 320-327, http://dx.doi.org/10.1016/J.ADAJ.2015.12.014. [49]

McLaws, M. (2015), "The relationship between hand hygiene and health care-associated infection: it's complicated.", *Infection and drug resistance*, Vol. 8, pp. 7-18, http://dx.doi.org/10.2147/IDR.S62704. [80]

McNulty, C. et al. (2018), "CTX-M ESBL-producing Enterobacteriaceae: estimated prevalence in adults in England in 2014", *Journal of Antimicrobial Chemotherapy*, Vol. 73/5, pp. 1368-1388, http://dx.doi.org/10.1093/jac/dky007. [6]

Melnyk, A., A. Wong and R. Kassen (2015), "The fitness costs of antibiotic resistance mutations.", *Evolutionary applications*, Vol. 8/3, pp. 273-83, http://dx.doi.org/10.1111/eva.12196. [91]

Morgan, D. et al. (2011), "Non-prescription antimicrobial use worldwide: a systematic review.", *The Lancet. Infectious diseases*, Vol. 11/9, pp. 692-701, https://doi.org/10.1016/S1473-3099(11)70054-8. [65]

Mostofsky, E., M. Lipsitch and G. Regev-Yochay (2011), "Is methicillin-resistant Staphylococcus aureus replacing methicillin-susceptible S. aureus?", *The Journal of antimicrobial chemotherapy*, Vol. 66/10, pp. 2199-214, http://dx.doi.org/10.1093/jac/dkr278. [39]

Nadimpalli, M. et al. (2018), "Combating Global Antibiotic Resistance: Emerging One Health Concerns in Lower- and Middle-Income Countries", *Clinical Infectious Diseases*, Vol. 66/6, pp. 963-969, http://dx.doi.org/10.1093/cid/cix879. [55]

Nelson, M. and S. Levy (2011), "The history of the tetracyclines", *Annals of the New York Academy of Sciences*, Vol. 1241/1, pp. 17-32, http://dx.doi.org/10.1111/j.1749-6632.2011.06354.x. [28]

Newton, P. et al. (2006), "Counterfeit anti-infective drugs", *The Lancet Infectious Diseases*, Vol. 6/9, pp. 602-613, https://doi.org/10.1016/S1473-3099(06)70581-3. [15]

Ni, Z. et al. (2017), "Antibiotic Resistance Determinant-Focused Acinetobacter baumannii Vaccine Designed Using Reverse Vaccinology.", *International journal of molecular sciences*, Vol. 18/2, http://dx.doi.org/10.3390/ijms18020458. [79]

OECD (2017), *Low-value health care with high stakes: Promoting the rational use of antimicrobials, published as Chapter 3 as part of the OECD publication Tackling Wasteful Spending on Health*, OECD Publishing, Paris, http://dx.doi.org/10.1787/9789264266414-en. [57]

OECD, WHO, FAO, OIE (2017), *Tackling Antimicrobial Resistance Ensuring Sustainable R&D*, http://www.oecd.org/g20/summits/hamburg/Tackling-Antimicrobial-Resistance-Ensuring-Sustainable-RD.pdf (accessed on 27 April 2018). [19]

Office of National Statistics (2018), *The 21st century mortality files - deaths dataset, England and Wales - Office for National Statistics*, https://www.ons.gov.uk/peoplepopulationandcommunity/birthsdeathsandmarriages/deaths/datasets/the21stcenturymortalityfilesdeathsdataset (accessed on 13 June 2018). [5]

Okeke, I. et al. (2005), "Antimicrobial resistance in developing countries. Part I: recent trends and current status", *The Lancet Infectious Diseases*, Vol. 5/8, pp. 481-493, http://dx.doi.org/10.1016/S1473-3099(05)70189-4. [16]

Paget, J. et al. (2017), *Antimicrobial resistance and causes of non-prudent use of antibiotics in human medicine in the EU*, http://dx.doi.org/ISBN 978-92-79-66537-0. [58]

Parekh, P., L. Balart and D. Johnson (2015), "The Influence of the Gut Microbiome on Obesity, Metabolic Syndrome and Gastrointestinal Disease", *Clinical and Translational Gastroenterology*, Vol. 6/6, pp. e91-e91, http://dx.doi.org/10.1038/ctg.2015.16. [26]

Popovich, K., R. Weinstein and B. Hota (2008), "Are Community-Associated Methicillin-Resistant Staphylococcus aureus (MRSA) Strains Replacing Traditional Nosocomial MRSA Strains?", *Clinical Infectious Diseases*, Vol. 46/6, pp. 787-794, http://dx.doi.org/10.1086/528716. [38]

Price, L. et al. (2012), "Staphylococcus aureus CC398: host adaptation and emergence of methicillin resistance in livestock.", *mBio*, Vol. 3/1, pp. e00305-11, http://dx.doi.org/10.1128/mBio.00305-11. [45]

Rampling, A. et al. (2001), "Evidence that hospital hygiene is important in the control of methicillin-resistant Staphylococcus aureus", *Journal of Hospital Infection*, Vol. 49/2, pp. 109-116, http://dx.doi.org/10.1053/jhin.2001.1013. [81]

Rappuoli, R., D. Bloom and S. Black (2017), "Deploy vaccines to fight superbugs", *Nature*, Vol. 552/7684, pp. 165-167, http://dx.doi.org/10.1038/d41586-017-08323-0. [72]

Riiser, A. (2015), "The human microbiome, asthma, and allergy.", *Allergy, asthma, and clinical immunology : official journal of the Canadian Society of Allergy and Clinical Immunology*, Vol. 11, p. 35, http://dx.doi.org/10.1186/s13223-015-0102-0. [25]

Rubin, R. (1993), "Fungal and bacterial infections in the immunocompromised host.", *European journal of clinical microbiology & infectious diseases : official publication of the European Society of Clinical Microbiology*, Vol. 12 Suppl 1, pp. S42-8, http://www.ncbi.nlm.nih.gov/pubmed/8477762 (accessed on 23 May 2018). [86]

Safrany, N. and D. Monnet (2012), "Antibiotics obtained without a prescription in Europe", *The Lancet Infectious Diseases*, Vol. 12/3, pp. 182-183, https://doi.org/10.1016/S1473-3099(12)70017-8. [70]

Salmenlinna, S., O. Lyytikäinen and J. Vuopio-Varkila (2002), "Community-Acquired Methicillin-Resistant <i>Staphylococcus aureus,</i> Finland", *Emerging Infectious Diseases*, Vol. 8/6, pp. 602-607, http://dx.doi.org/10.3201/eid0806.010313. [54]

Spellberg, B. et al. (2016), "Antibiotic Resistance in Humans and Animals", *National Academy of Medicine Discussion Paper*, https://nam.edu/wp-content/uploads/2016/07/Antibiotic-Resistance-in-Humans-and-Animals.pdf (accessed on 14 June 2018). [41]

Steinke, D. et al. (2000), "Practice factors that influence antibiotic prescribing in general practice in Tayside.", *The Journal of antimicrobial chemotherapy*, Vol. 46/3, pp. 509-12, http://www.ncbi.nlm.nih.gov/pubmed/10980184 (accessed on 23 May 2018). [60]

Strati, F. et al. (2017), "New evidences on the altered gut microbiota in autism spectrum disorders", *Microbiome*, Vol. 5/1, p. 24, http://dx.doi.org/10.1186/s40168-017-0242-1. [27]

Tacconelli, E. et al. (2018), "Discovery, research, and development of new antibiotics: the WHO priority list of antibiotic-resistant bacteria and tuberculosis.", *The Lancet. Infectious diseases*, Vol. 18/3, pp. 318-327, https://doi.org/10.1016/S1473-3099(17)30753-3. [37]

Takahashi, Y. et al. (2016), "Social network analysis of duplicative prescriptions: One-month analysis of medical facilities in Japan.", *Health policy (Amsterdam, Netherlands)*, Vol. 120/3, pp. 334-41, http://dx.doi.org/10.1016/j.healthpol.2016.01.020. [67]

Teixeira Rodrigues, A. et al. (2013), "Understanding physician antibiotic prescribing behaviour: a systematic review of qualitative studies", *International Journal of Antimicrobial Agents*, Vol. 41/3, pp. 203-212, http://dx.doi.org/10.1016/j.ijantimicag.2012.09.003. [64]

UNEP (2017), *Frontiers 2017 Emerging Issues of Environmental Concern*, United Nations Environment Programme, Nairobi, https://www.unenvironment.org/resources/frontiers-2017-emerging-issues-environmental-concern. [52]

Van Boeckel, T. et al. (2015), "Global trends in antimicrobial use in food animals", *Proceedings of the National Academy of Sciences*, Vol. 112/18, pp. 5649-5654, http://dx.doi.org/10.1073/pnas.1503141112. [42]

Van Boeckel, T. et al. (2017), "Reducing antimicrobial use in food animals.", *Science (New York, N.Y.)*, Vol. 357/6358, pp. 1350-1352, http://dx.doi.org/10.1126/science.aao1495. [44]

van Buul, L. et al. (2012), "Antibiotic Use and Resistance in Long Term Care Facilities", *Journal of the American Medical Directors Association*, Vol. 13/6, pp. 568.e1-568.e13, http://dx.doi.org/10.1016/j.jamda.2012.04.004. [48]

Vazquez-Lago, J. et al. (2012), "Attitudes of primary care physicians to the prescribing of antibiotics and antimicrobial resistance: a qualitative study from Spain", *Family Practice*, Vol. 29/3, pp. 352-360, http://dx.doi.org/10.1093/fampra/cmr084. [61]

Wachter, D., M. Joshi and B. Rimal (1999), "Antibiotic dispensing by drug retailers in Kathmandu, Nepal.", *Tropical medicine & international health : TM & IH*, Vol. 4/11, pp. 782-8, http://www.ncbi.nlm.nih.gov/pubmed/10588773 (accessed on 27 April 2018). [33]

Wazana, A. (2000), "Physicians and the pharmaceutical industry: is a gift ever just a gift?", *JAMA*, Vol. 283/3, pp. 373-80, http://www.ncbi.nlm.nih.gov/pubmed/10647801 (accessed on 23 May 2018). [69]

WHO (2017), "Antimicrobial Resistance", http://www.euro.who.int/__data/assets/pdf_file/0005/348224/Fact-sheet-SDG-AMR-FINAL-07-09-2017.pdf (accessed on 15 May 2018). [12]

WHO (2017), "WHO | The burden of health care-associated infection worldwide", http://www.who.int/infection-prevention/publications/burden_hcai/en/ (accessed on 23 May 2018). [87]

WHO (2014), *Antimicrobial resistance: global report on surveillance 2014*, World Health Organization, Geneva, http://www.who.int/drugresistance/documents/surveillancereport/en/. [36]

WHO (2001), *Water Treatment and Pathogen Control*, http://apps.who.int/iris/bitstream/handle/10665/42796/9241562552.pdf;jsessionid=8CC25CEBDE5644821ACA8E5D9CF4031D?sequence=1 (accessed on 22 May 2018). [84]

World Bank (2017), *Drug-Resistant Infections: A Threat to Our Economic Future*, World Bank, Washington, D.C., http://www.worldbank.org/en/topic/health/publication/drug-resistant-infections-a-threat-to-our-economic-future. [18]

Wright, G. (2010), "Q&A: Antibiotic resistance: where does it come from and what can we do about it?", *BMC Biology*, Vol. 8/1, p. 123, http://dx.doi.org/10.1186/1741-7007-8-123. [35]

Xu, J. and J. Gordon (2003), "Honor thy symbionts", *Proceedings of the National Academy of Sciences*, Vol. 100/18, pp. 10452-10459, http://dx.doi.org/10.1073/pnas.1734063100. [34]

Yang, F. et al. (2017), "Protective Efficacy of the Trivalent Pseudomonas aeruginosa Vaccine Candidate PcrV-OprI-Hcp1 in Murine Pneumonia and Burn Models", *Scientific Reports*, Vol. 7/1, p. 3957, http://dx.doi.org/10.1038/s41598-017-04029-5. [78]

Young, V. (2017), "The role of the microbiome in human health and disease: an introduction for clinicians.", *BMJ (Clinical research ed.)*, Vol. 356, p. j831, http://dx.doi.org/10.1136/BMJ.J831. [23]

Zaffiri, L., J. Gardner and L. Toledo-Pereyra (2012), "History of Antibiotics. From Salvarsan to Cephalosporins", *Journal of Investigative Surgery*, Vol. 25/2, pp. 67-77, http://dx.doi.org/10.3109/08941939.2012.664099. [1]

Zhang, Y. et al. (2015), "Impacts of Gut Bacteria on Human Health and Diseases", *International Journal of Molecular Sciences*, Vol. 16/12, pp. 7493-7519, http://dx.doi.org/10.3390/ijms16047493. [22]

Chapter 3. Trends in antimicrobial resistance in OECD countries

Tiago Cravo Oliveira and Michael Padget

Antimicrobial resistance (AMR) proportions have evolved very differently across countries and antibiotic-bacterium combinations in the last decade. This chapter looks at the challenges involved in defining and measuring resistance internationally, along with the methodology used to estimate historic and future resistance proportions. The chapter presents predicted resistance proportions for 52 countries for 2015, along with the rate of change since 2005 (averaged across eight priority antibiotic-bacterium pairs). The chapter then provides data on the projected resistance proportions across the same countries up to 2030. Factors contributing to the wide variability in the predicted resistance proportions between antibiotic-bacterium pairs within and across different countries are explored. The chapter concludes by looking at the problem of increasing resistance to second and third-line antimicrobials and highlights steps needed to achieve better empirical research and more targeted policy actions.

The statistical data for Israel are supplied by and under the responsibility of the relevant Israeli authorities. The use of such data by the OECD is without prejudice to the status of the Golan Heights, East Jerusalem and Israeli settlements in the West Bank under the terms of international law.

Note by Turkey:

The information in this document with reference to "Cyprus" relates to the southern part of the Island. There is no single authority representing both Turkish and Greek Cypriot people on the Island. Turkey recognises the Turkish Republic of Northern Cyprus (TRNC). Until a lasting and equitable solution is found within the context of the United Nations, Turkey shall preserve its position concerning the "Cyprus issue".

Note by all the European Union Member States of the OECD and the European Union:

The Republic of Cyprus is recognised by all members of the United Nations with the exception of Turkey. The information in this document relates to the area under the effective control of the Government of the Republic of Cyprus.

Key findings

- Antimicrobial resistance (AMR) in high-priority bacteria has increased in the last decade in a majority of countries. It is estimated that average resistance proportions for eight antibiotic-bacterium combinations, across OECD countries, grew from 14% in 2005 to 17% in 2015. Resistance could grow further to 18% by 2030 if current trends continue into the future. These figures mask significant variation across countries and regions, as well as antibiotic-bacterium pairs.
- In OECD countries, in 2015, the highest average resistance proportions predicted (around 35% in Turkey, Korea and Greece) were seven times higher than the lowest proportions (around 5% in Iceland, the Netherlands and Norway). Outside OECD countries, in India, the People's Republic of China and the Russian Federation, for example, average rates were estimated to be in excess of 42%. In certain countries and with certain antibiotic-bacterium combinations, four out of every five infections were due to resistant bacteria. The estimated average resistance proportions in G20) countries and OECD Key Partners were 30% and 41% respectively.
- The majority of countries in the OECD, European Union (EU) and G20 are estimated to have experienced both reductions and increases in resistance proportions for different antibiotic-bacterium pairs between 2005 and 2015, suggesting marked differences in the evolution of resistance across countries, bacteria and antibiotic agents.
- While growth in drug resistance proportions could slow down in the coming decades, there are reasons for concern. The recent progress in reducing methicillin-resistant *Staphylococcus aureus (*MRSA) could be halted, or even reversed in some countries, and growth of resistance in difficult to treat enterococcal infections is projected to accelerate. Consumption of second-line antibiotic therapies will grow if current trends persist, potentially further promoting resistance and limiting options for treatment. With populations growing and ageing, the number at risk of infection will also increase.
- Differences in resistance proportions across countries and antibiotic-bacterium combinations are likely associated with differences in antimicrobial consumption, infection prevention and control, as well as use of health care services, but not only. Differences in measurement methods, as well as in probable correlates and drivers (including animal health, sanitation, migration, urbanisation, etc.) are likely relevant, but a lack of internationally comparable and reliable data on these factors hinders empirical research and robust policy-making. Surveillance and monitoring of all facets of AMR are needed.

3.1. Measuring and understanding international data on AMR is challenging

AMR is an umbrella term that includes many different types of drug resistance. While reports typically refer to broader classes of microorganisms and antimicrobial agents (e.g. third-generation cephalosporin-resistant *Enterobacteriaceae*), resistance is, in practice, defined and measured at the level of a specific microorganism (e.g. *Klebsiella pneumoniae*) and a specific antimicrobial drug (e.g. ceftriaxone, which is a third-generation cephalosporin). Ensuring data on AMR are internationally comparable is difficult for a number of reasons including the existence – and varying use – of multiple drugs, standards, guidelines, methods and equipment in different parts of the world (see Box 3.1). Cross-country differences in how individual-level results are aggregated to produce population-level measures (e.g. proportions, incidence) further limit comparability.

The development and more widespread use of guidelines have facilitated the collection and aggregation of international data on AMR. This collation and reporting of cross-country estimates can promote further discussion around how to tackle the significant difficulties that remain. The Center for Disease Dynamics, Economics & Policy (CDDEP), for example, started collating data on resistance proportions in 2010 and publishing them in a web-based set of visualisations called ResistanceMap[1]. The current version provides data on resistance proportions for up to 49 countries for different combinations of up to 12 organisms and 17 antibiotic groups as well as antibiotic consumption for different groups of agents for up to 75 countries, from 2000 to 2015. ResistanceMap[1] provides country-level yearly resistance data (number of isolates tested and proportion found to be resistant) primarily collected from international surveillance networks, like EARS-Net and CEASAR.[2]

The antibiotic-bacterium combinations included in this analysis were selected based on: a) significance of the burden of disease in OECD countries and the EU, both in the health care sector and the community; b) policy priority for OECD, G20 and EU countries (Cecchini, Langer and Slawomirski, 2015[1]); c) data availability (namely availability from CDDEP and networks such as EARS-Net); and d) inclusion in the World Health Organization (WHO) global priority list of antibiotic-resistant bacteria to guide research and development of new antibiotics (WHO, 2017[2]).

According to the latest figures from the surveillance networks included in ResistanceMap[1] and OECD analyses (see Box 3.2) the unweighted average of estimated resistance proportions, across eight specific antibiotic-bacterium combinations, was 17% in OECD countries in 2015 (see Table 3.1). Iceland, Netherlands and Norway had the lowest predicted average resistance proportions, around 5%, while in Turkey, Korea and Greece more than 35% of infections were estimated to be due to resistant bacteria, on average, across all eight antibiotic-bacterium combinations. India, China and the Russian Federation all had average resistance proportions in excess of 42% and, for some antibiotic-bacterium pairs, over 80% of infections were from resistant bacteria.

Box 3.1. The challenge of defining and measuring drug resistance

International comparisons of AMR typically rely on data from national and international surveillance networks which aggregate antimicrobial susceptibility test results from multiple laboratories. Results are often presented in annual surveillance reports such as those published by the European Centre for Disease Prevention and Control (ECDC) (2017[3]), WHO (2014[4]) and the Australian Commission on Safety and Quality in Health Care (2017[5]). Multiple factors can affect the accuracy or comparability of the statistics reported in these publications, including:

- **In the community**: Antimicrobial susceptibility test results may never reach a surveillance network if patients: 1) do not seek care, 2) self-medicate, for example with leftover antibiotics (OECD, 2017[6]), or 3) seek treatment from informal care providers. Given that severe infections (such as those caused by resistant bacteria) should eventually lead to formal health care utilisation and testing, it is likely that the number of susceptible infections in networks is conservative and resistance proportions are overestimated.
- **In the clinic/hospital**: Even when patients seek care from a formal health care provider, test results may never make it to a surveillance network. A patient with an infection caused by a bacterium susceptible to antimicrobial treatment may not be tested if the physician prescribes treatment and the symptoms subside. Again, this should lead to an underestimation of infections from bacteria that are susceptible to treatment and an overestimation of resistance proportions. Even if a test is ordered, the clinic/hospital may work with a laboratory that is not part of a surveillance network. The sample may also be contaminated leading to inaccurate test results.
- **In the laboratory**: Different laboratories may use different testing standards, guidelines and equipment, all of which could potentially affect the final outcome (i.e. whether a bacterium is considered resistant). Technical decisions that could affect the outcome include the choice of growth media, measurement method (e.g. phenotypic or genotypic), incubation conditions, and precision of different concentrations of antimicrobial agents (Turnidge and Paterson, 2007[7]; Hindler and Stelling, 2007[8]). Even phenotypic test results from the same laboratory can be categorised differently depending on the choice of breakpoints used (Kassim et al., 2016[9]; van der Bij et al., 2012[10]; Wolfensberger et al., 2013[11]).
- **In the surveillance network**: Some surveillance networks only report results for certain types of samples (ECDC, 2017[3]) while others report on all samples (WHO, 2017[12]). Furthermore, some networks discard repeated measurements (i.e. tests that are conducted more than once a year when patients have recurring infections). Studies that include all tests generally find higher resistance proportions than those that do not (Hindler and Stelling, 2007[8]).

There is no gold standard in the definition and measurement of AMR (unlike, for example, with blood pressure) making many of the decisions described above equally valid. Little is known about the direction and magnitude of some of these biases (Turnidge and Paterson, 2007[7]) making it very difficult to adjust published estimates. Surveillance networks help achieve comparability in that they set common standards and guidelines, but it is important to understand how different networks pool their data.

Table 3.1. Resistance proportions for eight priority antibiotic-bacterium pairs in 2015

COUNTRY	3GCRKP	FREC	CRPA	MRSA	3GCREC	PRSP	VRE	CRKP	AVERAGE
India*	85.4	78.6	52.9	45.8	81.1	44.4	9.1	59.2	57.1
China*	69.9	66.2	49.8	57.0	51.4	31.2	16.3	8.1	43.7
Russian Federation	95.0	60.0	46.8	22.0	77.0	31.9	3.2	7.0	42.9
Romania	72.0	31.0	69.0	57.0	27.0	39.0	12.2	34.0	42.6
Indonesia*	59.6	51.5	38.9	70.5	50.5	15.4	20.6	8.7	39.5
Peru*	54.9	68.9	28.3	53.8	55.6	24.3	23.3	4.2	39.2
Turkey	68.0	48.0	32.0	25.0	51.0	47.3	9.3	30.0	38.8
Greece	71.0	31.0	44.0	39.0	21.0	23.8	8.4	63.0	37.7
Saudi Arabia*	68.4	39.9	43.8	37.7	35.2	33.4	14.5	23.7	37.1
Korea*	53.8	58.6	32.5	56.9	34.5	22.3	14.2	8.7	35.2
Mexico	53.0	62.0	35.0	31.0	58.0	11.4	8.5	14.0	34.1
Brazil*	44.6	61.8	32.5	44.5	30.9	27.7	15.0	13.0	33.8
Colombia*	50.2	51.6	35.8	43.9	42.3	20.6	15.7	9.9	33.8
Slovak Republic	68.0	46.0	58.0	28.0	32.0	21.3	5.4	2.0	32.6
Argentina	48.0	30.0	55.0	45.0	17.0	25.0	19.2	14.0	31.6
Italy	57.0	46.0	26.0	34.0	31.0	12.0	4.2	36.0	30.8
Costa Rica*	39.4	59.2	31.9	45.1	35.6	10.4	10.8	5.5	29.7
South Africa*	63.4	31.6	44.7	30.4	20.0	29.6	4.4	4.4	28.6
Bulgaria	76.0	38.0	27.0	13.0	40.0	23.0	4.2	3.0	28.0
Cyprus	44.0	46.0	21.0	43.0	29.0	8.1	10.7	13.0	26.8
Israel*	33.2	35.7	28.6	44.8	22.5	13.8	5.2	19.1	25.4
Poland	65.0	30.0	43.0	16.0	13.0	24.0	8.0	1.0	25.0
Croatia	48.0	25.0	43.0	25.0	13.0	19.0	8.8	4.0	23.2
Portugal	43.0	31.0	24.0	47.0	17.0	11.0	7.7	4.0	23.1
United States*	21.0	34.9	18.0	43.8	16.1	12.7	29.2	8.2	23.0
Chile*	30.3	31.6	25.1	26.4	24.6	11.9	10.2	8.1	21.0
Japan*	7.1	36.6	21.0	53.7	30.0	6.2	3.7	5.1	20.4
Malta	18.0	40.0	23.0	49.0	12.0	6.6	7.6	7.0	20.4
Hungary	37.0	29.0	38.0	25.0	17.0	7.0	4.2	1.0	19.8
Lithuania	52.0	21.0	32.0	9.0	16.0	16.0	9.9	0.0	19.5
Latvia	49.0	29.0	25.8	6.0	19.0	9.0	8.5	2.0	18.5
Spain	21.0	32.0	27.0	25.0	12.0	24.0	1.1	4.0	18.3
Czech Republic	56.0	24.0	23.0	14.0	16.0	3.0	3.7	1.0	17.6
Ireland	17.0	24.0	16.0	18.0	12.0	18.0	27.1	1.0	16.6
France	32.0	21.0	21.0	16.0	12.0	23.0	0.3	1.0	15.8
New Zealand*	21.0	10.2	9.9	36.4	7.8	19.0	17.6	3.1	15.6
Canada*	12.6	21.3	26.4	18.8	8.2	8.6	13.3	3.8	14.1
Slovenia	23.0	25.0	23.0	9.0	14.0	9.0	2.4	2.0	13.4
Luxembourg	28.0	25.0	13.9	9.0	13.0	8.5	5.6	0.0	12.9
Estonia	25.0	16.0	21.6	4.0	12.0	3.0	1.6	0.0	10.4
Germany	11.0	21.0	18.0	11.0	11.0	6.0	4.4	0.0	10.3
Belgium	21.0	27.0	7.0	12.0	11.0	1.0	1.0	1.0	10.1
Australia	6.0	13.0	3.5	18.0	11.0	6.0	21.4	0.0	9.9
Austria	10.0	21.0	15.0	8.0	10.0	6.0	1.2	1.0	9.0
United Kingdom	12.0	16.0	3.0	11.0	12.0	8.0	10.1	0.0	9.0
Switzerland	7.0	17.0	10.0	4.0	10.0	3.8	0.2	0.0	6.5
Denmark	9.0	15.0	7.0	2.0	9.0	5.0	1.7	0.0	6.1
Finland	4.0	12.0	9.0	2.0	7.0	13.0	0.0	0.0	5.9
Sweden	4.0	14.0	9.0	1.0	7.0	10.0	0.0	0.0	5.6
Norway	7.0	11.0	13.0	1.0	7.0	5.0	0.0	0.0	5.5
Netherlands	9.0	14.0	9.0	1.0	6.0	2.0	0.5	0.0	5.2
Iceland	0.0	7.0	7.9	0.0	2.0	5.6	5.3	0.0	3.5
OECD COUNTRIES	29.0	26.6	21.6	19.6	17.0	12.1	7.1	6.1	17.4
EU28 COUNTRIES	33.2	26.7	24.2	18.7	16.0	12.3	5.7	6.0	17.8
ALL COUNTRIES	35.2	31.2	25.8	25.7	20.8	14.6	8.6	7.4	21.2
G20 COUNTRIES	45.7	42.0	31.6	35.4	33.6	21.2	11.6	12.9	29.2
OECD KEY PARTNERS	64.6	57.9	43.8	49.6	46.8	29.7	13.1	18.7	40.5

Note: * indicates country is missing more than 50% of observations, across all eight antibiotic-bacterium pairs for 2015. The colour scheme is based on a two-point scale (minimum in light grey, maximum in blue, points in between coloured proportionally). Countries (and country groupings) are sorted top to bottom from highest to lowest average resistance proportions (across antibiotic-bacterium combinations). Antibiotic-bacterium combinations are sorted left to right from highest to lowest average resistance proportions (across countries). FREC: fluoroquinolone-resistant *E. coli*, VRE: vancomycin-resistant *E. faecalis* and *E. faecium*, 3GCREC: third-generation cephalosporin-resistant *E. coli*, CRKP: carbapenem-resistant *K. pneumoniae*, 3GCRKP: third-generation cephalosporin-resistant *K. pneumoniae*, CRPA: carbapenem-resistant *P. aeruginosa*, MRSA: methicillin-resistant *S. aureus*, PRSP: penicillin-resistant *S. pneumoniae*.
Source: OECD analyses of data from surveillance networks included in ResistanceMap[1].

Resistance proportions in countries outside the OECD (estimated at an average 29%, across all eight antibiotic-bacterium combinations) were significantly higher than those in member states in 2015. Members of the EU had average rates (18%) comparable to OECD countries and member states of the G20 had predicted resistance proportions of 30%. The highest average resistance proportions, an estimated 41%, were in key partners of the OECD (i.e. countries that contribute to the OECD's work in a sustained and comprehensive manner but are not formal members).

Box 3.2. Methodology used to estimate historic and future resistance proportions

Historical and future resistance proportions were estimated using a combination of statistical techniques and models seeking to make use of as much publicly available, internationally comparable, data as possible, while explicitly accounting for uncertainty in the underlying data, models and assumptions. The approach sought to fill data gaps using best guesses from theoretically-hypothesised and empirically-tested relationships with correlates.

Resistance and consumption data were collected from ResistanceMap[1]. The primary sources of resistance data in ResistanceMap[1] are public and private laboratory networks – such as EARS-Net – that routinely collect antimicrobial susceptibility test results. Data on antibiotic consumption were sourced from IMS Health's MIDAS and XPonent databases. Data on a wide range of topics (from health and sanitation to agricultural and livestock production) were collected from the World Bank, WHO, the Food and Agriculture Organization (FAO), the United Nations World Population Prospects (UN WPP), the United States Department of Agriculture, and the OECD's own databases.

Producing complete estimates of resistance proportions for eight antibiotic-bacterium combinations (third-generation cephalosporin-resistant *E. coli*, fluoroquinolones-resistant *E. coli*, penicillin-resistant *S. pneumoniae*, methicillin-resistant *S. aureus*, carbapenem-resistant *K. pneumoniae*, third-generation cephalosporin-resistant *K. pneumoniae*, carbapenem-resistant *P. aeruginosa*, and vancomycin-resistant *E. faecalis* and *E. faecium*) in 52 countries from 2000 to 2030, including uncertainty, involved the following procedures:

1. multiple imputation of missing historical values using all relevant information from observed relationships with correlates
2. forecasting of potential correlates of resistance proportions using external forecasts (e.g. UN WPP) and internal forecasts of antibiotic consumption using exponential smoothing with an additive damped trend
3. forecasts of resistance proportions using an ensemble of three models, equally weighted, to capture different aspects of the underlying phenomena (a mixed-effects linear regression, exponential smoothing with an additive damped trend, and a random forest)
4. incorporation of uncertainty from various sources, namely imputations of missing values, model selection and specification, and some model parameters. The final estimates are described using means and 95% uncertainty intervals (e.g. see Figure 3.8).

Forecasts do not incorporate future policy actions or interventions.

3.2. Predicted resistance proportions increased between 2005 and 2015 in a majority of countries and for most antibiotic-bacterium combinations

Between 2005 and 2015, predicted resistance proportions for eight antibiotic-bacterium combinations in OECD countries, increased, on average, by 3 percentage points from 14%

in 2005 to 17% in 2015 (see Table 3.3). In seven countries (Switzerland, United Kingdom, Japan, Belgium, Germany, Iceland and Canada), resistance proportions went down, on average across all antibiotic-bacterium-country combinations, by 2.5 percentage points. In the majority of countries, however, average resistance proportions across all eight antibiotic-bacterium pairs increased, by as much as 13 percentage points in OECD countries (e.g. Slovak Republic and Italy), but potentially even more in Brazil, the Russian Federation and China (around 17 percentage points). However, these averages mask significant variation within countries across antibiotic-bacterium combinations.

Despite average reductions in a few countries, it is estimated that in no country have resistance proportions for all eight antibiotic-bacterium combinations gone down between 2005 and 2015. In contrast, in eight countries (Brazil, China, Peru, Argentina, Colombia, Saudi Arabia, Israel and the Russian Federation) resistance proportions increased for all eight antibiotic-bacterium pairs. However, for the majority of countries, both increases and reductions were predicted, in some cases quite extreme.

In France, for example, the proportion of *Klebsiella pneumoniae* (*K. pneumoniae*) resistant to third-generation cephalosporins increased by an estimated 27 percentage points (from 5% to 32%, a growth rate of 540%) while the proportion of *Streptococcus pneumoniae* (*S. pneumoniae*) resistant to penicillin went down by a predicted 13 percentage points (from 36% to 23%, a growth rate of -36%) over the same ten years. In Mexico while the proportion of *Staphylococcus Aureus* (*S. aureus*) resistant to oxacillin (i.e. MRSA) went down by a predicted 21 percentage points (from 52% to 31%, a growth rate of -40%), the proportion of *Escherichia Coli* (*E. coli*) resistant to third-generation cephalosporins increased by an estimated 18 percentage points (from 40% to 58%, a growth rate of 45%).

Using resistance proportions in 2005 as the base value, growth rates (change in resistance proportions as a percentage of the 2005 base proportions) across countries and antibiotic-bacterium combinations are very heterogeneous. Across OECD countries, compared to 2005 values and using averages of country growth rates, resistance proportions for MRSA went down the most, by an estimated 17%, while the proportion of *E. coli* resistant to third-generation cephalosporins increased by a predicted 222% between 2005 and 2015. Among OECD countries, Italy and the United States had some of the biggest predicted growth rates in resistance proportions, more than 140% higher in 2015 compared to 2005, on average across all eight antibiotic-bacterium combinations. Resistance proportions in non-OECD members Croatia and Romania were more than 200% higher than estimates for ten years before. Belgium and Portugal had the biggest reductions in estimated resistance proportions compared to 2005, 10% and 2% respectively. Across all countries and antibiotic-bacterium combinations, predicted resistance proportions in 2015 were between 100% lower and 1 200% higher than in 2005, a very significant range of variation.

It is likely that differences in baseline resistance proportions and rates of change across countries and antibiotic-bacterium combinations are associated with differences in antimicrobial use, infection prevention and control, as well as the use of health care services (ECDC, 2017[3]), not to mention differences in measurement. However, the problem goes beyond the human health sector with links to the animal sector and the environment. The list of potential correlates and drivers of resistance is long, ranging from human and animal health and sanitation, agricultural and livestock production, urbanisation and population density, migration and trade, economic growth and governance, and population structure. Studies seeking to empirically test the direction and magnitude of these relationships have been hampered by two broad yet intertwined challenges: a lack of data and a limited understanding of how all these factors are related, to each other and to drug resistance.

Table 3.2. Percentage point changes in resistance proportions for eight priority antibiotic-bacterium combinations between 2005 and 2015 in select countries

COUNTRY	FREC	3GCRKP	3GCREC	CRPA	CRKP	VRE	PRSP	MRSA	AVERAGE
Russian Federation*	28.8	34.9	42.5	17.8	1.1	0.8	12.2	4.9	17.9
China*	39.0	34.5	18.5	13.5	3.4	4.5	19.8	8.8	17.8
Brazil*	42.4	27.5	12.4	12.8	8.3	5.6	14.4	15.6	17.4
Peru*	42.6	28.1	14.9	10.1	1.6	4.2	13.3	0.6	14.4
Slovak Republic	32.0	26.8	24.0	25.9	-3.2	1.9	-10.8	12.0	13.6
Italy	17.0	37.0	22.0	2.4	32.7	-4.0	3.0	-3.0	13.4
Argentina*	16.2	13.8	3.5	36.4	4.7	10.4	8.4	12.3	13.2
Colombia*	31.5	20.7	17.6	13.1	4.8	2.1	7.6	4.8	12.8
Saudi Arabia*	27.5	29.0	7.4	9.3	3.4	7.5	1.0	8.9	11.7
Costa Rica*	32.3	31.6	10.7	5.1	3.7	3.0	2.2	-1.7	10.9
Israel*	20.1	18.1	13.0	10.4	7.9	1.8	4.9	10.0	10.8
Romania	20.0	-7.7	9.0	23.4	31.2	8.2	-2.0	-3.0	9.9
Indonesia*	21.1	15.9	7.1	12.0	7.0	0.3	-2.6	1.1	7.7
Greece	18.0	9.0	12.0	0.0	32.0	-6.5	-4.5	-3.0	7.1
Korea*	25.4	17.6	9.3	0.4	-3.1	2.9	1.8	0.0	6.8
Lithuania*	8.9	24.3	9.8	13.7	-2.2	5.0	-1.7	-5.8	6.5
South Africa*	17.3	11.8	10.1	3.4	-1.0	-0.1	12.3	-3.2	6.3
Croatia	16.0	2.0	12.0	17.0	4.0	6.4	2.0	-12.0	5.9
India*	1.9	6.4	2.9	13.1	24.0	-0.6	4.1	-6.1	5.7
New Zealand*	6.2	19.0	6.8	3.2	3.1	3.7	5.9	-3.4	5.6
Turkey*	16.6	16.9	22.7	-9.8	16.8	1.8	-1.6	-19.3	5.5
Hungary	7.0	9.0	13.0	15.0	1.0	4.2	-14.0	5.0	5.0
Cyprus	14.0	19.8	13.0	-0.6	4.6	-1.3	3.2	-13.0	5.0
Slovenia	13.0	4.0	12.0	7.0	2.0	2.4	-2.0	-1.0	4.7
Chile*	11.6	18.2	1.9	4.7	2.7	2.5	1.7	-6.3	4.6
Czech Republic	4.0	24.0	14.0	-8.0	1.0	-0.2	-1.0	1.0	4.4
Spain	3.0	14.0	4.0	8.0	4.0	0.0	-1.0	-2.0	3.7
Latvia	18.2	4.2	11.5	-0.3	-5.6	4.4	9.0	-14.0	3.4
Poland	10.0	-1.0	8.0	10.5	1.0	3.9	1.6	-8.0	3.3
Australia*	7.0	3.8	9.2	-2.6	-2.0	5.1	1.7	0.2	2.8
Malta	9.0	13.0	11.0	3.0	5.0	-11.9	-0.8	-7.0	2.7
United States*	14.9	8.0	12.1	1.0	7.2	6.5	-18.3	-10.2	2.7
Estonia	10.0	17.0	9.0	-16.4	-2.1	0.3	1.0	2.0	2.6
Ireland	7.0	10.0	8.0	0.9	-0.7	11.7	7.0	-24.0	2.5
France	7.0	27.0	9.0	0.0	1.0	-0.3	-13.0	-11.0	2.5
Netherlands	4.0	5.0	3.0	3.0	0.0	0.1	1.0	0.0	2.0
Denmark	10.0	-0.7	7.0	0.6	-2.6	0.1	1.0	0.0	1.9
Norway	5.0	3.0	5.0	-1.0	-1.0	0.0	3.0	1.0	1.9
Bulgaria	9.0	23.0	12.0	-11.0	3.0	1.9	-10.0	-16.0	1.5
Finland	4.0	1.0	5.0	-6.0	0.0	0.0	6.0	-1.0	1.1
Austria	1.0	3.0	6.0	2.0	1.0	0.2	1.0	-6.0	1.0
Mexico	11.0	0.0	18.0	5.1	7.0	-8.9	-5.1	-21.0	0.8
Portugal	2.0	19.3	5.0	2.6	-7.8	-4.5	-6.0	0.0	0.7
Sweden	5.0	3.0	5.0	10.0	-4.1	-0.3	6.0	0.0	0.6
Luxembourg	6.0	6.9	8.0	-3.4	-6.3	-1.6	-3.5	-4.0	0.3
Canada*	6.4	1.7	2.7	0.2	-3.2	3.7	-8.2	-1.5	0.2
Iceland	4.0	-3.7	2.0	1.3	-4.0	-2.5	-2.4	0.0	-0.7
Germany	-4.0	3.0	9.0	-12.0	-2.0	-0.4	2.0	-10.0	-1.8
Belgium	10.0	8.3	7.0	-6.8	3.2	-3.3	-11.0	-19.0	-2.5
Japan*	-6.9	0.7	4.2	-5.5	2.0	-1.4	-1.8	-13.0	-2.7
United Kingdom	-1.0	-1.0	6.0	-6.0	0.0	-4.8	4.0	-33.0	1.6
Switzerland*	-4.6	-4.1	2.0	-9.7	-6.8	-2.5	0.2	-16.9	-5.3
OECD COUNTRIES	8.6	9.7	9.1	0.4	1.7	0.6	-1.2	-5.7	2.9
EU28 COUNTRIES	17.9	15.4	11.4	6.6	4.2	2.4	3.4	-1.6	7.5
ALL COUNTRIES	11.5	11.3	9.3	3.0	3.2	1.0	-0.1	-4.9	4.3
G20 COUNTRIES	11.8	11.1	9.2	3.1	1.9	1.0	0.2	-4.0	4.3
OECD KEY PARTNERS	8.6	9.7	9.1	0.4	1.7	0.6	-1.2	-5.7	2.9

Note: * indicates country is missing more than 50% of observations, across all eight antibiotic-bacterium pairs, for both 2005 and 2015. The colour scheme is based on a two-point scale (minimum in light grey, maximum in blue, points in between coloured proportionally). Countries (and country groupings) are sorted top to bottom from highest to lowest average resistance proportions (across antibiotic-bacterium combinations). Antibiotic-bacterium combinations are sorted left to right from highest to lowest average resistance proportions (across countries). FREC: fluoroquinolone-resistant *E. coli*, VRE: vancomycin-resistant *E. faecalis* and *E. faecium*, 3GCREC: third-generation cephalosporin-resistant *E.* coli, CRKP: carbapenem-resistant *K. pneumoniae*, 3GCRKP: third-generation cephalosporin-resistant *K. pneumoniae*, CRPA: carbapenem-resistant *P. aeruginosa*, MRSA: methicillin-resistant *S. aureus*, PRSP: penicillin-resistant *S. pneumoniae*.
Source: OECD analyses of data from surveillance networks included in ResistanceMap[1].

Comprehensive, comparable and reliable data on many of these factors are lacking. Even ignoring the difficulties in ensuring surveillance data are comparable across countries or regions (see Box 3.1), many low and middle-income countries either do not have national surveillance systems in place or surveillance is conducted in private hospitals and the resulting data not shared with international organisations. In high-income countries, where surveillance data from the human health sector are more widely available, there are still regional gaps and statistics in the animal sector are limited. While there has been progress, for example in determining what should be measured and monitored, important data gaps remain, making it difficult to set priorities and identify policy options (Wernli et al., 2017[13]).

A second difficulty is that drivers of resistance can interact, forming a complex web of relationships in which the same variable can have both direct and indirect, as well as non-linear, effects on the emergence and spread of resistance. The empirical literature is full of examples of these intricate associations. For example, it is widely acknowledged that both the underuse and overuse of antibiotics can lead to drug resistance (Mendelson et al., 2016[14]), which would suggest a non-linear relationship. Out-of-pocket spending in low and middle-income countries is positively correlated with AMR, a relationship that Alsan and colleagues (2015[15]) posit is due to high co-payments inducing patients to seek treatment from less well-regulated private providers with financial incentives to prescribe inappropriately. Collignon and co-authors (2015[16]) find that governance and corruption at the national-level are better predictors of antibiotic resistance than economic output or even antibiotic consumption, while Rönnerstrand and Lapuente (2017[17]) show that corruption is, in fact, a good predictor of antibiotic consumption.

3.3. The emergence and spread of AMR is a complex phenomenon with multiple interrelated causes and drivers

There is wide variation in the predicted resistance proportions for 2015 (Table 3.1) and rates of change between 2005 and 2015 (Table 3.2) across countries and antibiotic-bacterium combinations. For the reasons previously mentioned, it is difficult to say what factors are behind these differences but it is possible to identify broad patterns of drug resistance, not only by sex and age, but also by level of antibiotic consumption and economic development.

Across six antibiotic-bacterium combinations for which surveillance data are available from EARS-Net, the estimated incidence rates of all infections (i.e. the sum of infections caused by resistant and susceptible bacteria) exhibit a similar age pattern: children less than one year old and adults over 50 years old are more likely to be infected (see Figure 3.1). The population over 80 years old exhibit the highest rates of infection. This pattern is likely associated with the development of immune responses with age, starting with an immature immune system at birth, which develops with time and then declines in old age (Simon,

Hollander and McMichael, 2015[18]). Furthermore, infants and the elderly are at a higher risk of being admitted to hospital, and thus at a higher risk of acquiring a hospital infection.

Figure 3.1. Incidence rates for six bacteria and proportion that are resistant to specific antibiotics, by age and sex, in all EARS-Net countries combined in 2015

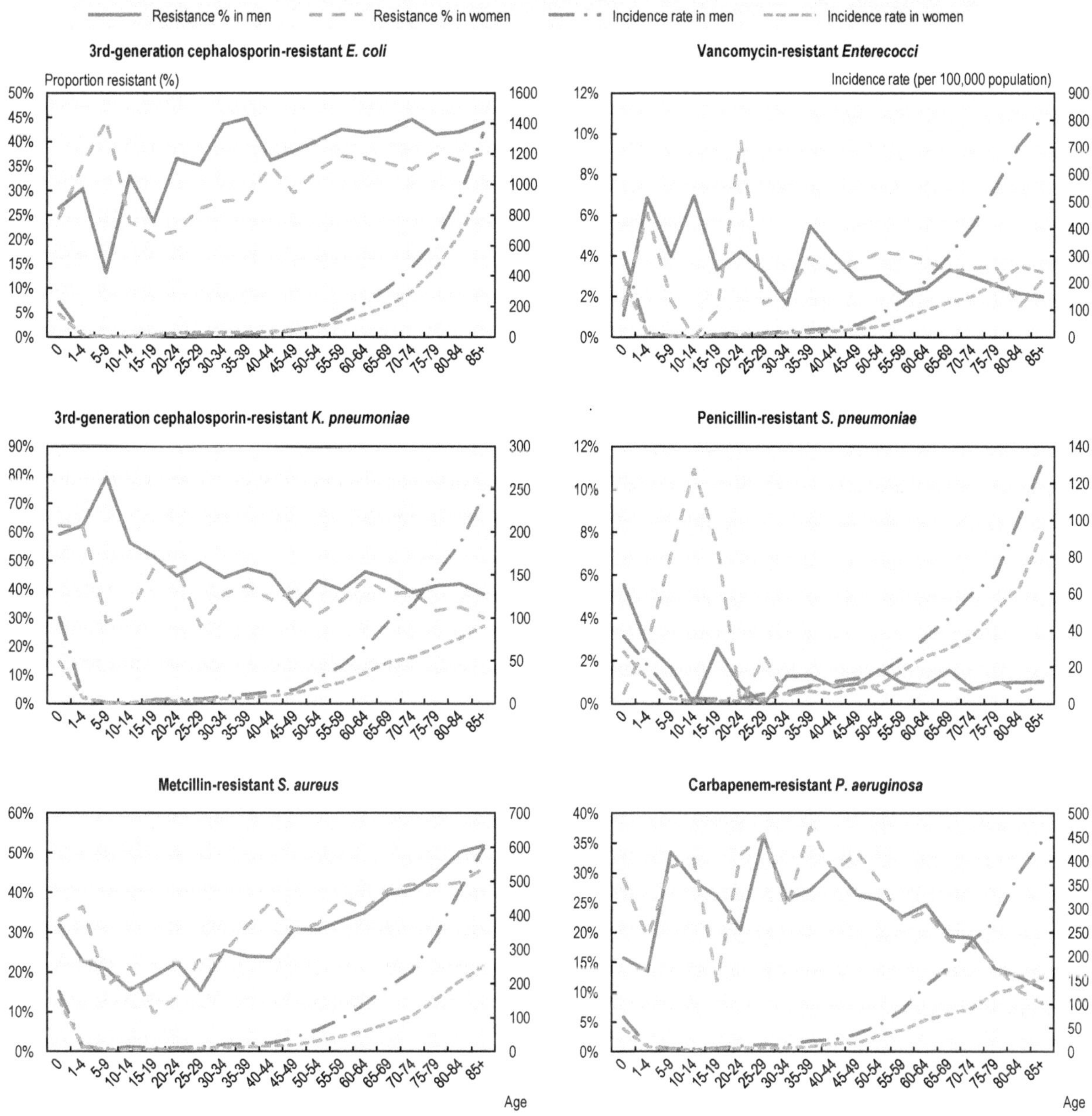

Note: Incidence rates estimated using total number of infections in the EU/EEA (from EARS-Net) and age-specific population from the United States Census Bureau.
Source: OECD analyses of surveillance data from EARS-Net.

StatLink http://dx.doi.org/10.1787/888933854706

Men are significantly more likely than women to become infected. This is in line with other studies that have found men are more susceptible than women to many infections, a difference that has been tentatively associated with sex steroid hormones. These hormones are believed to both lower immunocompetence in men and affect genes and behaviours that influence their susceptibility and resistance to infection (Klein, 2000[19]).

While there are clear differences in incidence of infections across age and gender, the proportion of infections that are caused by bacteria resistant to antibiotics exhibit no discernible age-sex-pattern across different antibiotic-bacterium combinations (see Figure 3.1). With the exception of third-generation cephalosporin-resistant *E. coli*, resistance proportions in men and women are similar. Older people seem to be more likely to become infected with *S. aureus* resistant to antibiotic treatment (methicillin in this case) than younger people, while the reverse is true for those infected with *P. aeruginosa* (for which the antibiotic is carbapenems). Differences in resistance proportions by age may be due to both measurement and underlying factors. For example, resistance proportions may be higher for older populations due to increased exposure to antimicrobials and health care, both of which are risk factors for drug resistance. Similarly, younger people might put off care for less severe infections so that once an antimicrobial susceptibility test is conducted there is a higher chance that resistant bacteria will be found. The interplay between these and other factors might explain the age patterns observed for *S. aureus* and *P. aeruginosa.*

For six bacteria, both the incidence of infections and the proportion resistant to antimicrobials, show notably different patterns across body sites (see Figure 3.2). Differences in the number of certain types of infections stem from the characteristics of bacteria (e.g. whether they are predominately found in health care or community settings, their transmission mechanisms, what parts of the body they naturally colonise, etc.). For example, *E. coli* and *K. pneumoniae* are found in the human gut and are a common cause of urinary tract infections, while *S. pneumoniae* is often carried in the human respiratory tract or sinuses and is a leading cause of pneumonia (see Box 2.3 in Chapter 2)

There are also differences in the proportions resistant to antibiotic treatment (see Figure 3.2). As with age and sex, these differences could be due to both measurement biases and underlying resistance mechanisms. Drug concentrations can differ between different body sites yet clinical breakpoints used in many antimicrobial susceptibility tests are based on bloodstream concentrations (Turnidge and Paterson, 2007[7]), potentially adjusted in some cases where concentrations are known to be different (e.g. in the urinary tract). Differences in concentration could affect both measurement and underlying resistance.

As previously reported by Albrich et al., (2004[20]), there is a positive correlation between antibiotic consumption and the proportion of infections that are due to bacteria resistant to antibiotic treatment for certain antibiotic-bacterium combinations in specific years (see the panels for *S. pneumoniae* and *S. aureus* in Figure 3.3). However, the existence of outliers suggests antibiotic consumption is not the only factor associated with resistance. In Mexico, MRSA is higher than expected given how low the consumption of broad-spectrum penicillins is. In Belgium, the proportion of *S. pneumoniae* resistant to penicillins is much lower than expected given the relatively high level of consumption, yet this is likely associated with the use of different breakpoints, as explained by Goossens and colleagues (2013[21]), a reminder of how much measurement issues matter. Even when total antibiotic consumption is used in place of specific antibiotic groups, these outliers persist (data not shown). For carbapenem-resistant *P. aeruginosa*, the relationship between total antibiotic consumption and resistance appears to be non-existent (see Figure 3.3). Non-linear relationships between consumption and resistance proportions were explored but not found (data not shown). Other studies have also found a lack of a relationship between consumption and resistance for certain antibiotic-bacterium combinations (ECDC/EFSA/EMA, 2017[22]).

Figure 3.2. Incidence rates for six bacteria and proportion resistant to specific antibiotics, by type of infection, in all EARS-Net countries in 2015

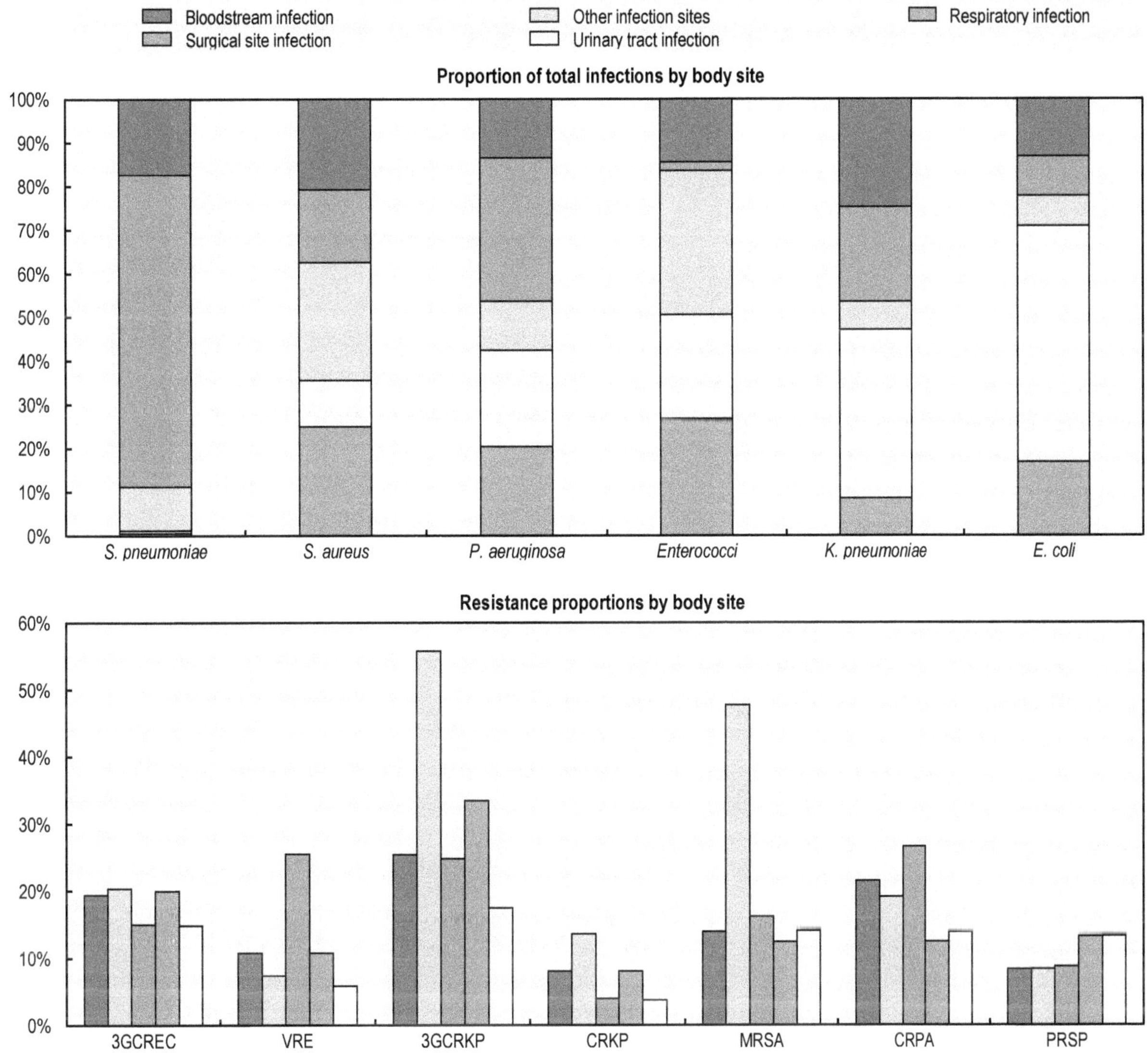

Note: FREC: fluoroquinolone-resistant *E. coli*, VRE: vancomycin-resistant *E. faecalis* and *E. faecium*, 3GCREC: third-generation cephalosporin-resistant *E. coli*, CRKP: carbapenem-resistant *K. pneumoniae*, 3GCRKP: third-generation cephalosporin-resistant *K. pneumoniae*, CRPA: carbapenem-resistant *P. aeruginosa*, MRSA: methicillin-resistant *S. aureus*, PRSP: penicillin-resistant *S. pneumoniae*.
Source: OECD analyses of data from (Cassini et al., 2018[23]).

StatLink http://dx.doi.org/10.1787/888933854725

Figure 3.3. Associations between antibiotic consumption and resistance proportions for four antibiotic-bacterium combinations in 2015

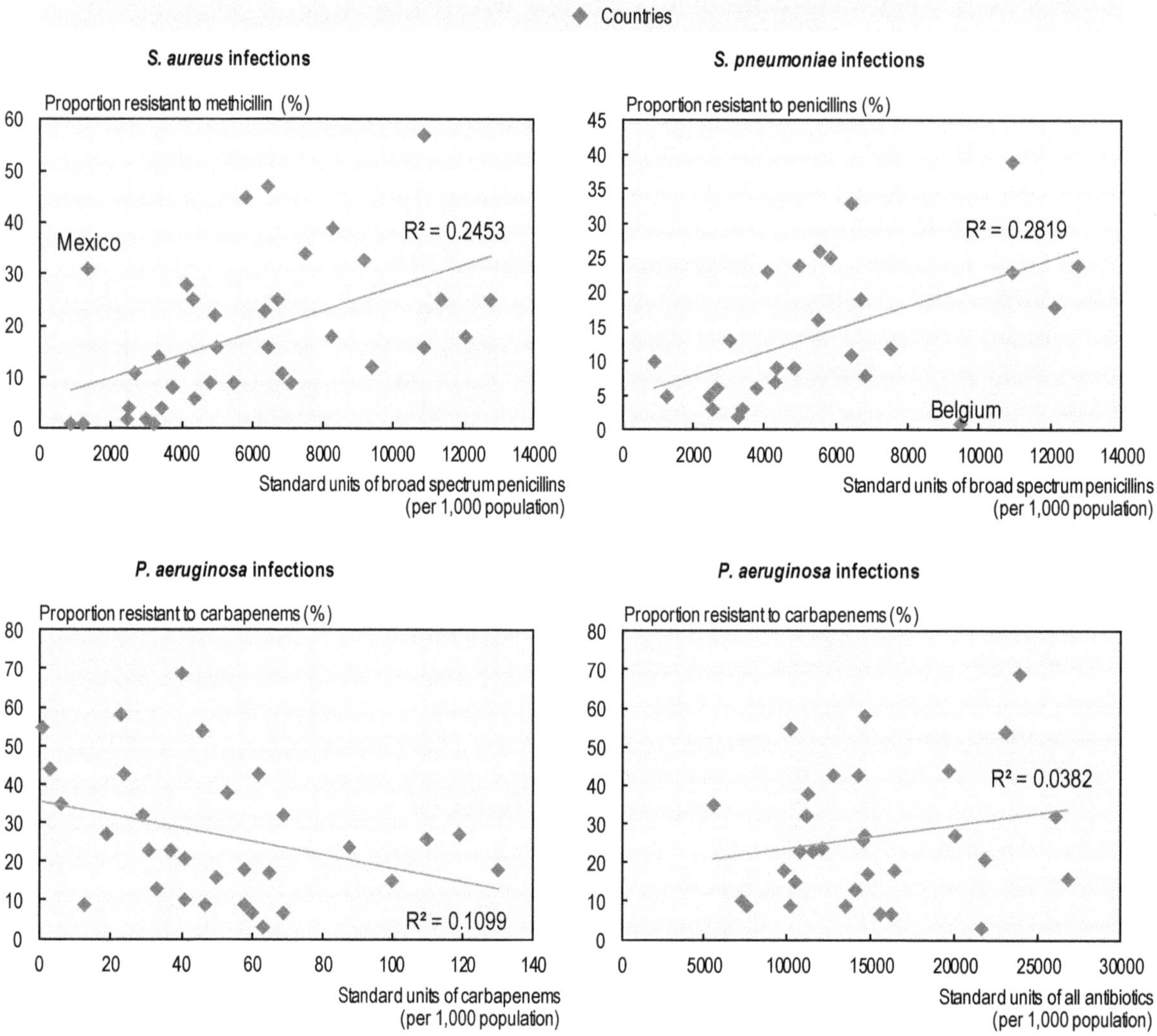

Source: OECD analyses of data from surveillance networks included in ResistanceMap[1].

StatLink http://dx.doi.org/10.1787/888933854744

While the patterns shown in Figure 3.3 could be partly due to measurement issues, there are at least two other non-mutually-exclusive explanations. One is that it is not so much the quantity of antibiotics prescribed but the appropriateness of consumption that is associated with drug resistance (Zilberberg et al., 2017[24]). This would be in line with observations that both low and high consumption of antibiotics can be associated with higher resistance, and might potentially explain why countries with low consumption of antibiotics exhibit such a high proportion of infections from resistant bacteria. The second potential explanation is that antibiotic consumption is merely one of a number of determinants and correlates of drug resistance.

There are, as previously mentioned, many factors thought to be associated with drug resistance, from infection prevention and control, to antibiotic consumption in the animal sector (see Box 3.3), access to health care, trade in goods and services, and migration, to mention just a few. Some of these factors could be associated with drug resistance in some, but possibly not all, countries and for certain antibiotic-bacterium combinations only. Some of these relationships are illustrated in Figure 3.5.

Box 3.3. Antimicrobial consumption in the animal sector

Globally, the bulk of antimicrobials is, in fact, not consumed by humans, but rather given to animals, mostly food-producing animals such as poultry and cattle. In the United States, it was estimated that around 80% of all antibiotic consumption is in the animal sector (Van Boeckel et al., 2015[25]). In the 28 EU/EEA member states that collect both animal and human consumption data, OECD analyses indicate 70% of the active substance of antimicrobials was sold for use in food-producing animals (ECDC/EFSA/EMA, 2017[22]). Antimicrobial agents are used in food-producing animals for a number of reasons including treating sick animals and preventing the spread of infectious diseases, but also, in some countries, to increase growth rates and feed efficiency (Cecchini, Langer and Slawomirski, 2015[11]). Demand for animal protein is rising worldwide driving up the consumption of antimicrobials in the livestock sector. If current trends continue and no effective policy action is put in place, between 2010 and 2030, the global consumption of antimicrobials in food-producing animals is projected to increase by about 67% (Van Boeckel et al., 2015[25]).

Figure 3.4. Associations between combined antibiotic consumption in animals and humans, and proportion of *E. coli* resistant to specific antibiotics in 2015 in the EU28

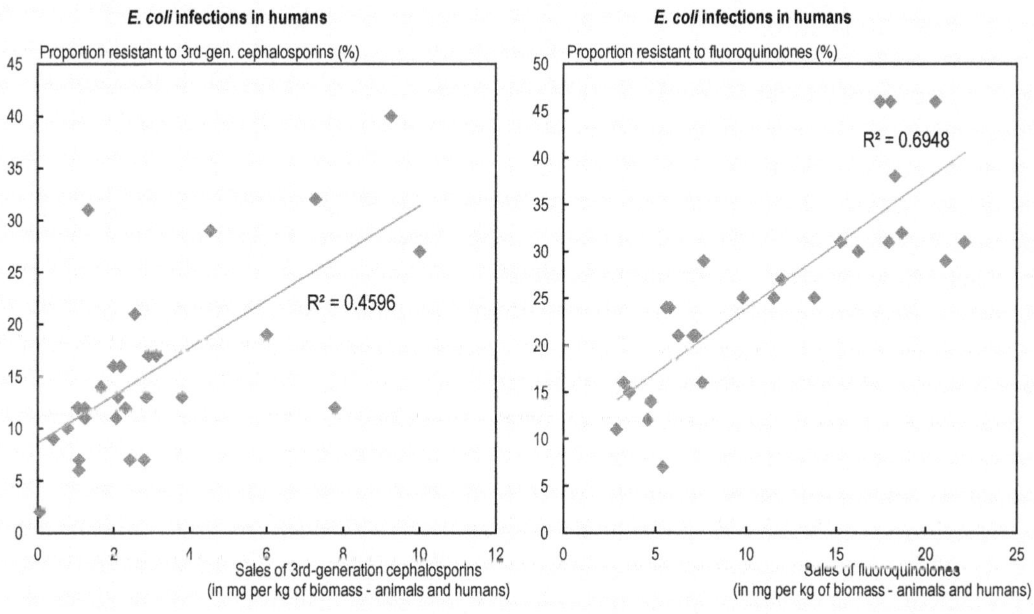

Note: it is considered the average human being weighs 62.5 kg.
Source: OECD analyses of data from surveillance networks included in ResistanceMap[1], ECDC and ESVAC.

StatLink http://dx.doi.org/10.1787/888933854763

Antimicrobial consumption in animals favours AMR in ways that are similar to consumption in humans, so that more consumption may lead to more resistance. When animals develop resistant infections these may spread to humans through food, the environment (e.g. water and soil), or through direct contact between animals and humans (Tang et al., 2017[26]). Figure 3.4 illustrates the positive correlation that exists between combined consumption of antibiotics in the human and animal sectors and the proportion of infections in humans that are resistant to specific antibiotic treatments. The association between consumption and antibiotic-resistant *E. coli* is visibly stronger when taking into account animal use, besides human consumption only, even though recent analyses have found no direct link between antibiotic use in animals and resistance in *E. coli* in humans (ECDC, EFSA and EMA, 2017[27]).

Efforts to measure drug resistance should include measurement of antimicrobial consumption and resistance in animals. While monitoring and surveillance in the animal sectors are currently limited, international organisations are increasingly promoting not only measurement (ECDC/EFSA/EMA, 2017[22]), but also good governance in the veterinary sector, adoption of international standards, and antimicrobial stewardship (OIE, 2016[28]).

Per capita gross domestic product (GDP) is well correlated with the proportion of *P. aeruginosa* resistant to carbapenems (countries with a higher GDP per capita have lower proportions of infections caused by resistant bacteria), but less well correlated with rates of third-generation cephalosporin-resistant *E. coli* (data not shown). Resistance proportions for third-generation cephalosporin-resistant *E. coli* are more strongly associated with agricultural value added as a percentage of GDP (the higher the agricultural value added the higher the proportion of resistant infections).

In line with previous research (Alsan et al., 2015[15]), out-of-pocket health spending (as a percentage of total health expenditure) is positively associated with proportion of third-generation cephalosporin-resistant *K. pneumoniae*, but less well correlated with penicillin-resistant *S. pneumoniae* (relationship not shown). The number of doctors' consultations per capita is well correlated with the proportion of *S. aureus* resistant to methicillin when disregarding observations for Mexico and Portugal, which have higher than expected resistance proportions given the low number of consultations in these countries. Mexico is often an outlier in these relationships, exhibiting higher than expected resistance proportions given levels of antibiotic consumption, doctors' appointments and agricultural value added.

Another factor that has been shown to correlate well with drug resistance is governance (see Figure 3.6). The World Bank Worldwide Governance Indicators capture the views of thousands of stakeholders globally on six dimensions of governance: voice and accountability; political stability and absence of violence/terrorism; government effectiveness; regulatory quality; rule of law; and control of corruption (Kaufmann, Kraay and Mastruzzi, 2011[29]). The average country scores for these six dimensions are consistently well correlated with resistance proportions for six antibiotic-bacterium combinations, a relationship that is generally in agreement with Collignon and co-authors' study (2015[16]) of the connection between poor governance and AMR. As illustrated below in Figure 3.6, the average score of the Worldwide Governance Indicators does a better job of explaining high resistance proportions in Mexico than the number of doctor appointments, value added from agriculture or even antibiotic consumption.

The average Worldwide Governance Indicators score is better correlated with resistance proportions than any other factor, including consumption of antibiotics (it is likely that the Worldwide Governance Indicators scores are associated antimicrobial use and misuse as well as infection and prevention control). However, the relationship between governance and drug resistance also has outliers. Ghana and Thailand exhibit much lower than expected rates of antibiotic-resistant infections (carbapenem-resistant *P. aeruginosa* in Ghana and carbapenem-resistant *K. pneumoniae* in Thailand) than suggested by their average governance scores, again suggesting there are multiple factors at play.

Figure 3.5. Associations between potential correlates of drug resistance and resistance proportions for four antibiotic-bacterium combinations in 2015

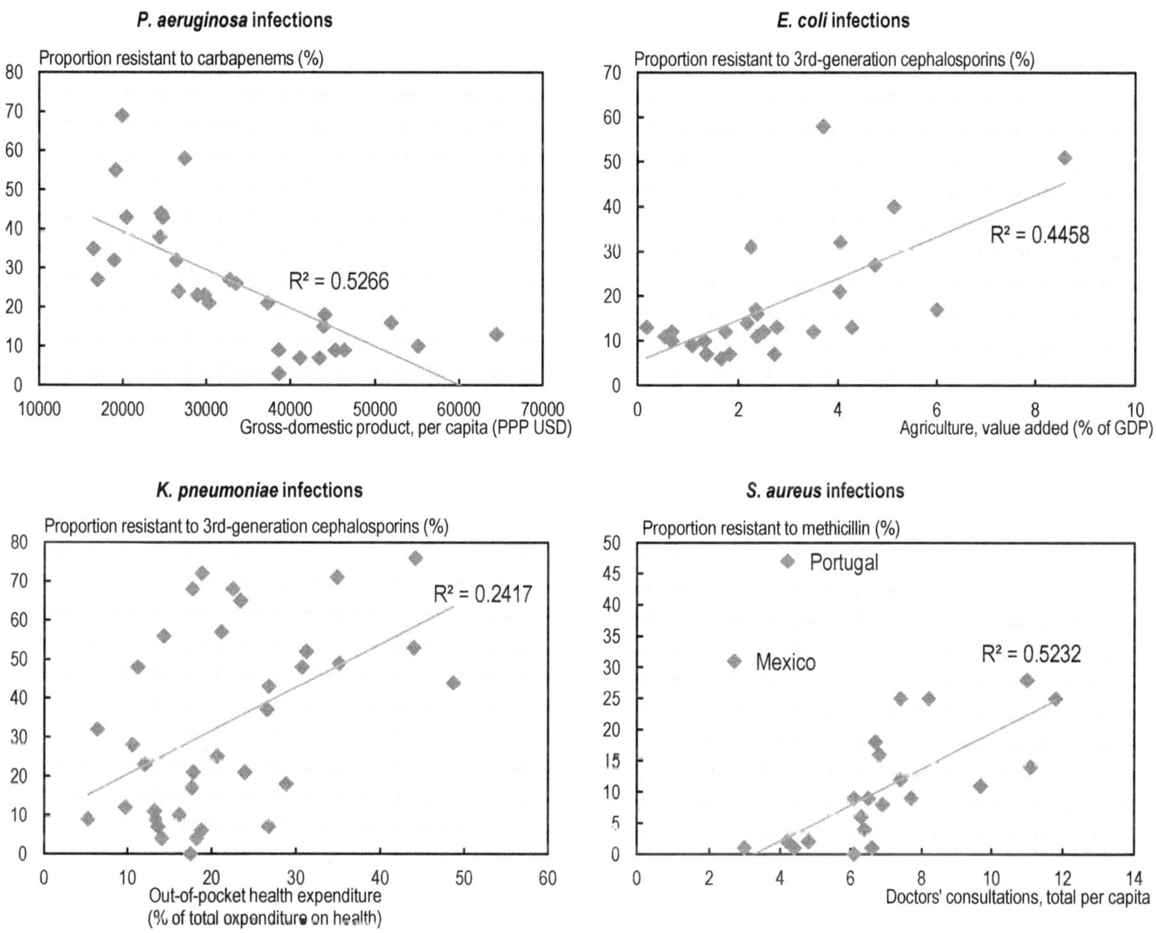

Note: Agriculture corresponds to ISIC divisions 1-5 and includes forestry, hunting, and fishing, as well as cultivation of crops and livestock production. The R-squared statistic for the bottom-right panel (*S. aureus*) excludes outliers Portugal and Mexico.

Source: OECD analyses of data from surveillance networks included in ResistanceMap[1], and data from World Bank and OECD databases.

StatLink http://dx.doi.org/10.1787/888933854782

Figure 3.6. Associations between average scores of worldwide governance indicators and proportion of infections caused by antibiotic-resistant bacteria in 2015

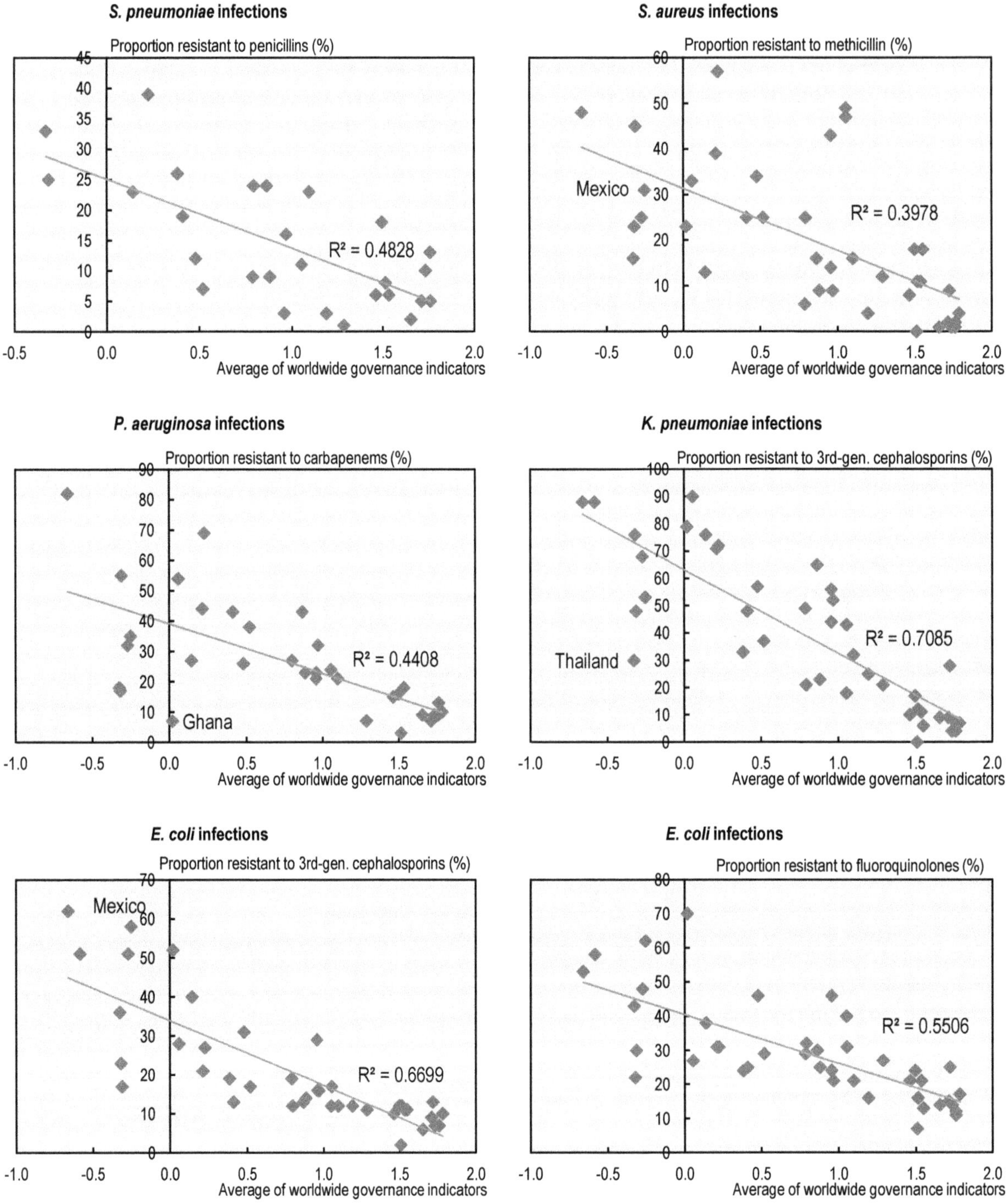

Source: OECD analyses of data from surveillance networks included in ResistanceMap[1] and World Bank data.

StatLink http://dx.doi.org/10.1787/888933854801

While this analysis is merely illustrative (and while correlation is not causation), it suggests that even though some dimensions (e.g. governance, GDP, out-of-pocket health expenditure, value-added agriculture, among others) may be associated with AMR rates, there is no single major correlate or driver of drug resistance. The emergence and spread of AMR is a complex phenomenon with multiple interrelated causes and consequences. It exhibits many of the characteristics of complex adaptive systems (Plsek and Greenhalgh, 2001[30]), such as non-linear relationships, feedback loops and co-evolution of multiple systems (e.g. human, animal and environment). For such a complex phenomenon, simple linear cause-effect relationships, even when part of multivariate models, will have limited value (Rutter et al., 2017[31]). As Wernli and colleagues (2017[13]) suggest, more and better data need to be collected and aggregated to inform more sophisticated analyses of determinants and correlates of AMR.

3.4. Should current trends continue into the future, resistance proportions will grow moderately in most countries, but there will be significant heterogeneity

The consequences of growing drug resistance, in terms of the future health and economic burden of AMR, have been used as a call for action. Some analyses concluded that, by 2050, the world could lose (Adeyi et al., 2017[32]; O'neill, 2016[33]): 10 million lives every year, 3.8% of its annual GDP, USD 1.2 trillion annually in additional health care expenditures, and an additional 28.3 million people to extreme poverty. These figures are based on hypothetical scenarios of the evolution of incident infections and the proportion resistant to antimicrobial treatment (KPMG LLP, 2014[34]). Motivated by the availability of internationally comparable data on resistance proportions (from surveillance networks included in ResistanceMap1) and by calls to make estimates more empirically driven (de Kraker, Stewardson and Harbarth, 2016[35]), the OECD projected resistance proportions for eight antibiotic-bacterium combinations for 52 countries (including members, accession and key partners of the OECD, as well as members of the G20 and countries in the European Economic Area) up to 2030 (see Box 3.2 for a description of the forecasting methodology used).

In OECD countries, average resistance proportions across eight antibiotic-bacterium combinations are estimated to have increased from 14% (range: 3-33%) in 2005 to 17% (range: 3-39%) in 2015, and may go up further to 18% (range: 6-40%) by 2030 if current trends in resistance, and correlates of resistance, continue into the future, and no policy actions are taken (see Figure 3.7). Growth in resistance proportions is thus projected to continue, though moderately, in OECD countries and beyond, under a business-as-usual scenario. Between 2005 and 2015, the predicted proportion of infections from resistant bacteria grew much faster than projected for the period 2015-2030, however these averages mask significant heterogeneity across countries and antibiotic-bacterium combinations.

Of the 52 countries in the analyses, the average resistance proportions for eight antibiotic-bacterium combinations could increase in 37 countries and decrease in 13 countries (see Table 3.3). Despite average reductions in a few countries, no country is projected to reduce resistance proportions for all eight antibiotic-bacterium combinations. On the contrary, five countries (Bulgaria, Luxembourg, Iceland, Slovenia and Denmark) could see resistance proportions increase for all eight combinations. The majority of countries could see both increases and reductions. Resistance proportions could increase in 64% of country-antibiotic-bacterium combinations (on average, proportions could grow in these country-antibiotic-bacterium combinations by 42%, when taking 2015 rates as base values), and could decrease in 36% of combinations (on average, proportions could drop by 9%, compared to proportions in 2015).

Figure 3.7. Average proportion of infections caused by bacteria resistant to antimicrobial treatment for eight antibiotic-bacterium combinations in 2005, 2015 and 2030

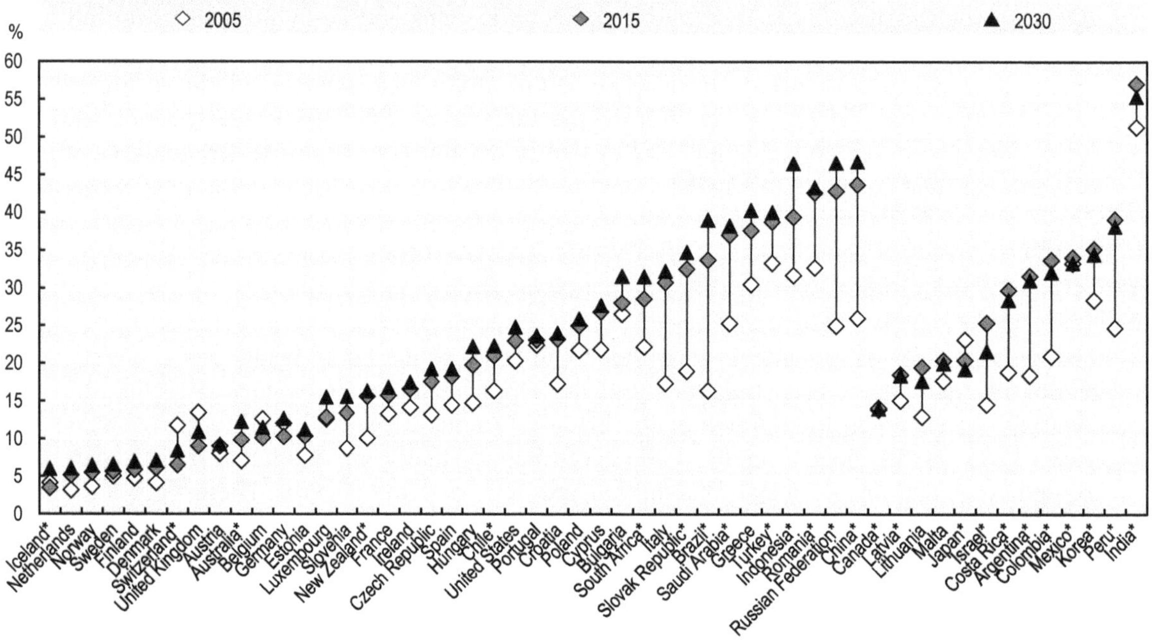

Note: * indicates country is missing more than 50% of observations, across all eight antibiotic-bacterium pairs, between 2005 and 2015. For countries on the left of this graph, resistance proportions will be higher in 2030, compared to 2015. For countries on the right, rates will be lower in 2030. Otherwise, countries are sorted left to right based on ascending resistance proportions in 2015.

Source: OECD analyses of data from surveillance networks included in ResistanceMap[1].

StatLink http://dx.doi.org/10.1787/888933854820

In OECD countries, growth rates of resistance proportions for third-generation cephalosporin-resistant *E. coli* and *K. pneumoniae*, using the average of country-specific growth rates, are projected to slow down significantly from 163% between 2005 and 2015 to 16% between 2015 and 2030. On the other hand, the proportion of infections caused by vancomycin-resistant *E. faecium* and *E. faecalis* are projected to grow at a rate of 31% between 2015 and 2030 in OECD countries, compared to a growth rate of 5% between 2005 and 2015 (the same trend is projected in G20 countries). Different regions could see very different progressions. While OECD countries could see proportions of penicillin-resistant *S. pneumoniae* grow faster in the coming decades, the opposite is true for EU countries. Conversely, rates of MRSA in OECD countries should continue to decline (if at a slower rate) but are expected to actually grow in EU countries between 2015 and 2030. Growth in carbapenem-resistant *K. pneumoniae* is projected to intensify in the coming years across all regions but especially in G20 countries and OECD key partners.

Table 3.3. Percentage point changes in resistance proportions for eight priority antibiotic-bacterium combinations between 2015 and 2030

COUNTRY	FREC	3GCREC	PRSP	3GCRKP	CRKP	VRE	MRSA	CRPA	AVERAGE
Indonesia*	15.7	7.9	11.6	18.9	1.7	0.5	-0.7	0.8	7.1
Brazil*	10.7	4.3	8.9	16.4	-0.2	3.3	0.2	-1.3	5.3
Russian Federation*	18.3	-1.9	5.9	-8.6	5.6	7.0	5.4	-1.6	3.8
Bulgaria	7.3	3.5	0.6	4.0	2.3	6.8	0.7	3.5	3.6
China*	3.5	10.1	9.8	1.3	6.2	-6.2	2.3	-2.7	3.1
South Africa*	11.4	2.9	6.3	-2.9	2.1	4.1	1.9	-2.2	3.0
Greece	5.5	8.4	-0.6	1.2	-5.1	0.5	6.6	4.9	2.7
Luxembourg	0.9	3.1	1.6	3.0	3.2	4.9	1.4	3.1	2.6
Iceland*	3.7	1.8	1.6	5.1	3.4	2.1	0.6	1.7	2.5
Hungary	4.5	5.7	-0.4	1.0	2.9	5.7	4.3	-4.3	2.4
Australia*	0.4	3.5	3.1	6.1	3.7	2.2	-4.5	4.7	2.4
Germany	3.2	5.0	-0.6	4.8	2.3	2.7	1.0	0.5	2.4
Slovak Republic*	9.9	0.8	1.5	-4.1	4.2	14.1	0.3	-9.2	2.2
Slovenia	0.9	2.9	1.9	3.2	1.1	3.2	0.9	3.1	2.2
United Kingdom	0.6	3.7	-0.7	-0.2	2.6	4.5	-1.0	5.8	1.9
Switzerland*	1.1	-0.9	1.3	3.1	3.5	1.5	2.5	3.2	1.9
United States	0.2	8.1	-3.6	9.3	3.8	-5.0	-1.2	2.9	1.8
Czech Republic	-0.1	0.2	2.5	-3.1	2.4	6.6	0.9	4.0	1.7
Italy	2.1	6.2	0.5	5.7	-9.7	0.6	3.3	3.2	1.5
Belgium	-0.2	2.6	2.4	-1.8	1.1	0.1	1.4	5.3	1.4
Chile*	5.6	-0.1	0.9	-0.5	0.8	3.0	0.6	-0.2	1.3
Turkey*	2.7	-1.3	6.2	0.8	-6.4	4.3	1.3	2.1	1.2
Saudi Arabia*	18.2	1.9	6.3	-2.9	-4.6	-5.2	-1.6	-2.8	1.2
Finland	1.9	-0.4	-0.4	0.5	1.3	1.3	1.2	3.0	1.0
Spain	-0.2	4.9	1.1	1.7	1.7	-0.1	1.7	-2.6	1.0
France	1.4	3.2	-0.6	1.4	1.4	-0.4	1.2	0.4	1.0
Denmark	2.3	0.7	0.9	1.4	1.4	0.9	0.2	0.1	1.0
Sweden	-0.5	1.0	1.0	1.1	1.4	1.8	0.9	0.5	0.9
Norway	2.1	2.4	0.0	-0.4	1.3	1.8	0.8	-1.1	0.9
Poland	7.9	2.7	-0.5	-5.4	3.7	6.8	-0.1	-8.0	0.9
Estonia	1.1	-1.2	1.4	-2.0	2.5	3.5	0.7	1.0	0.9
Cyprus	0.4	-0.3	3.8	-8.0	-0.3	-5.3	0.6	16.0	0.9
Netherlands	1.3	0.5	1.1	-0.8	1.4	2.6	1.1	-0.6	0.8
Ireland	2.3	2.9	0.6	1.1	2.3	2.1	-2.9	-1.8	0.8
Croatia	5.0	0.8	3.3	2.7	0.4	2.8	-2.2	-6.3	0.8
New Zealand*	2.5	6.3	-2.2	5.1	0.0	-4.3	-1.6	-0.1	0.7
Romania*	9.0	3.2	3.1	1.7	2.7	-4.9	0.6	-9.8	0.7
Portugal	1.0	3.6	-0.2	-4.1	3.3	-2.6	2.3	0.8	0.5
Austria	-0.5	0.8	-0.3	1.0	1.4	-1.3	0.8	-0.1	0.2
Canada*	2.4	2.7	0.6	-0.9	1.1	-1.2	-3.3	-2.1	-0.1
Latvia*	-5.0	-2.3	-1.1	1.7	2.1	4.3	-2.0	1.3	-0.1
Malta	-5.8	0.6	1.4	1.4	1.4	-2.9	1.7	-0.8	-0.4
Argentina*	6.3	2.4	0.0	2.5	-3.4	1.7	-2.6	-11.3	-0.6
Korea*	-8.4	-0.8	2.5	-2.2	4.4	-1.2	-1.2	1.4	-0.7
Mexico*	-6.9	2.0	4.6	-6.8	-2.3	4.0	0.5	-0.9	-0.7
Peru*	-5.3	-1.9	-1.7	8.6	2.4	-5.6	-3.4	-0.8	-1.0
Japan*	-3.2	-5.6	0.5	9.2	-0.1	-9.3	0.7	-1.4	-1.2
Costa Rica*	-1.6	-4.8	2.7	-3.5	2.1	-3.5	-0.8	-1.2	-1.3
Colombia*	1.3	1.5	-2.3	3.3	-1.0	-6.5	-3.0	-3.4	-1.6
India*	-4.5	-3.8	2.6	-3.2	-8.1	-1.0	5.8	-1.0	-1.7
Lithuania	-1.4	-3.8	-3.4	-2.4	2.0	0.4	-4.1	2.6	1.8
Israel*	-5.6	-3.6	-0.1	-4.3	-4.2	-8.2	2.2	-6.1	-3.7
OECD COUNTRIES	1.0	1.8	0.6	0.8	1.1	1.4	0.5	0.3	1.0
EU28 COUNTRIES	3.0	1.6	2.9	2.5	0.2	-1.1	0.0	-1.1	1.0
ALL COUNTRIES	1.6	1.7	1.2	0.7	0.9	0.5	0.4	-0.2	0.8
G20 COUNTRIES	3.9	2.7	3.4	2.6	0.0	0.3	0.4	-0.3	1.6
OECD KEY PARTNERS	1.0	1.8	0.6	0.8	1.1	1.4	0.5	0.3	1.0

Note: * indicates country is missing more than 50% of observations, across all eight antibiotic-bacterium pairs, between 2005 and 2015. The colour scheme is based on a two-point scale (minimum in light grey, maximum in blue, points in between coloured proportionally). Countries (and country groupings) are sorted top to bottom from highest to lowest average resistance proportions (across antibiotic-bacterium combinations). Antibiotic-bacterium combinations are sorted left to right from highest to lowest average resistance proportions (across countries). FREC: fluoroquinolone-resistant *E. coli*, VRE: vancomycin-resistant *E. faecalis* and *E. faecium*, 3GCREC: third-generation cephalosporin-resistant *E. coli*, CRKP: carbapenem-resistant *K. pneumoniae*, 3GCRKP: third-generation cephalosporin-resistant *K. pneumoniae*, CRPA: carbapenem-resistant *P. aeruginosa*, MRSA: methicillin-resistant *S. aureus*, PRSP: penicillin-resistant *S. pneumoniae*.
Source: OECD analyses of data from surveillance networks included in ResistanceMap[1].

Predicted historic and future resistance proportions for different antibiotic-bacterium combinations in selected OECD countries from 2000 to 2030 are illustrated in Figure 3.8. The heterogeneity in resistance proportions across countries, antibiotic-bacterium combinations and years, as well as the evolution of resistance proportions over time, is striking. The panels also illustrate data gaps and their impact on uncertainty in the estimation.

When considering all country-antibiotic-bacterium combinations together, resistance proportions could grow on average 23% between 2015 and 2030. However, this average masks significant heterogeneity in growth rates across countries and antibiotic-bacterium pairs. In OECD countries, the largest projected growth rate in resistance proportions is 50% for penicillin-resistant *S. pneumoniae* in the Slovak Republic (an increase of 14 percentage points, from 28% in 2015 to 42% in 2030). However, in the same country, resistance proportions for carbapenem-resistant *P. aeruginosa* could go down by 10 percentage points (from 58% to 49%, a growth rate of -16%). The largest projected reduction in resistance proportions is -27% for carbapenem-resistant *K. pneumoniae* in Italy (a drop of 10 percentage points, from 36% to 26%). However, the resistance proportions for third-generation cephalosporins-resistant *E. coli* in Italy could go up by 6 percentage points (from 31% to 37%, a growth rate of 20%).

Figure 3.8. Predicted historic and future resistance proportions for eight priority antibiotic-bacterium combinations in selected OECD countries from 2000 to 2030

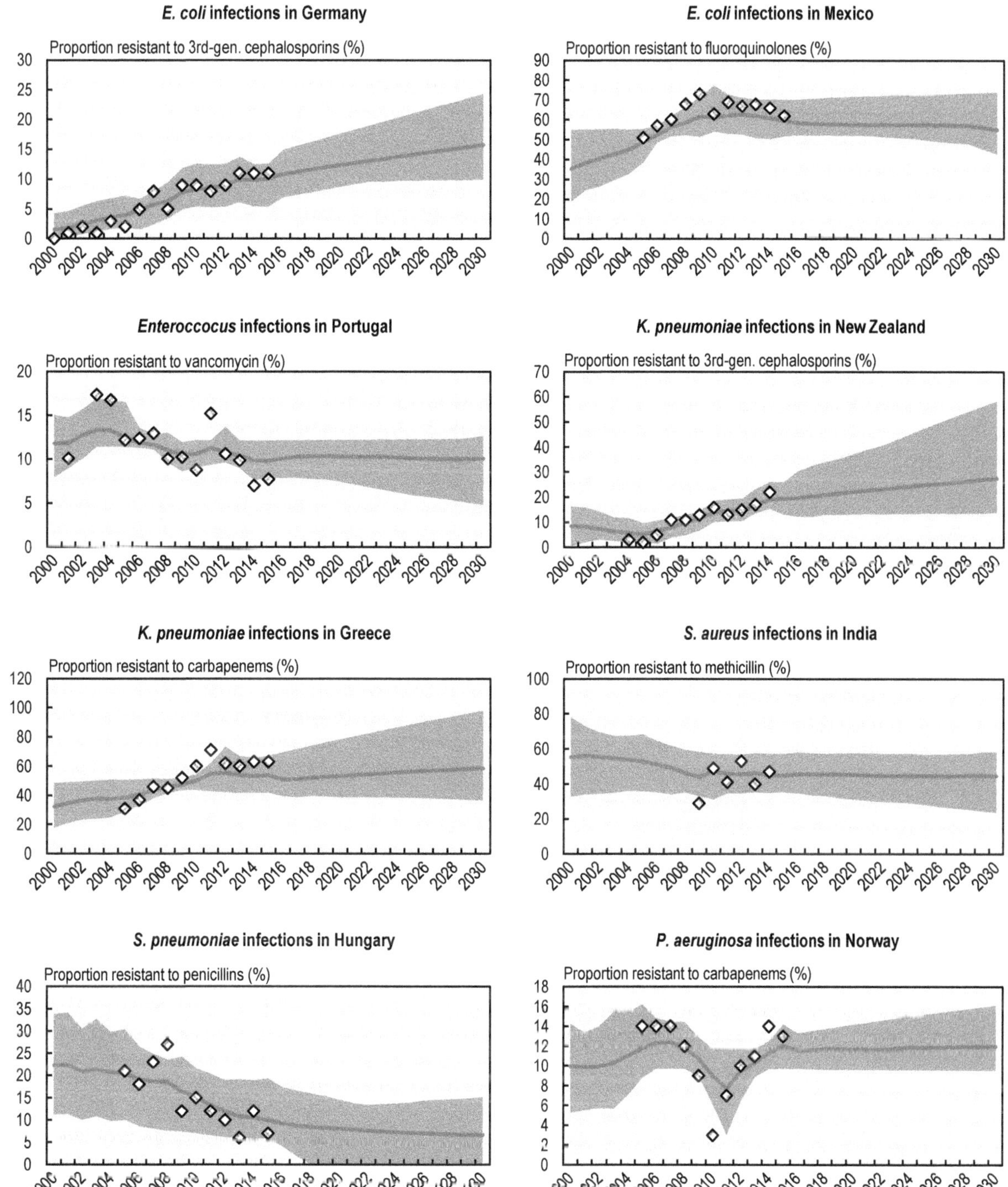

Note: Points are original data, lines are means and bands are 95% uncertainty intervals.
Source: OECD analyses of data from surveillance networks included in ResistanceMap[1].

3.5. Growing resistance to third-line treatments and difficult-to-treat microorganisms are a concern for the coming years

Growth of resistance proportions for fluoroquinolone-resistant *E. coli* and third-generation cephalosporin-resistant *E. coli* and *K. pneumoniae* are projected to slow down from 2015 to 2030. In part, this waning growth could be due to a slowing of growth rates in the consumption of fluoroquinolones and third-generation cephalosporins in a large majority of countries for the period 2015-2030 compared to 2005-15. Furthermore, consumption of third-generation cephalosporins could decrease in half of the countries analysed here. However, the use of fluoroquinolones could still grow by 27%, on average across all countries, by 2030. More than a fifth of *E. coli* in OECD countries, and close to half in G20 countries, were already resistant to fluoroquinolones in 2015, and resistance proportions for this antibiotic-bacterium combination are projected to keep growing up to 2030. The proportions of *E. coli* and *K. pneumoniae* infections resistant to third-generation cephalosporins are also projected to increase (see Figure 3.9).

Figure 3.9. Average proportions of *E. coli* and *K. pneumoniae* resistant to third-generation cephalosporins and carbapenems (only *K. pneumoniae*) in 2015

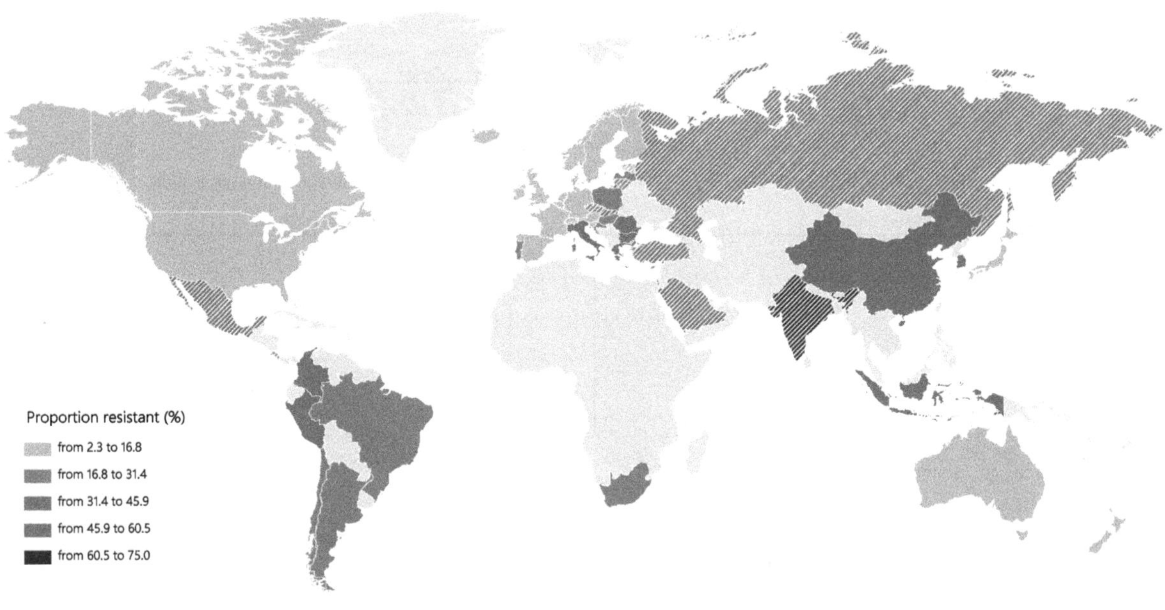

Note: Stripes indicate average resistance for these antibiotic-bacterium combinations is projected to decrease up to 2030.
Source: OECD analyses of data from surveillance networks included in ResistanceMap[1].

These trends are concerning as both third-generation cephalosporins and fluoroquinolones are generally used as second-line treatments. Growing resistance to these antimicrobials could lead to increased use of third-line treatments like carbapenems, promoting the emergence and spread of carbapenem-resistant bacteria (ECDC, 2017[3]). WHO (2017[2]) considers the urgency of need for new antibiotics to treat carbapenem and third-generation cephalosporin-resistant *Enterobacteriaceae* (including *E. coli* and *K. pneumoniae*) is critical, and while proportions of carbapenem-resistant *K. pneumoniae* were relatively low in 2015, they are projected to increase (see Figure 3.10).

Figure 3.10. Trends in antimicrobial resistance in selected regions and country groups among high-priority antibiotic-bacterium combinations, by line of treatment

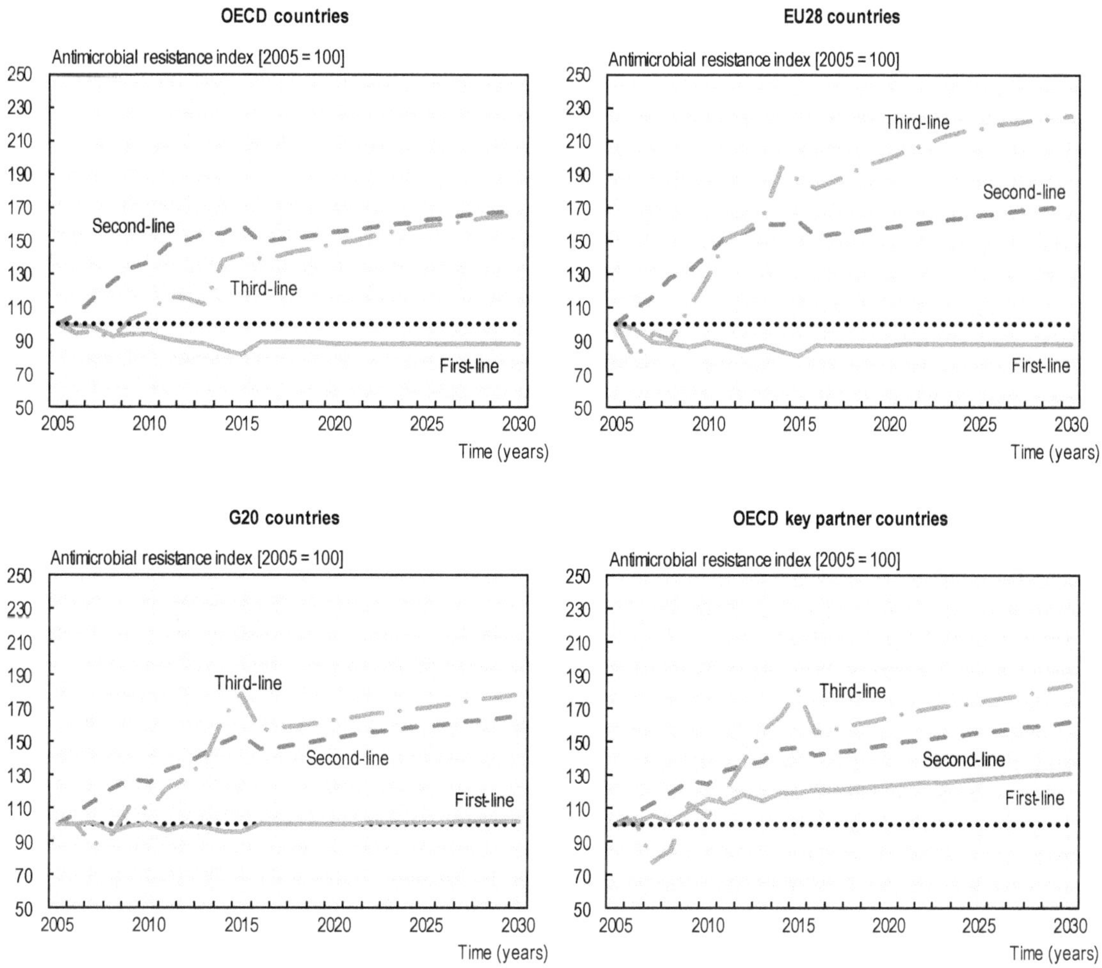

Note: Data were normalised to average antimicrobial resistance in 2005 (equal to 100) for each treatment line (e.g. a value of 150 for resistance to second-line treatments in 2015 in G20 countries means that resistance to second-line treatments is 50% higher than it was in 2005 in G20 countries). Resistance to first-line treatments is defined as the average of the proportions of penicillin-resistant *S. pneumoniae* and MRSA. Resistance to second-line treatments is the average of the proportions of *E. coli* and *K. pneumoniae* resistant to third-generation cephalosporins and of *E. coli* resistant to fluoroquinolones. Resistance to third-line treatments is defined as the proportion of *K. pneumoniae* resistant to carbapenems.
Source: OECD analyses of data from surveillance networks included in ResistanceMap[1].

In EU28 and G20 countries, as well as OECD key partners, resistance proportions to third-line treatments are now growing faster than those of second-line treatments (markedly so in the EU28). The only options that will be left to treat infections with bacteria resistant to third-line treatments like carbapenems will be older antimicrobial agents with lower efficacy, such as polymyxins (e.g. colistin), or combination therapy. In certain countries with high resistance proportions, like Greece and Italy, resistance to polymyxins is already emerging with potentially disastrous consequences, as these remain one of the few last options for treatment (ECDC, 2015[36]).

Resistance among difficult to treat microorganisms like *Enterococci* (e.g. *E. faecalis* and *E. faecium*) and *P. aeruginosa* is also worrisome. These bacteria are intrinsically resistant to several antimicrobial agents and are challenging to contain in health care settings (ECDC, 2015[36]). Close to two-thirds of *P. aeruginosa* were already resistant to carbapenems in Romania and the Slovak Republic in 2015. In some countries with already high resistance (e.g. Greece, Turkey or Bulgaria), the proportion of carbapenem-resistant *P. aeruginosa* is projected to rise. Vancomycin-resistant *E. faecalis* and *E. faecium* is projected to rise in 36 countries while consumption of glycopeptides (e.g. vancomycin) could grow in 40 countries. Growing consumption might not be a problem in itself (as discussed in previous sections), but it is important to balance access to antimicrobial therapies with prudent and appropriate use (stewardship). As discussed in Chapter 5, stringent interventions for infection control are also essential to prevent further emergence and spread of resistance.

Proportions of MRSA dropped considerably across the majority of OECD countries between 2005 and 2015 but further progress could be slow, based on projected trends up to 2030. In some EU countries, reductions in AMR rates could be reversed altogether. Moreover, in the Slovak Republic, Hungary, the Russian Federation and the Czech Republic, the proportions of resistant bacteria have actually increased in recent years and should continue to rise in the coming decades. In some countries (e.g. South Africa, Croatia and Bulgaria), reductions in resistance proportions could be reversed, in line with projected growth in the consumption of penicillins. Despite recent trends, MRSA remains high in certain countries and the transfer of health care-associated clones into the community suggests comprehensive cross-sector policies are needed (ECDC, 2017[37]).

Conclusion: More and better data needed for robust policy making

The proportion of infections that are resistant to antimicrobial therapies will continue to grow, if moderately, in a majority of OECD, EU and G20 countries in the coming decades, if current trends in antimicrobial consumption, economic and population growth, and health spending continue into the future, and no policy action is taken. While some progress has been achieved in slowing down, or even reducing, resistance for MRSA, projections indicate these gains could be halted or reversed in the coming years, if no effective action is put in place. For other pathogens, the growth in resistance proportions of the last 10 to 15 years will likely persist, even if more moderately. There is significant variation across countries, bacteria and antibiotics, suggesting previous forecasting efforts assuming a single growth rate are not corroborated by available data. The reasons behind this variation remain, unfortunately, difficult to pinpoint with any certainty.

Data-driven models of AMR have limited explanatory power, as illustrated by wide confidence intervals (see Figure 3.8). There are important gaps in both data and understanding and these are naturally intertwined. The data that do exist are potentially biased and often not comparable due to challenges in defining and measuring drug resistance (see Box 3.1). More primary research and data collection are needed on the many facets of AMR, from the human health sector, to food and veterinary sectors, to travel, governance and general economic development. There are already some suggestions for what should be monitored, from access to sanitation and safe drinking water, to non-prescription availability and misuse of antibiotics, as well as the economic and health burden of drug resistant infections (Wernli et al., 2017[13]). There are innovative approaches to data collection such as citizen science initiatives in which samples are crowd-sourced from populations directly (Freeman et al., 2016[38]), and some pharmaceutical companies collect global surveillance data (Ashley et al., 2018[39]). Initiatives such as the WHO Global Antimicrobial Resistance Surveillance System (GLASS) and surveillance networks like EARS-Net are important as they set guidelines and standards that are shared by all participating partners. Countries should continue to promote the collection and dissemination of data on all aspects related to AMR.

More and better data are essential to producing high-quality estimates that, in turn, can inform robust policies in addressing growing drug resistance. Still, it is important not to delay action while surveillance and monitoring systems are being set up. While, as discussed in Chapter 5, a number of OECD countries have already put in place policies to tackle inappropriate consumption, as populations grow and age, more people will be at risk of infection and more antimicrobials will be consumed. Policy needs to go further, as the costs of inaction may be very significant as discussed in following chapter.

Notes

1 ResistanceMap aggregates data from international surveillance networks like EARS-Net, CEASER, GLASS, and others, which in turn aggregate data from national surveillance networks.

2 The European Antimicrobial Resistance Surveillance Network (EARS-Net) is the largest publicly funded system for antimicrobial resistance surveillance in Europe. Participating countries include Austria, Belgium, Bulgaria, Croatia, Cyprus, Czech Republic, Denmark, Estonia, Finland, France, Germany, Greece, Hungary, Iceland, Ireland, Italy, Latvia, Lithuania, Luxembourg, Malta, Netherlands, Norway, Poland, Portugal, Romania, Slovak Republic, Slovenia, Spain, Sweden, and the United Kingdom. The Central Asian and Eastern European Surveillance of Antimicrobial Resistance (CAESAR) network includes all countries of the WHO European Region that are not part of EARS-Net, namely: Albania, Armenia, Azerbaijan, Belarus, Bosnia and Herzegovina, Georgia, Kazakhstan, Kyrgyzstan, Montenegro, the Republic of Moldova, the Russian Federation, Serbia, Switzerland, Tajikistan, the former Yugoslav Republic of Macedonia, Turkey, Turkmenistan, Ukraine and Uzbekistan, as well as Kosovo (in accordance with United Nations Security Council resolution 1244 (1999)).

References

Adeyi, O. et al. (2017), *Drug-resistant infections : a threat to our economic future (Vol. 2) : final report (English)*, http://documents.worldbank.org/curated/en/323311493396993758/final-report (accessed on 16 January 2018). [32]

Albrich, W., D. Monnet and S. Harbarth (2004), "Antibiotic selection pressure and resistance in Streptococcus pneumoniae and Streptococcus pyogenes.", *Emerging infectious diseases*, Vol. 10/3, pp. 514-7, http://dx.doi.org/10.3201/eid1003.030252. [20]

Alsan, M. et al. (2015), "Out-of-pocket health expenditures and antimicrobial resistance in low-income and middle-income countries: an economic analysis", *The Lancet Infectious Diseases*, Vol. 15/10, pp. 1203-1210, https://doi.org/10.1016/S1473-3099(15)00149-8. [15]

Ashley, E. et al. (2018), "An inventory of supranational antimicrobial resistance surveillance networks involving low- and middle-income countries since 2000", *Journal of Antimicrobial Chemotherapy*, Vol. 73/7, pp. 1737-1749, http://dx.doi.org/10.1093/jac/dky026. [39]

Australian Commission on Safety and Quality in Health Care (2017), *AURA 2017: Second Australian report on antimicrobial use and resistance in human health*, Australian Commission on Safety and Quality in Health Care, Sydney, https://www.safetyandquality.gov.au/wp-content/uploads/2018/01/AURA-2017-Second-Australian-report-on-Antimicrobial-Use-and-Resistance-in-human-health.pdf (accessed on 16 January 2018). [5]

Cassini, A. et al. (2018), "Attributable deaths and disability-adjusted life-years caused by infections with antibiotic-resistant bacteria in the European Union and the European Economic Area in 2015: a population-level health estimate", *Lancet Infectious Disease*, http://dx.doi.org/10.1016/S1473-3099(18)30605-4. [23]

Cecchini, M., J. Langer and L. Slawomirski (2015), "Antimicrobial Resistance in G7 Countries and Beyond: Economic Issues, Policies and Options for Action", OECD, Paris, http://www.oecd.org/els/health-systems/Antimicrobial-Resistance-in-G7-Countries-and-Beyond.pdf (accessed on 16 January 2018). [1]

Collignon, P. et al. (2015), "Antimicrobial Resistance: The Major Contribution of Poor Governance and Corruption to This Growing Problem", *PLOS ONE*, Vol. 10/3, p. e0116746, http://dx.doi.org/10.1371/journal.pone.0116746. [16]

de Kraker, M., A. Stewardson and S. Harbarth (2016), "Will 10 Million People Die a Year due to Antimicrobial Resistance by 2050?", *PLOS Medicine*, Vol. 13/11, p. e1002184, http://dx.doi.org/10.1371/journal.pmed.1002184. [35]

ECDC (2017), *Antimicrobial resistance surveillance in Europe 2016. Annual Report of the European Antimicrobial Resistance Surveillance Network (EARS-Net).*, ECDC, Stockholm, http://dx.doi.org/10.2900/296939. [3]

ECDC (2017), *TESSy -The European Surveillance System: Antimicrobial resistance (AMR) reporting protocol 2017: European Antimicrobial Resistance Surveillance Network (EARS-Net) surveillance data for 2016.*, ECDC, Stockholm, https://ecdc.europa.eu/sites/portal/files/documents/EARS-Net-reporting-protocol-2017.pdf (accessed on 12 February 2018). [37]

ECDC (2015), *Antimicrobial resistance surveillance in Europe 2015. Annual Report of the European Antimicrobial Resistance Surveillance Network (EARS-Net).*, ECDC, Stockholm, https://ecdc.europa.eu/sites/portal/files/media/en/publications/Publications/antimicrobial-resistance-europe-2015.pdf (accessed on 13 February 2018). [36]

ECDC/EFSA/EMA (2017), "ECDC/EFSA/EMA second joint report on the integrated analysis of the consumption of antimicrobial agents and occurrence of antimicrobial resistance in bacteria from humans and food- producing animals", *EFSA Journal*, Vol. 15/7, http://dx.doi.org/10.2903/j.efsa.2017.4872. [22]

ECDC, EFSA and EMA (2017), *ECDC/EFSA/EMA second joint report on the integrated analysis of the consumption of antimicrobial agents and occurrence of antimicrobial resistance in bacteria from humans and food-producing animals Joint Interagency Antimicrobial Consumption and Resistance Analysis (JIACRA) Report*, http://dx.doi.org/10.2903/j.efsa.2017.4872. [27]

Freeman, S. et al. (2016), "Crowdsourced Data Indicate Widespread Multidrug Resistance in Skin Flora of Healthy Young Adults.", *Journal of microbiology & biology education*, Vol. 17/1, pp. 172-82, http://dx.doi.org/10.1128/jmbe.v17i1.1008. [38]

Goossens, M., B. Catry and J. Verhaegen (2013), "Antimicrobial resistance to benzylpenicillin in invasive pneumococcal disease in Belgium, 2003-2010: the effect of altering clinical breakpoints.", *Epidemiology and infection*, Vol. 141/3, pp. 490-5, http://dx.doi.org/10.1017/S0950268812001057. [21]

Hindler, J. and J. Stelling (2007), "Analysis and Presentation of Cumulative Antibiograms: A New Consensus Guideline from the Clinical and Laboratory Standards Institute", *Clinical Infectious Diseases*, Vol. 44/6, pp. 867-873, http://dx.doi.org/10.1086/511864. [8]

Kassim, A. et al. (2016), "Comparison of Clinical Laboratory Standards Institute and European Committee on Antimicrobial Susceptibility Testing guidelines for the interpretation of antibiotic susceptibility at a University teaching hospital in Nairobi, Kenya: a cross-sectional study", *Annals of Clinical Microbiology and Antimicrobials*, Vol. 15/1, p. 21, http://dx.doi.org/10.1186/s12941-016-0135-3. [9]

Kaufmann, D., A. Kraay and M. Mastruzzi (2011), "The Worldwide Governance Indicators: Methodology and Analytical Issues", *Hague Journal on the Rule of Law*, Vol. 3/02, pp. 220-246, http://dx.doi.org/10.1017/S1876404511200046. [29]

Klein, S. (2000), "The effects of hormones on sex differences in infection: from genes to behavior", *Neuroscience & Biobehavioral Reviews*, Vol. 24/6, pp. 627-638, https://doi.org/10.1016/S0149-7634(00)00027-0. [19]

KPMG LLP (2014), *The global economic impact of anti-microbial resistance*, KPMG LLP, https://home.kpmg.com/content/dam/kpmg/pdf/2014/12/amr-report-final.pdf (accessed on 16 January 2018). [34]

Mendelson, M. et al. (2016), "Maximising access to achieve appropriate human antimicrobial use in low-income and middle-income countries", *The Lancet*, Vol. 387/10014, pp. 188-198, https://doi.org/10.1016/S0140-6736(15)00547-4. [14]

OECD (2017), *Tackling Wasteful Spending on Health*, OECD Publishing, Paris, https://doi.org/10.1787/9789264266414-en. [6]

OIE (2016), *The OIE Strategy on Antimicrobial Resistance and the Prudent Use of Antimicrobials*, OIE, http://www.oie.int/fileadmin/Home/eng/Media_Center/docs/pdf/PortailAMR/EN_OIE-AMRstrategy.pdf (accessed on 14 February 2018). [28]

O'neill, J. (2016), *Tackling drug-resistant infections globally: Final report and recommendations*, https://amr-review.org/sites/default/files/160525_Final%20paper_with%20cover.pdf (accessed on 13 February 2018). [33]

Plsek, P. and T. Greenhalgh (2001), "Complexity science: The challenge of complexity in health care.", *BMJ (Clinical research ed.)*, Vol. 323/7313, pp. 625-8, http://www.ncbi.nlm.nih.gov/pubmed/11557716 (accessed on 16 January 2018). [30]

Rönnerstrand, B. and V. Lapuente (2017), "Corruption and use of antibiotics in regions of Europe", *Health Policy*, Vol. 121/3, pp. 250-256, http://dx.doi.org/10.1016/J.HEALTHPOL.2016.12.010. [17]

Rutter, H. et al. (2017), "The need for a complex systems model of evidence for public health.", *Lancet*, Vol. 390/10112, pp. 2602-2604, https://doi.org/10.1016/S0140-6736(17)31267-9. [31]

Simon, A., G. Hollander and A. McMichael (2015), "Evolution of the immune system in humans from infancy to old age.", *Proceedings. Biological sciences*, Vol. 282/1821, p. 20143085, http://dx.doi.org/10.1098/rspb.2014.3085. [18]

Tang, K. et al. (2017), "Restricting the use of antibiotics in food-producing animals and its associations with antibiotic resistance in food-producing animals and human beings: a systematic review and meta-analysis", *The Lancet Planetary Health*, Vol. 1/8, pp. e316-e327, https://doi.org/10.1016/S2542-5196(17)30141-9. [26]

Turnidge, J. and D. Paterson (2007), "Setting and revising antibacterial susceptibility breakpoints.", *Clinical microbiology reviews*, Vol. 20/3, pp. 391-408, table of contents, http://dx.doi.org/10.1128/CMR.00047-06. [7]

Van Boeckel, T. et al. (2015), "Global trends in antimicrobial use in food animals", *Proceedings of the National Academy of Sciences*, Vol. 112/18, pp. 5649-5654, http://dx.doi.org/10.1073/pnas.1503141112. [25]

van der Bij, A. et al. (2012), “Clinical breakpoint changes and their impact on surveillance of antimicrobial resistance in Escherichia coli causing bacteraemia”, *Clinical Microbiology and Infection*, Vol. 18/11, pp. E466-E472, http://dx.doi.org/10.1111/j.1469-0691.2012.03996.x. [10]

Wernli, D. et al. (2017), “Antimicrobial resistance: The complex challenge of measurement to inform policy and the public”, *PLOS Medicine*, Vol. 14/8, p. e1002378, http://dx.doi.org/10.1371/journal.pmed.1002378. [13]

WHO (2017), *Global antimicrobial resistance surveillance system (GLASS) report: early implementation 2016-2017*, World Health Organization, Geneva, http://apps.who.int/iris/bitstream/10665/259744/1/9789241513449-eng.pdf?ua=1 (accessed on 12 February 2018). [12]

WHO (2017), *Prioritization of pathogens to guide discovery, research and development of new antibiotics for drug-resistant bacterial infections, including tuberculosis.*, World Health Organisation, Geneva, http://www.who.int/medicines/areas/rational_use/PPLreport_2017_09_19.pdf?ua=1 (accessed on 12 February 2018). [2]

WHO (2014), *Antimicrobial resistance: global report on surveillance 2014*, http://apps.who.int/iris/bitstream/handle/10665/112642/9789241564748_eng.pdf;jsessionid=7896DA46F16714263D42D26A092CB051?sequence=1 (accessed on 09 October 2018). [4]

Wolfensberger, A. et al. (2013), “Change of Antibiotic Susceptibility Testing Guidelines from CLSI to EUCAST: Influence on Cumulative Hospital Antibiograms”, *PLoS ONE*, Vol. 8/11, p. e79130, http://dx.doi.org/10.1371/journal.pone.0079130. [11]

Zilberberg, M. et al. (2017), “Carbapenem resistance, inappropriate empiric treatment and outcomes among patients hospitalized with Enterobacteriaceae urinary tract infection, pneumonia and sepsis”, *BMC Infectious Diseases*, Vol. 17/1, p. 279, http://dx.doi.org/10.1186/s12879-017-2383-z. [24]

Chapter 4. Health and economic burden of antimicrobial resistance

Driss Ait Ouakrim, Tiago Cravo Oliveira and Mario Jendrossek

Antimicrobial resistance (AMR) is a major public health concern worldwide. The OECD has developed a micro-simulations model to produce comparable cross-country estimates of the health and economic impact of AMR, for a comprehensive set of infections susceptible to develop resistance. Individual analyses were performed for 33 OECD and European Union/European Economic Area (EU/EEA) member countries. The model estimates for the included countries show that the current burden of AMR is substantial but, at this point, still limited in comparison to the impact of other conditions. This chapter provides an overview of current economic studies on AMR, describes the findings of the main analyses, along with the major knowledge gaps in the current economic literature on AMR. The characteristics and results of the OECD AMR microsimulation model are then presented, followed by the results of a second analysis conducted by the OECD, focusing specifically on the potential health burden of AMR in the context of antimicrobial prophylaxis treatments. The final section of this chapter summarises the main findings and discusses their policy implications.

Note by Turkey:

The information in this document with reference to "Cyprus" relates to the southern part of the Island. There is no single authority representing both Turkish and Greek Cypriot people on the Island. Turkey recognises the Turkish Republic of Northern Cyprus (TRNC). Until a lasting and equitable solution is found within the context of the United Nations, Turkey shall preserve its position concerning the "Cyprus issue".

Note by all the European Union Member States of the OECD and the European Union:

The Republic of Cyprus is recognised by all members of the United Nations with the exception of Turkey. The information in this document relates to the area under the effective control of the Government of the Republic of Cyprus.

Key findings

- Large variations exist between countries. Across the 33 countries included, the model estimates that on average antimicrobial resistance (AMR) causes around 60 000 deaths per year. Of these, around 33 000 occur in the European Union (EU) and European Economic Area (EEA) countries, while 29 500 occur in the United States.
- Between 2015 and 2050, AMR will have caused around 2.4 million deaths in the included countries and 1.3 million in the EU/EEA region. With one million deaths over the 35 year period, the United States will experience the highest number of cumulative AMR deaths for an individual country.
- There are large differences between countries. In relative terms, southern European countries carry the heaviest burden of AMR. The situation of some of those countries is of particular concern. In Italy, for example, between 2015 and 2050, the model estimates that 500 000 people will die due to AMR. Over the same period, the model predicts that around 92 000 AMR deaths will occur in Germany.
- Each year, AMR results in around 1.75 million disability-adjusted life years (DALYs) lost across the modelled countries with 1 million DALYs lost in EU/EEA countries. In absolute terms, the largest countries experience the highest health burden of AMR. The United States comes first with 724 000 DALYs per year, followed by Italy, France, the United Kingdom, Germany and Spain with estimates ranging from 67 000 to 311 000 DALYs.
- Annually, AMR results in over 700 million extra hospital days (EHDs) across all the included countries and 568 million in the EU/EEA area. The country-specific estimates follow a pattern similar to the other outcomes. The highest number occurs in Italy with almost 2 300 EHDs per 100 000 persons due to AMR, followed by Portugal and France with around 1 250 EHDs per 100 000 persons.
- The effects of AMR cost the health systems of the countries included in the analysis around USD purchasing power parity (PPP) 3.5 billion per year. For EU/EEA countries, that estimate amounts to USD PPP 1.5 billion, per year, which means that in less than 10 years, the impact of AMR on health care expenditure has increased by 60%.
- Over the periode 2015-2050, AMR will have cost the health systems of EU/EEA countries a total of USD PPP 60 billion, while in the United States, Canada and Australia, this amount will reach a combined total of approximatly of USD PPP 74 billion.
- Around 439 000 additional postoperative infections and 307 000 post-intervention deaths would occur each year in the EU if no effective antimicrobial treatment was available for the eleven most common surgical and blood cancer chemotherapy interventions in the EU, which require prophylactic antibiotic treatment.
- Across the modelled countries, a scenario of absence of effective antimicrobial treatments would result in approximately 288 000 deaths per year and cost the different health systems a total of USD PPP 16.3 billion, annually. In the EU/EEA area, this scenario would result in 142 000 deaths per year for a cost of USD PPP 6.4 billion.

4.1. Quantifying the burden of AMR

Antimicrobials are an essential instrument in modern medicine. Their diffusion and widespread use in clinical care throughout the second half of the twentieth century markedly decreased the burden of infectious diseases, and lead to the development of many complex medical interventions such as organ transplantations, advanced surgery, chemotherapy and care for premature babies. AMR represents a direct threat to all these advances. Its rise and dissemination, if left unchecked, will inflict considerable damage to population health, and place a heavy burden on economies and society as a whole.

To address such a threat, it is important for policy makers to have accurate estimates of the health and economic burden of AMR, to inform the design of policies and regulations able to mitigate its current and long-term consequences.

The OECD developed a micro-simulations model to produce comparable cross-country estimates of the health and economic impact of AMR, for a comprehensive set of infections susceptible to develop resistance. Individual analyses were performed for 33 OECD and EU member countries. Three main areas were examined:

- the current health burden caused by AMR and its impact on expenditure and hospital cost
- the potential impact of the decreasing effectiveness of prophylactic antimicrobial therapies on common surgical and chemotherapeutic procedures in Europe
- the potential health and economic consequences of the so-called 'post-antibiotic' world, in which virtually no antibiotic would be effective. It should be noted that there is relative consensus that such an extreme scenario is unlikely to materialise (De Kraker, Stewardson and Harbarth, 2016[1]). Modelling its potential consequences is therefore mainly useful from a conceptual and theoretical point of view – in line with previous AMR models – to inform a benchmark for advocacy.

AMR is currently one of the world's leading public health concerns. It is a significant global threat that is particularly complex to apprehend from an analytical and economic perspective (see Box 4.1). Over the last decade, many studies have provided estimates of the potential economic impact of AMR. This chapter provides an overview of current economic studies. Their main findings are described, along with the major knowledge gaps in the current economic literature on AMR. The characteristics and results of the OECD AMR microsimulation model are presented. The results of a second model focusing specifically on the potential health burden of AMR in the context of antimicrobial prophylaxis treatments, and under different scenarios of treatment effectiveness, are presented. The final section of this chapter summarises the main findings and discusses their policy implications.

4.2. What does the current evidence tell us?

Quantifying the health and economic burden of antimicrobial resistance is challenging both because of the paucity of the data and the multi-dimensionality of the issue (Laxminarayan et al., 2016[2]). Many studies have investigated the burden of antimicrobial resistance, using a variety of approaches (Cohen et al., 2010[3]) (Sipahi, 2008[4]) (Tansarli et al., 2013[5]). Two of the first prominent analyses of the effects of AMR have been produced by the United States Centre for Disease Control and

Prevention (CDC, 2013[6]) and by a joint effort of the European Centre for Disease Prevention and Control (ECDC) and the European Medicines Agency (ECDC-EMEA, 2009[7]):

- The ECDC and EMEA estimated the burden of five resistant bacteria[1] in EU countries, Norway and Iceland. The report concludes that in 2007, over 386 000 people developed one of the included resistant infections in the bloodstream, respiratory tract, urinary tract or skin/soft tissue, which resulted in over 25 000 extra deaths and 2.5 million EHDs. The attributable health care costs and productivity losses associated with resistance were estimated at EUR 1.5 billion per year (ECDC-EMEA, 2009[7]).
- In 2013, the CDC concluded that each year, at least 2 million illnesses and 23 000 deaths are caused by AMR infections[2] in the United States. These estimates have a direct cost to the US health system of more than 20 billion dollars per year (CDC, 2013[6])

In the last five years, several other studies have attempted to provide global estimates of the health and economic burden of resistance. In high-income countries, with low prevalence of infectious diseases such as tuberculosis or malaria, healthcare-associated infections are a major concern. Health systems are heavily dependent on antimicrobials for many aspects of secondary health care such as cancer treatment or the prevention of iatrogenic infections during surgery. Studies in this category have therefore predominantly focused on assessing the health and economic burden of AMR from the hospital perspective. Some of the most prominent studies in this category include:

- A large retrospective cohort study estimated that patients with methicillin-resistant *Staphylococcus aureus* (MRSA) and cephalosporin-resistant *Enterobacteriaceae* bloodstream infections are, respectively, 2.4 and 1.8 times more likely to die after admission to hospital and have an excess length of stay in hospitals of 13.3 and 9.3 days compared to non-infected patients. The cost of each infection was estimated, respectively, at EUR 11 000 and 7 300 (Stewardson et al., 2016[8]).
- A study investigating the potential health consequences of increases in antibiotic resistance on the ten most common surgical procedures and immunosuppressing cancer chemotherapies that rely on antibiotic prophylaxis in the United States. The results showed that a 30% reduction in the efficacy of antibiotic prophylaxis for the included procedures would result on average, each year, in 120 000 additional post-treatment infections (ranging from 40 000 for a 10% reduction in efficacy to 280 000 for a 70% reduction in efficacy), and 6 300 infection-related deaths (ranging from 2 100 for a 10% reduction in efficacy, to 15 000 for a 70% reduction). A scenario of 100% reduction in efficacy would result in around 390 000 additional infections and 21 600 additional deaths per year, for the included procedures (Teillant et al., 2015[9]).

Box 4.1. AMR as a negative externality

In economic terms, AMR represents an externality (i.e. an activity causing an effect on third parties) resulting from the use of antimicrobials to treat infections. This means that the effect of antimicrobial use, in terms of selection pressure and subsequent drug resistance, may not initially be felt directly by the patient or the prescribing clinician but will ultimately have an impact on the overall welfare of other patients in the community and have adverse social and economic effects (Coast, Smith and Millar, 1996[10]). Determining the cost of resistance is a complex task due to lack of evidence and good quality data, and high parameter uncertainty related to the complex nature of the problem of resistance. Some of the challenges include the following:

- Cost of externalities are difficult to measure. In the case of antimicrobials neither the immediate consumer, nor the supplier or prescriber, has to bear the full cost of inappropriate usage, i.e. AMR.
- Precise cost estimates should take into account the specificity of each microorganism in terms of single or combined resistance, treatment procedures, and associated costs.
- AMR can undermine the safety of hospitals and that of many medical interventions, whose success relies on the existence of effective antimicrobial prophylaxis treatments. This in turn can push people not to undergo recommended procedures due the higher risk of infection and potential death, which can lead to increased morbidity and health care expenditure (Smith and Coast, 2013[11]).
- The effect of AMR goes beyond public health and has potential detrimental impacts on a number of social and economic sectors (e.g. the labour market, livestock industries, tourism industry). Assessing the economic burden of AMR implies that its associated costs, across various sectors of the economy, should be clearly identified and measured.

A second group of studies focus on the impact of AMR on the broader economy, usually reporting results in terms of impact on gross domestic product (GDP). The two main drivers used in these analyses to assess the impact on GDP are changes in population size and in the supply of labour force that might result from increased levels of AMR. Some of the most prominent studies in this category include:

- A study published by KPMG in 2014, estimated that by 2050, under a 100% resistance scenario, 700 million deaths would occur annually as a direct result of AMR[3], which would inflict a reduction of USD 1.4 trillion on the world economy (KPMG, 2014[12]).
- In a report commissioned in 2014 by the UK Independent Review on Antimicrobial Resistance (O'Neill, 2016[13]). Rand Europe estimated[4] that by 2050, under a 100% resistance scenario, the cumulative loss of people in productive age would range from 11 million to 444 million, which would correspond to a cumulative GDP loss to the global economy between USD 5.8 trillion and USD 49.4 trillion (Jirka et al., 2014[14]).

- Finally, the Word Bank (World Bank, 2016[15]) provided estimates based on two potential scenarios low and high prevalence of AMR. The analysis projects that by 2050, annual global GDP would likely fall by 1.1%, relative to a base-case scenario with no AMR effects; the GDP shortfall would exceed USD 1 trillion annually after 2030. In the high AMR-impact scenario, the world will lose 3.8% of its annual GDP by 2050, with an annual shortfall of USD 3.4 trillion by 2030.

Overall, the findings from most published burden of disease studies and health economic analyses, consistently suggest that AMR is a major and global public health issue and a critical challenge faced by health systems worldwide. These studies are based on a variety of methodologies, accounting systems, diseases included, and often reach very different estimates (see Annex 4.A), which cannot be directly compared. Despite this heterogeneity, however, they systematically highlight the urgent need for policies to contain resistance.

A common limitation of most existing evaluations is their focus on usually small sets of resistant infections and an analytical approach that does not take into account the broader potential effects of AMR on other conditions and the health care system in general. To a large extent, this is due to the complex nature of the problem of resistance. A second issue concerns the fact that most economic studies on AMR – including the one described above – tend to consider the costs and health outcomes due to resistance without comparison. They provide valuable and detailed descriptive information in terms of cost and health consequences of resistance. This kind of descriptive work is very important but does not provide a complete picture of the problem of AMR in terms of either costs or effects (see Chapter 6).

4.3. The OECD Strategic Public Health Planning for AMR (SPHeP-AMR) model

The OECD developed a health economic model to evaluate the burden of AMR and provide estimates of the current and long-term effects on the population health and health system finances of a selected number of OECD and EU/EEA countries (see Box 4.2). The main aim of the SPHeP-AMR model is to address some of the knowledge gaps and limitations of the current health economic literature described above. The model has two complementary objectives:

1. design a base case model to estimate the current health and economic effects of AMR and to calculate the projections of those effects into the future
2. develop a cost-effectiveness model to assess the impact of selected AMR prevention policies by comparing the potential effects of their implementation to the base case scenario.

The rest of this chapter describes the findings and implications of the first objective. The methodology and findings of the second objective are discussed in Chapter 6.

Box 4.2. The OECD Strategic Public Health Planning for AMR (SPHeP-AMR) model

The OECD SPHeP-AMR model is designed as a first order Monte Carlo Markov microsimulation. Based on a dynamic population, it simulates the natural history of AMR and the evolution of its impact on health and economic outcomes between 2015 and 2050 (Figure 4.1). The model includes ten possible and mutually exclusive states. Transition probabilities (derived from current estimates of prevalence and incidence of included pathogens, rates of resistance or non-resistance, mortality and other parameters) allow movement between the health states during yearly cycles. Costs and health outcomes are assigned to each state and transition.

The model projects the population, number of deaths, disability-adjusted life years (DALYs), health expenditure and extra hospital days (EHDs) associated with each pathogen into the future under the following assumptions:

- No co-infections: subjects cannot develop multiple infections at the same time.
- The evolution of AMR incidence was based on estimates from the model described in Chapter 3.
- Transmission from infected to healthy subjects is exogenous to the model and relies on estimates from the model described in Chapter 3.
- Subjects with a history of AMR have the same risk of an AMR infection as those with no previous diagnosis.
- All other resistant infections other that the antibiotic-bacterium combinations included in the model are considered as susceptible.

Individual models were run separately for 33 countries: the 28 members of the European Union (EU28), along with Norway, Iceland, Australia, Canada and the United States, taking into account national characteristics, including functioning of the health care system (e.g. probability of admittance to a hospital, average length of stay, etc.), demography and prevalence of hospital and community infections. All analyses were conducted from the health care system perspective.

Figure 4.1. Structure of the AMR model

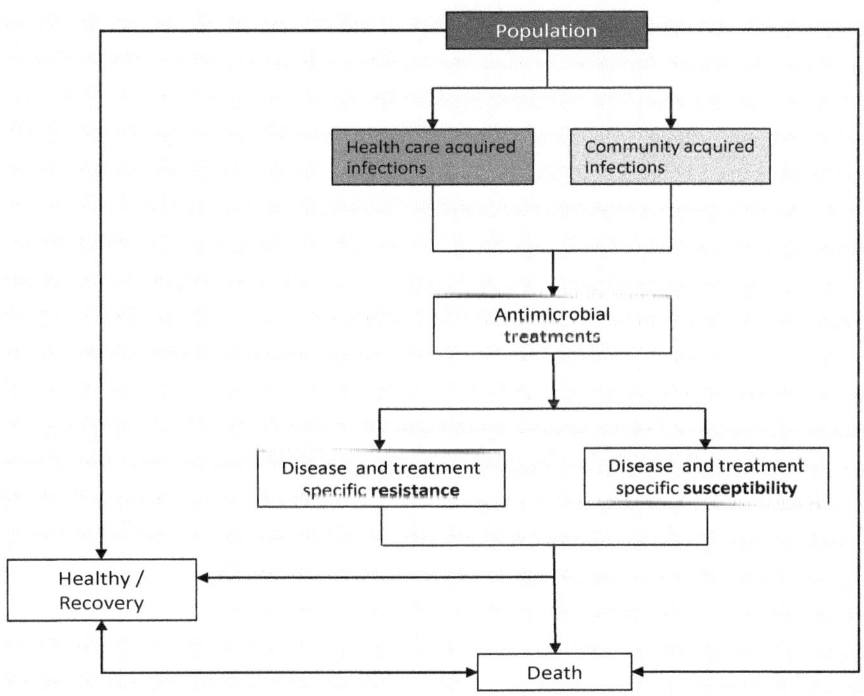

The model accounts for 8 bacteria and a total of 17 antibiotic-bacterium combinations and simulates resistant and susceptible infections occurring in five body sites: bloodstream, respiratory system, urinary tract, surgical site, and other. The selection of the infective agents included in the analysis was based on ECDC experts' advice following three main criteria: i) significance of the burden of disease in OECD countries and the EU, both in the health care sector and the community; ii) policy priority for OECD and EU countries; and iii) data availability. Table 4.1 shows the full list of antibiotic-bacterium combinations included in the microsimulation.

Table 4.1. Pathogens included in the model

Species	Strain-characteristics	Setting	
		Health care	Community
Acinetobacter spp.	*Acinetobacter spp* excluding those with resistance to carbapenem and/or fluoroquinolones and/or colistin	X	
	Acinetobacter spp with resistance to carbapenem	X	
	Acinetobacter spp with resistance to fluoroquinolones	X	
	Acinetobacter spp with resistance to colistin	X	
Streptococcus pneumoniae (*S. p pneumoniae*)	*S. pneumoniae* excluding single penicillin resistance and combined resistance to penicillins and macrolides		X
	penicillin-resistant *S. pneumoniae* (excluding macrolide resistant isolates)		X
	S. pneumoniae with combined penicillin and macrolide resistance		X
Staphylococcus aureus (*S. aureus*)	*S. aureus* excluding MRSA-positive isolates	X	X
	Methicillin-resistant *S. aureus*	X	X
Escherichia coli (*E. coli*)	*E. coli* excluding those with resistance to third-generation cephalosporins and/or carbapenem and/or colistin.	X	X
	E. coli with resistance to third-generation cephalosporins excluding carbapenem and colistin	X	X
Klebsiella pneumoniae (*K. pneumoniae*)	*K. pneumoniae* excluding isolates with resistance to third-generation cephalosporins and/or carbapenems and/or colistin.	X	X
	K. pneumoniae with resistance to third-generation cephalosporins excluding carbapenem and colistin resistance.	X	X

	K. pneumoniae with carbapenem resistance excluding colistin resistance	X
	K. pneumoniae with colistin resistance.	X
Pseudomonas aeruginosa (*P. aeruginosa*)	*P. aeruginosa* excluding carbapenem resistance and/or colistin resistance and/or resistance to three or more of piperacillin ±tazobactam, fluoroquinolone, ceftazidime and aminoglycosides	X
	P. aeruginosa with carbapenem resistance (not resistant to colistin)	X
	P. aeruginosa with multidrug resistance (i.e. three or more of piperacillin ±tazobactam, fluoroquinolone, ceftazidime and aminoglycosides) excluding carbapenem and colistin.	X
	P. aeruginosa with colistin resistance.	X
Enterococcus faecalis (*E. faecalis*) & *Enterococcus faecium* (*E. faecium*)	*E. faecalis* and *E. faecium* excluding vancomycin-resistant isolates	X
	Vancomycin-resistant *E. faecalis* and *E. faecium*	X

Data to model the epidemiology of infections in EU and EEA countries, by 5-year age categories was made available by the ECDC. A detailed description of the methodology used by the ECDC to derive the AMR incidence estimates used in the SPHeP-AMR model for different countries and body sites is provided elsewhere (Cassini et al., 2018[16]).

Estimates of the number of incident cases for Australia, Canada and the United States were provided by the projection model described in Chapter 3. Other input data to model the health impact of infections (e.g. the increased risk of death for resistant infections) and their impact on use of health care services, including case fatality, length of stay associated with the development of an infection were extracted from extensive reviews of the literature conducted by the ECDC (Cassini et al., 2018[16]).

The economic data and approach is largely based on the WHO-CHOICE methodology (WHO, 2003[17]). The hospital costs are calculated as the product of the average cost for a hospital day in a given country (as provided by WHO (Johns, Baltussen and Hutubessy, 2003[18])) multiplied by the average length of stay for each pathogen as found in the literature. The advantages and limitations of this approach have been described elsewhere (Graves et al., 2010[19]). All cost estimates are expressed in 2017 USD PPP.

Health outcomes are expressed in terms of DALYs. These were calculated following the standard WHO approach for cost-effectiveness analysis described in previous OECD publications (Cecchini, Devaux and Sassi, 2015[20]). Disability weights – specific to the pathogens and body sites considered in this study – were provided by the ECDC (Cassini et al., 2018[16]).

The uncertainty around the key model parameters was assessed with a probabilistic sensitivity analysis approach, where all parameters are varied simultaneously, with multiple sets of parameter values being sampled from a priori-defined probability distribution (Briggs, Claxon and Sclulpher, 2006[21]). This approach was also used to derive 95% uncertainty intervals for each model outcome estimate.

4.4. The heavy burden of AMR on population health

4.4.1. Mortality

Figure 4.2 presents the OECD model estimates of mortality due AMR infections for the countries included in the simulation. Large variations exist between countries. Across all 33 countries in the model, the model estimates that on average AMR causes around 60 000 deaths per year. Of these, around 33 000 occur in the EU/EEA counties, while 29 500 occur in the United States. With an average of 18.1 deaths per 100 000 persons due to AMR each year, Italy has the highest mortality rate among the included countries, followed by Greece, Portugal, the United States and France with 14.8, 11.3, 8.9 and 8.6 AMR deaths per 100 000 persons, respectively. For the rest of the countries the estimated rates range from around 7 deaths for Cyprus to 0.3 for Iceland, per 100 000 persons. Figure 4.3 shows the cumulative number of AMR deaths over the 35 years of the simulation. The model estimates that by 2050, AMR will have caused around 2.4 million deaths in the included countries and 1.3 million in the EU/EEA region. The United States will experience the highest number of cumulative AMR deaths for an individual country. Estimates for Europe show large differences between countries. With almost 500 000 AMR deaths over the simulation period Italy is in stark contrast to the rest of Europe, as the estimate for France – the second country with the highest projected cumulative mortality – is around 238 000 deaths.

These estimates are substantially lower than results reported by some of the recently published analyses described above. The RAND model, for example, estimated that by 2050, with an assumption of stable resistance rates, AMR would cause around 2.1 million deaths per year for the working age population in the OECD-EU-EEA region. It is, however, difficult, if not impossible to compare this finding to the OECD model estimates due to major differences in methodology and analytical scope. For example, the RAND model has a strong focus on low and middle-income countries (LMICs) and therefore included AMR in the context of HIV, tuberculosis and malaria, given the high burden of these diseases in LMICs. The OECD model, on the other hand, deals primarily with health-care associated resistant infections, which are the current priority of high-income countries. Other differences can be identifies with the RAND model and all of the studies mentioned earlier. These methodological differences are similarly reflected in model outputs.

Figure 4.2. Average annual number of deaths due to AMR – 2015-2050

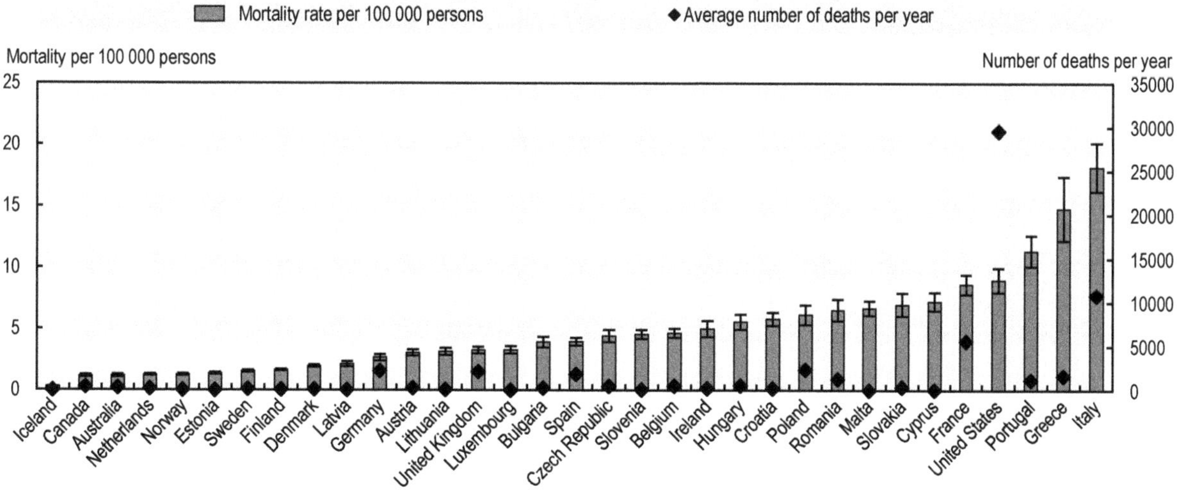

Note: For EU/EEA countries, AMR incidence and fatality parameters used in the model were provided by the ECDC (Cassini et al., 2018[16]).
Source: OECD analysis based on the OECD SPHeP-AMR model.

StatLink http://dx.doi.org/10.1787/888933854858

Figure 4.3. Cumulative number of AMR deaths – 2015-2050

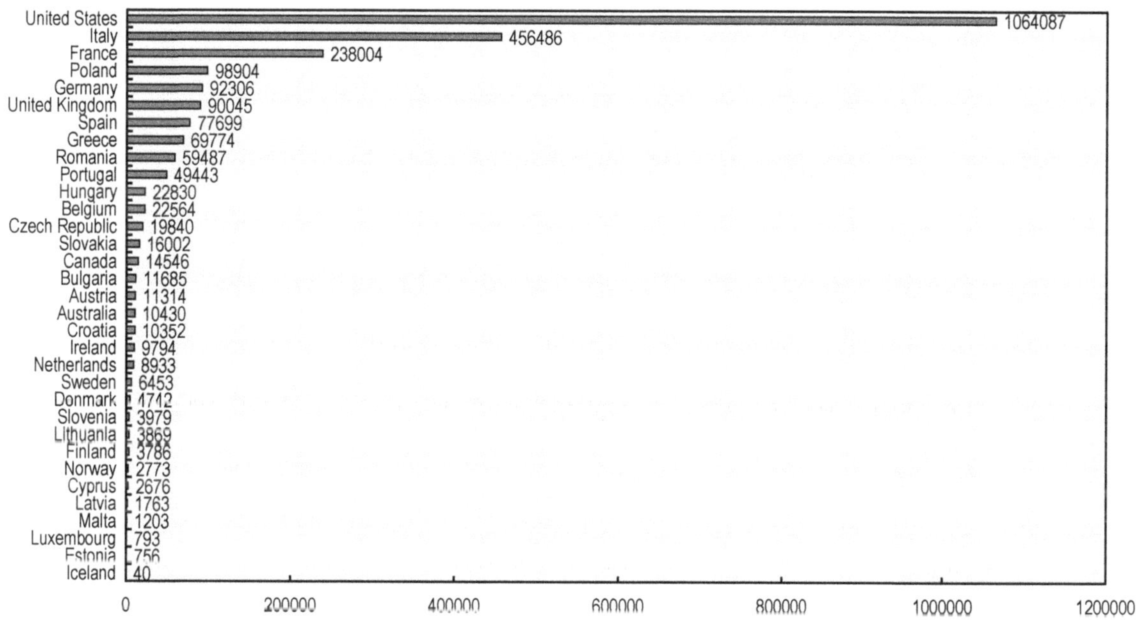

Note: For EU/EEA countries, AMR incidence and fatality parameters used in the model were provided by the ECDC (Cassini et al., 2018[16]).
Source: OECD analysis based on the OECD SPHeP-AMR model.

StatLink http://dx.doi.org/10.1787/888933854877

4.4.2. Disease burden of AMR

In terms of burden of disease, the OECD model estimates that each year AMR results in total of 1.75 million and 1 million DALYs lost across the all the modelled countries and EU/EEA countries, respectively. Generally, southern European countries experience the highest burden. Figure 4.4 shows the average annual number of DALYs per 100 000 persons, attributable to AMR. Italy is the hardest hit with an estimated average of 524 DALYs lost each year due to AMR. Five other southern European countries (with the exception of Romania) follow, namely: Greece, Romania, Portugal, Cyprus and France, with estimates ranging between 221 and 376 DALYs per 100 000. Again, in absolute terms, the largest countries experience the highest health burden of AMR. The United States comes first with 724 000 DALYs per year, followed by Italy, France, the United Kingdom, Germany and Spain with estimates ranging from 67 000 to 311 000 DALYs.

Figure 4.4. Average annual burden of AMR in DALYs – 2015-2050

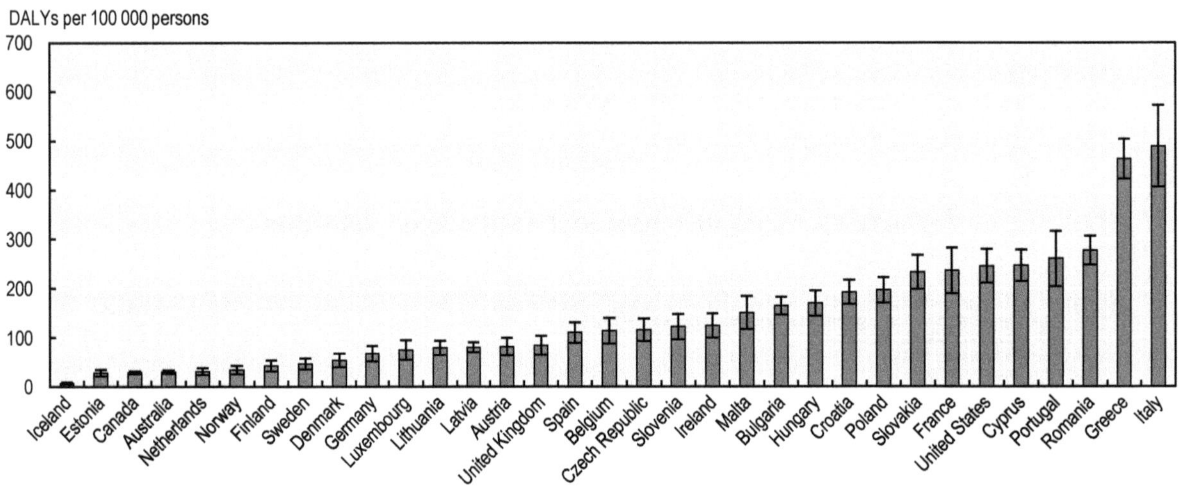

Source: OECD analysis based on the OECD SPHeP-AMR model
Note: For EU/EEA countries, AMR incidence parameters used in the model were provided by the ECDC (Cassini et al., 2018[16]).

StatLink http://dx.doi.org/10.1787/888933854896

4.5. Impact on hospital resources and health care expenditure

The impact of AMR on health system finances is substantial in a tight fiscal environment and a context of high-cost pressure on the health care sector.

4.5.1. Stretched hospital resources

The OECD analysis estimates that, each year, AMR results in over 700 million EHDs across all the included countries and 568 million in the EU/EEA area. The country-specific estimates follow a pattern similar to the other outcomes. The highest number occurs in Italy with almost 2 300 EHDs per 100 000 persons due to AMR, followed by Portugal and France with around 1 250 EHDs per 100 000 persons. Figure 4.5 shows the distribution of EHDs across different age categories in the population. For all countries, over 60% of the EHDs occur in populations aged over 50 years, while a third occurs in children aged 9 years or under. In this age category, more than 90% of the EHDs are experienced by children under the age of 12 months. Teenagers and adults aged between 9 and 50 years, experience 10-15% of EHDs attributable to AMR. This age-group distribution is to be expected given that the risk of acquiring a resistant infection is partly driven by contact with hospital services. This distribution is strongly reflected in the OECD model, as it includes health care acquired rather than community-acquired infections.

Figure 4.5. Average annual number of extra hospital days associated AMR – 2015-2050

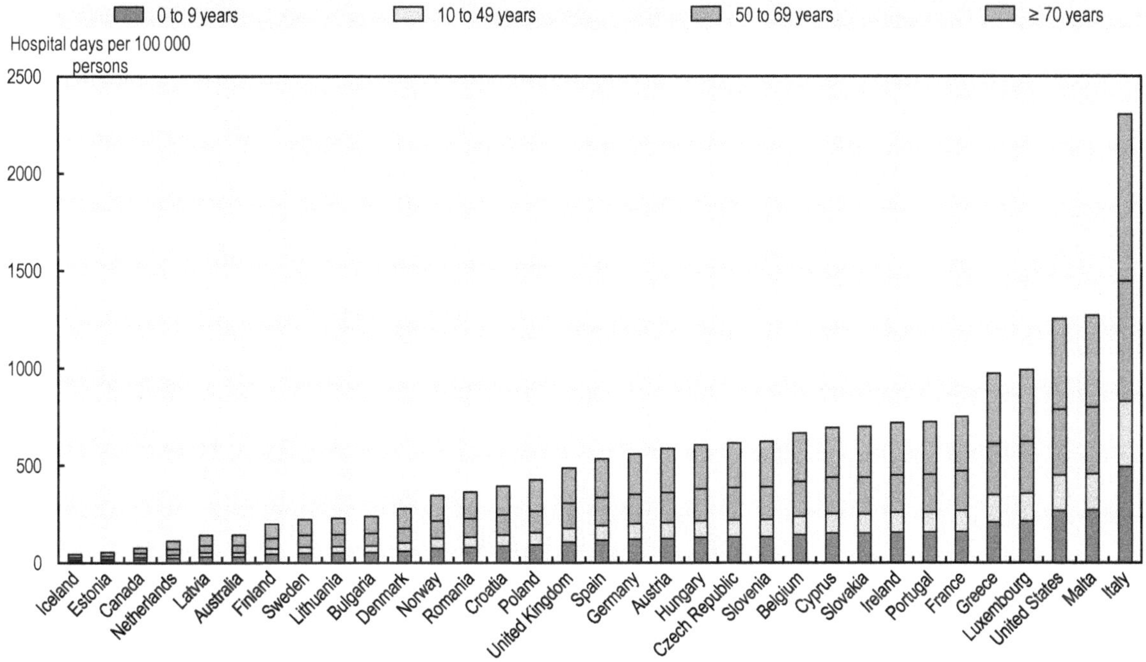

Note: EHD parameters used in the model were provided by the ECDC as well as AMR incidence data for EU/EEA countries (Cassini et al., 2018[16]).

Source: OECD analysis based on the OECD SPHeP-AMR model.

StatLink http://dx.doi.org/10.1787/888933854915

4.5.2. Health care expenditure

The effects of AMR costs the health systems of the countries included in the analysis around USD PPP 3.5 billion per year. In EU/EEA countries that estimate amounts to USD PPP 1.5 billion, per year. Figure 4.5 shows the cost estimates per 100 000 persons for each country. Again, Italy has the highest cost with USD PPP 662 000 per 100 000 persons, followed by Malta and the United States, Luxembourg and Greece with annual cost estimates between USD PPP 559 000 and USD PPP 645 000 per 100 000 persons. In absolute terms, the United States tops the list of the included countries, with annual health expenditure for AMR estimated at around USD PPP 2 billion. Italy and France are second and third with, respectively, USD PPP 393 million and USD PPP 342 million spent each year by the health system as a result of AMR. Far behind these countries come the other large European countries. Germany, the United Kingdom, Spain and Poland spend less than half the amount spent by France with annual estimates for these countries ranging from USD PPP 88 million to USD PPP 157 million per year. Figure 4.6 shows the cumulative cost over the simulation period. The model estimates that by 2050, AMR will have cost the health systems of EU/EEA countries a total of USD PPP 60 billion, while in the United States, Canada and Australia, this amount will reach around USD PPP 74 billion.

These estimates are, overall, consistent with findings from previous studies methodologically close to the OECD model in terms of scope and focus on health care expenditure. For example, the 2009 ECDC analysis of the economic burden of antibiotic resistance (ECDC-EMEA, 2009[7]) estimated, based on 2007 data, that AMR results in EUR 900 million of additional hospital costs per year. A crude comparision of this estimate to the OECD results means that, in less than 10 years, the impact of AMR on the health care budgets of the EU/EEA counties has increased by 60%.

Similarly, for the United States, a recent study, based on the analysis of data from the Medical Expenditure Panel Survey, estimated the total national costs of treating resistant infections at USD 2.2 billion annually, which is in line the OECD model estimate.

Figure 4.6. Annual health care expenditure associated with AMR – 2015-2050

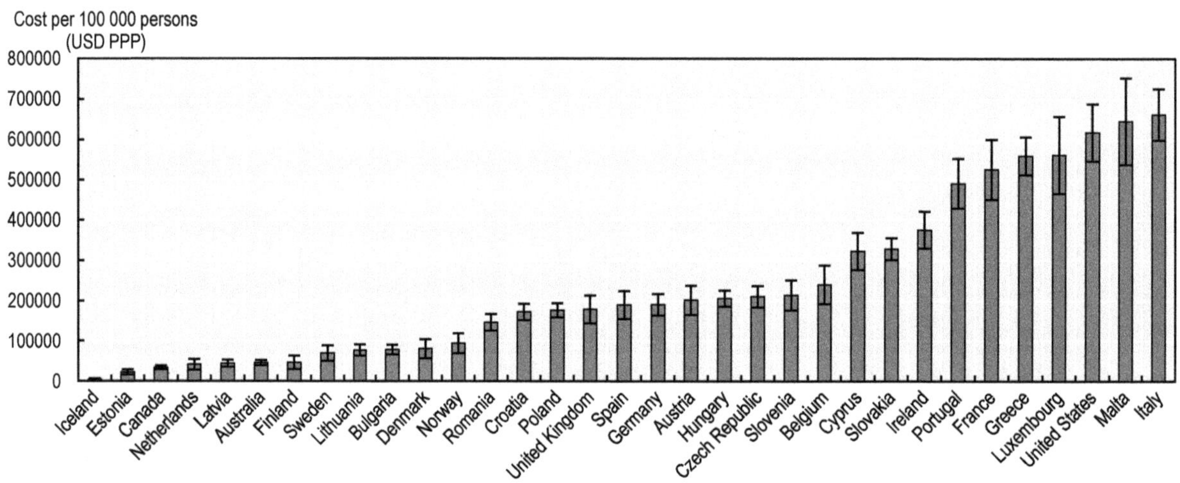

Source: OECD analysis based on the OECD SPHeP-AMR model.

StatLink http://dx.doi.org/10.1787/888933854934

Figure 4.7. Health care expenditure associated with AMR over-time

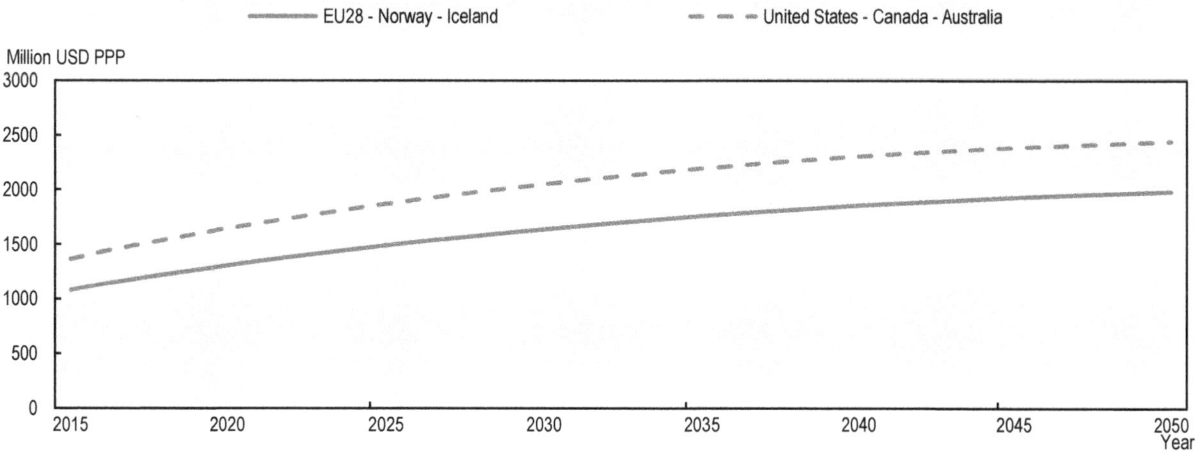

Note: Future impact on health care expenditure is discounted at a 3% rate.
Source: OECD analysis based on the OECD SPHeP-AMR model.

StatLink http://dx.doi.org/10.1787/888933854953

4.6. AMR jeopardises the safety of many medical procedures

One of the key objectives of the OECD evaluation of the impact of AMR, and the full health system approach adopted, is to assess its potential effects on medical interventions and procedures that rely on effective antimicrobials. The rational for this question is based on the hypothesis that the largest health and economic impact of AMR might come from the impossibility of performing many routine medical interventions due to the high risk of infection that would result from the declining efficacy of current antimicrobials (Smith and Coast, 2013[11]).

Currently, surgical site infections (SSIs) already represent an important public health issue. They are the second most common cause of health care-associated infections (HCAIs) accounting for 20% of all HCAIs (ECDC, 2013[22]). They also constitute a considerable burden in terms of mortality, morbidity, and poor quality of life for patients (Pinkney et al., 2013[23]). Annually, around 800 000 SSIs occur in Europe, leading to over 16 000 deaths (Cassini et al., 2016[24]). The treatment costs for a patient with an SSI is on average three times higher than that of a non-infected patient (Edwards et al., 2008[25]). In Europe, this represents a total annual extra cost to health systems estimated between EUR 1.5 billion and EUR 19 billion (Badia et al., 2017[26]) (Leaper et al., 2004[27]). Considerable and ongoing efforts in terms of infection control in hospitals have been put in place in many countries to prevent SSIs (ECDC, 2017[28]). AMR threatens these efforts, and consequently the safety and feasibility of many invasive procedures.

There is almost no empirical assessment of the potential effects of AMR for the treatment of SSIs. The study by Teillant et al. (2015[9]), mentioned earlier, is to date the only available analysis that has attempted to measure the potential "collateral" effects of AMR in terms of SSIs and associated deaths in the United States. Using a similar approach (see Box 4.3) the OECD investigated the effect of AMR on the risk of infection and death associated with surgical procedures and blood cancer chemotherapy - for which antibiotic prophylaxis treatment is recommended – for individual countries of the EU/EEA area.

Box 4.3. Estimating the effects of AMR in the context of prophylaxis

The Eurostat and EUCAN databases were used to identify the ten most common surgical and blood cancer chemotherapies procedures performed in Europe for which antibiotic prophylaxis is recommended by current guidelines. The included procedures are:

- Cataract surgery
- Caesarean section
- Hip replacement
- Appendectomy
- Knee replacement
- Hysterectomy
- Spinal surgery
- Transurethral prostatectomy
- Colorectal surgery
- Cholecystectomy
- Chemotherapy for blood cancers

PubMed was consulted to identify meta-analyses of randomised controlled trials reporting estimates of the absolute risk reduction of infections associated with antibiotic prophylaxis for the included procedures.

4.6.1. AMR threatens the safety of many medical procedures

The OECD analysis shows that the potential adverse impact of AMR on the outcomes of some of the most commonly performed surgical procedures in Europe is severe. The 11 surgeries and blood cancer chemotherapies included in the analysis represent approximately 9.5 million procedures performed annually in the EU/EEA area. Figure 4.8 and Figure 4.9 show the additional number of infections and deaths under the different scenarios of efficacy reduction for the counties included in the analysis.

Across the included countries, between 44 000 and 439 000 additional postoperative infections would occur each year under scenarios of 10% and 100% reduction in the effectiveness of antibiotic prophylaxis. This corresponds, respectively, to increases of 5% and 50% in postoperative infections relative to current estimates (ECDC, 2017[29]). In terms of mortality, under a 10% effectiveness reduction scenario, around 3 000 additional deaths would occur each year in the EU/EEA countries, which represents an 18% increase, compared to 2016 estimates. Under the worst-case scenario of resistance, the total number of deaths in the EU/EEA area would amount to around 30 700 per year. This represents an almost 200% increase in deaths due to postoperative infections when compared to current estimates.

Figure 4.8. Annual number of additional post-intervention infections associated with different scenarios of reduced effectiveness of prophylactic antimicrobial therapy

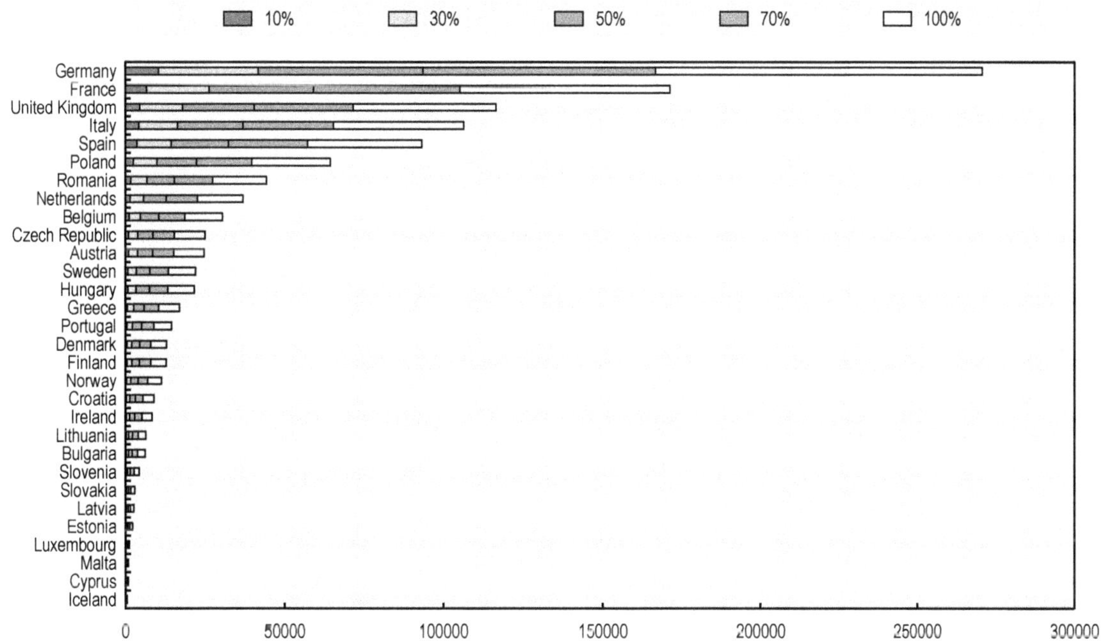

Source: OECD analysis based on cited sources.

StatLink http://dx.doi.org/10.1787/888933854972

Figure 4.9. Annual number of additional post-intervention deaths associated with different scenarios of reduced effectiveness of prophylactic antimicrobial therapy

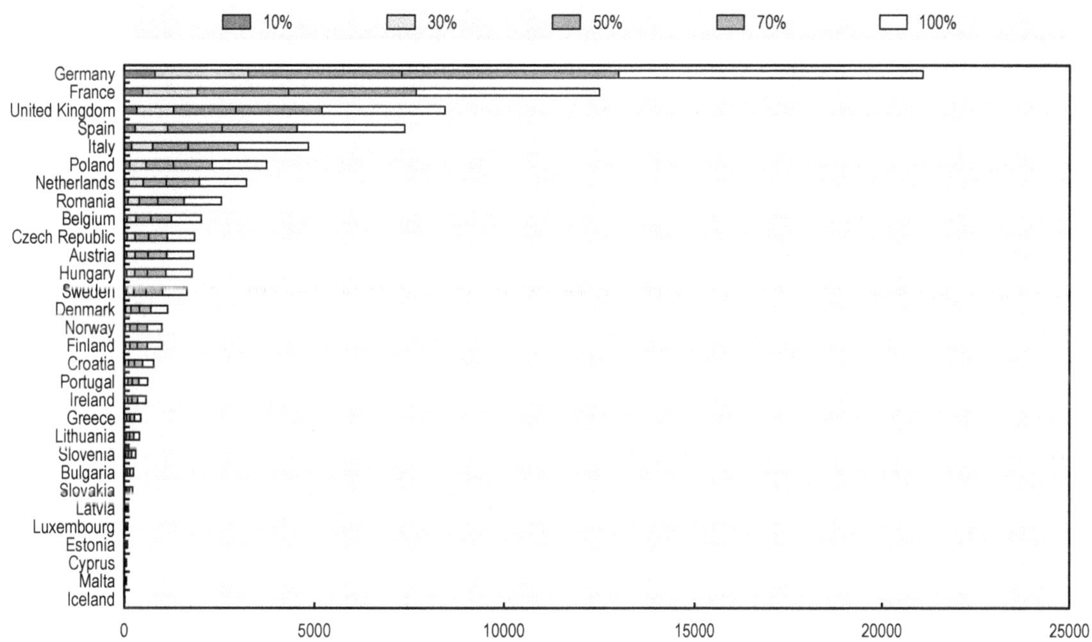

Source: OECD analysis based on cited sources.

StatLink http://dx.doi.org/10.1787/888933855257

4.7. What is the worst-case scenario for AMR?

The OECD model was used to estimate the consequences of a hypothetical worst-case scenario in which no antimicrobial treatment is effective. Figure 4.10 and Figure 4.11 report the effects on mortality and health expenditure, respectively. Across the modelled countries, a scenario of absence of effective antimicrobial treatment would result in approximately 288 000 deaths per year and cost the different health systems a total of USD PPP 16.3 billion. In the EU/EEA area, this scenario would result in 142 000 deaths per year for a cost of USD PPP 6.4 billion.

These results are considerably lower than previous analyses that have modelled the potential effects of a hypothetical worst-case scenario for AMR. The RAND study, for example, evaluated that such a scenario would cause around 8 million deaths per year (relative to a 0% resistance scenario) in the OECD/EU/EEA area. As noted previously, a direct comparison between this figure and the OECD estimates cannot be made due to differences in methodology and scope. A potential explanation of the relatively conservative estimates of the OECD analysis, even under an extreme scenario of absolute resistance, might be the fact that the OECD model is based on a much more granular analytical approach (i.e. microsimulation) than previous studies. In addition, the epidemiological model for EU/EEA countries are based on the most reliable and detailed estimates of AMR incidence currently available. These estimates were provided by the ECDC through the European Antimicrobial Resistance Surveillance Network (EARS-Net), which is the largest and most comprehensive system of AMR surveillance (Cassini et al., 2018[16]). As such, the OECD model is more data driven and its outputs are therefore likely to be more realistic.

It is important to acknowledge that a debate exists around the notion of a worst-case scenario analysis for AMR. While in theory it is possible to imagine a world in which antimicrobials are not effective, critics of previous attempts to model such a scenario point to the lack of empirical evidence and the fragility of the assumptions necessary to perform such analyses (De Kraker, Stewardson and Harbarth, 2016[1]).

The scientific limitations of this kind of scenario analyses are acknowledged. Nonetheless, from a public policy and economic perspective, modelling extreme situations, even if the probability of their realisation is small, provides useful indicators and tolls to stimulate research and debate. The findings can also help raise awareness about a threat such as AMR, encourage its prevention, and potentially inform the design of crisis response strategies.

Figure 4.10. Deaths associated with AMR under a 100% resistance scenario

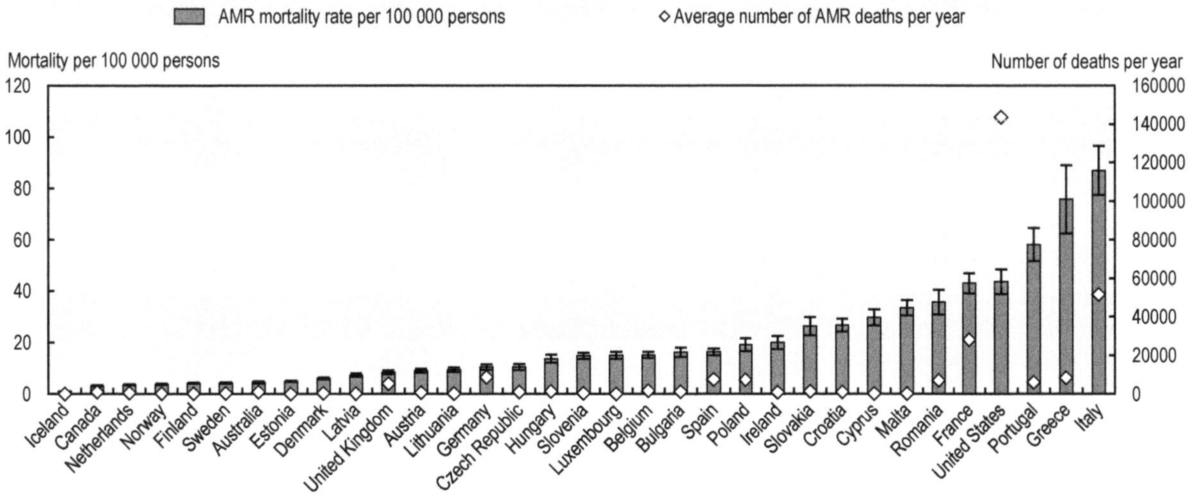

Source: OECD analyses based on the OECD SPHeP-AMR model.

StatLink http://dx.doi.org/10.1787/888933854991

Figure 4.11. Average annual health care expenditure associated with AMR under 100% resistance scenario

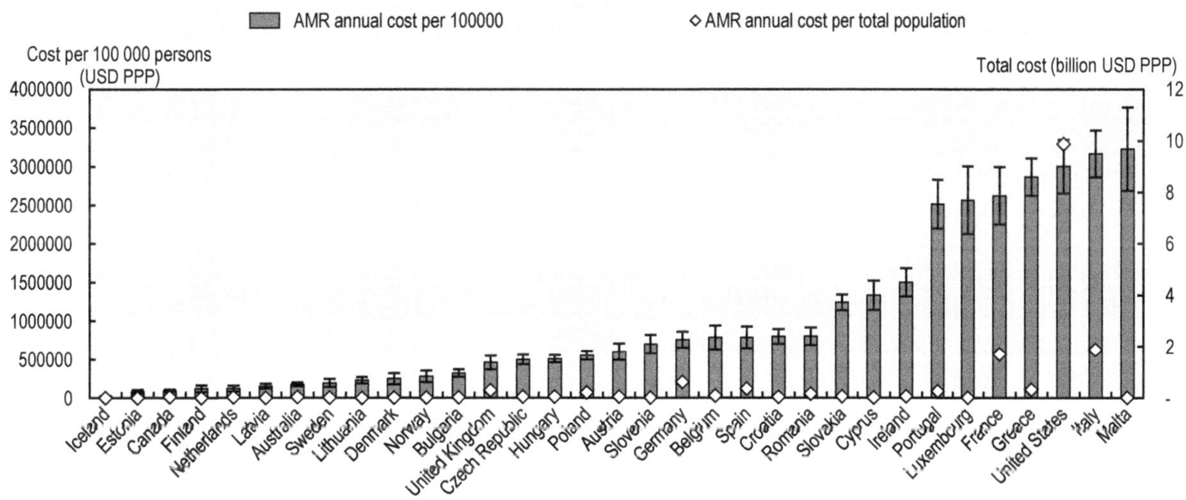

Source: OECD analyses based on the OECD SPHeP-AMR model.

StatLink http://dx.doi.org/10.1787/888933854839

Conclusion: still time to react!

AMR is now widely acknowledged as a global threat and a pressing health issue that requires rapid and coordinated international action. It took the efforts of many researchers, analysts and a variety of stakeholders, over many years, to bring AMR to the global stage and to convince the international community of its relevance and the need to act. The available evidence documents part of the potential impact and unpredictable effects of AMR on many sectors of society. But it also highlights many knowledge gaps, the scarcity of data and the fact that our current understanding of AMR – in terms of aetiology, epidemiology and economics – is relatively limited. By developing the microsimulation model described in this chapter, the OECD's aim is to contribute, from a public policy and economics perspective, to the knowledge-generating work currently underway to better identify and apprehend the challenges of AMR.

The main message that can be derived from the results of the OECD model is that the current health burden of AMR and its cost to health care systems are substantial but still relatively limited. However, the economic impact of AMR on the health care system is set to grow significantly over the next 35 years if no effective action is promptly put in place. There are also large differences between countries, with southern European countries carrying the heaviest burden of AMR. These differences are driven by local characteristics in terms of AMR epidemiology, but also by the existence (or absence thereof) and quality of AMR national action plans. The model estimates are broadly in line with the trends reported by previous studies, even though the specific results for each model output are not directly comparable to most of the existing estimates.

This analysis is conducted from a health care system perspective and evaluates, therefore, the health burden and expenditure directly incurred by health systems as a result of AMR. It is also based on a microsimulation approach, which allows a more refined analysis and is likely to produce more precise estimates of the impact of AMR. The model, however, does not assess the costs of AMR that might occur outside of the health care system (i.e. indirect costs). This differs from the approaches used by most of the recent macro-economic studies, whose results include indirect costs based on the analysis of the potential disturbances to the labour market and productivity in the global economy resulting from AMR.

The OECD model estimates, both in terms of the cost and health burden of AMR, are not necessarily large, particularly in comparison to the impact of other public health issues. For example the estimate of USD 1.5 billion in annual health care expenditure due to AMR in EU/EEA countries is dwarfed by the EUR 51 billion spent each year in the EU on cancer care (Luengo-Fernandez et al., 2013[30]). Treatment of lung cancer alone (around EUR 4.2 billion per year) represents almost three times the health care cost of AMR. In terms of mortality, the 33 000 AMR deaths per year compare to the 30 000 annual deaths due to oesophageal cancer – the sixth most common cause of cancer death in the EU (Ferlay et al., 2015[31]).

These comparisons, however, should not convey any sense of reassurance or diminish the urgency with which AMR should be tackled. The current health and economic burden of AMR is indeed currently lower than that of chronic conditions such as cancer, cardiovascular disease or mental health. Yet, in the long run, AMR represents a much bigger threat due to its complexity and potentially far-reaching and enduring health and economic consequences. The specificity of AMR is that it occurs in the realm of infectious diseases. It is caused by a multitude of different bacteria that can be transmitted, evolve constantly, and are genetically designed to ultimately adapt to treatment. Therefore, its evolution and effects are particularly difficult to characterise epidemiologically, and even more challenging to translate in terms of economic and public health impact.

The danger of AMR for high-performing health systems comes from this complexity and the fact that even high-income countries with low AMR infection rates and strong prevention systems in place, can be severely impacted by the spread of resistant bacteria that have developed in a different part of the world and for which no treatment is available. Another source of danger is the potential of AMR to undermine the safety of many invasive and complex medical procedures – i.e. the very characteristics of an advanced and high-performing health system – as shown by the analysis of AMR in the context of prophylaxis.

The reported results should be interpreted with caution and regarded as conservative. It is also important to bear in mind that the OECD model faces several limitations. For example, despite its wide scope in terms of infections and antibiotic-bacterium combinations covered in the analysis, the model does not include many other resistant infections due to lack of data and time constraints. Several assumptions were made to circumvent the many evidence gaps in the current scientific literature on AMR. For example, the assumption of non-transmission prevents the model from fully taking into account the potential effects of the rise in AMR seen in India or the People's Republic of China, on the modelled countries (see Chapter 3). Although, in the case of transmission, resistant infections dynamics, including transmission, are likely to be taken into account by the model through the ECDC incidence data, which reflect the transmission occurring in the population. Similarly, the potential long-term sequelae of AMR and associated costs were not taken into account in the model due to the limited available evidence.

The relatively contained health and cost impacts of AMR produced by the model are consistent with its focus on high-income countries. They confirm the argument made by previous analyses on the fact that most of the current impact of AMR is taking place in LMICs and set to continue to do so in the foreseeable future. The results likely also reflect the positive effects, in terms of AMR prevention, stemming from the efforts and policies put in place over the last ten years by many governments, health care providers and institutions at local and national levels, to reduce inappropriate use of antimicrobials and control the incidence of health care associated infections.

Overall, the OECD model shows existing efforts and initiatives to combat AMR need to be substantially amplified to reduce its current burden, but most importantly to prevent its future unpredictable and potentially catastrophic consequences. AMR is not a fatality. At this stage, the countries included in the model are in the best position to tackle it, as it still appears as a manageable health issue that can be addressed through the right set of policies and coordinated actions. The following chapters present an overview of the current international AMR policy landscape and provide a detailed assessment of the potential impact of selected AMR prevention policies in terms of effectiveness and cost-effectiveness.

Notes

[1] The bacteria included were: methicillin-resistant *Staphylococcus aureus* (MRSA), vancomycin-resistant *Enterococcus faecium* (VRE), third-generation cephalosporin-resistant *Escherichia coli* (C3EC) and *Klebsiella pneumoniae* (C3KP).

[2] The CDC classified the included resistant bacteria into three categories according to level of concern: i) Urgent: *Clostridium difficile*, carbapenem-resistant *Enterobacteriaceae* and drug-resistant *Neisseria gonorrhoeae*; ii) Serious: multidrug-resistant *Acinetobacter*, drug-resistant *Campylobacter*, fluconazole-resistant *Candida* (a fungus), extended spectrum β-lactamase producing *Enterobacteriaceae*, vancomycin-resistant *Enterococcus*, multidrug-resistant *Pseudomonas aeruginosa*, drug-resistant non-typhoidal *Salmonella*, drug-resistant *Salmonella typhi*, drug-resistant *Shigella*, methicillin-resistant *S. Aureus* (MRSA), drug-resistant *Streptococcus pneumonia*, drug-resistant tuberculosis; iii) Concerning: vancomycin-resistant *Staphylococcus aureus*, erythromycin-resistant Group A *Streptococcus*, clindamycin-resistant Group B *Streptococcus*

[3] The analysis includes: methicillin-resistant *S. Aureus* (MRSA), *Escherichia coli* (*E. Coli*) and *Klebsiella pneumonia* (KP) resistant to third generation cephalosporins, the human immunodeficiency virus (HIV), and tuberculosis (TB).

[4] The model includes: *Escherichia coli, Klebsiella pneumonia, Staphylococcus aureus*, HIV, Tuberculosis and Malaria.

References

Badia, J. et al. (2017), "Impact of surgical site infection on healthcare costs and patient outcomes: a systematic review in six European countries", *Journal of Hospital Infection*, Vol. 96, pp. 1-15, http://dx.doi.org/10.1016/j.jhin.2017.03.004. [26]

Briggs, A., K. Claxon and M. Sclulpher (2006), *Decision Modelling for Health Economic Evaluation*, Oxford University Press, https://global.oup.com/academic/product/decision-modelling-for-health-economic-evaluation-9780198526629?cc=fr&lang=en& (accessed on 07 September 2018). [21]

Cassini, A. et al. (2018), "Attributable deaths and disability-adjusted life-years caused by infections with antibiotic-resistant bacteria in the European Union and the European Economic Area in 2015: a population-level health estimate", *The Lancet Infectious Diseases*, http://dx.doi.org/10.1016/S1473-3099(18)30605-4. [16]

Cassini, A. et al. (2016), "Burden of Six Healthcare-Associated Infections on European Population Health: Estimating Incidence-Based Disability-Adjusted Life Years through a Population Prevalence Based Modelling Study", *PLoS Med*, Vol. 13, pp. 1-16, http://dx.doi.org/10.1371/journal.pmed.1002150. [24]

CDC (2013), *Antibiotic Resistance Threats in the United States, 2013*, U.S. Department of Health and Human Services, Atlanta, https://www.cdc.gov/drugresistance/threat-report-2013/pdf/ar-threats-2013-508.pdf (accessed on 24 July 2018). [6]

Cecchini, M., M. Devaux and F. Sassi (2015), "Assessing the impacts of alcohol policies: A microsimulation approach", *OECD Health Working Papers, No. 80, OECD Publishing,*, https://doi.org/10.1787/5js1qwkvx36d-en. [20]

Coast, J., R. Smith and M. Millar (1996), "Superbugs: should antimicrobial resistance be included as a cost in economic evaluation?", *Health Econ*, Vol. 5/3, pp. 217-226, https://doi.org/10.1002/(SICI)1099-1050(199605)5:3%3C217::AID-HEC200%3E3.0.CO;2-S. [10]

Cohen, B. et al. (2010), "Factors associated with variation in estimates of the cost of resistant infections", *Med Care*, Vol. 48/9, pp. 767-775, http://dx.doi.org/10.1097/MLR.0b013e3181e358b9. [3]

De Kraker, M., A. Stewardson and S. Harbarth (2016), "Will 10 Million People Die a Year due to Antimicrobial Resistance by 2050?", http://dx.doi.org/10.1371/journal.pmed.1002184. [1]

ECDC (2017), *Antimicrobial resistance surveillance in Europe 2015, Annual report of the European Antimicrobial Resistance Surveillance Network (EARS-Net)*, ECDC, https://ecdc.europa.eu/sites/portal/files/media/en/publications/Publications/antimicrobial-resistance-europe-2015.pdf. [29]

ECDC (2017), *Surveillance of surgical site infections and prevention indicators in European hospitals HAI-Net SSI protocol, version 2.2 Surveillance of surgical site infections and prevention indicators in European hospitals*, ECDC, http://dx.doi.org/10.2900/260119. [28]

ECDC (2013), *Systematic review and evidence-based guidance on perioperative antibiotic prophylaxis*. [22]

ECDC-EMEA (2009), *The bacterial challenge: time to react, ECDC/EMEA Joint Technical Report*, ECDC/EMEA, https://ecdc.europa.eu/sites/portal/files/media/en/publications/Publications/0909_TER_The_Bacterial_Challenge_Time_to_React.pdf. [7]

Edwards, C. et al. (2008), "Early infection after hip fracture surgery: risk factors, costs and outcome", *Journal of Bone and Joint Surgery - British Volume*, Vol. 90-B, pp. 770-777, https://doi.org/10.1302/0301-620X.90B6.20194. [25]

Ferlay, J. et al. (2015), "Cancer incidence and mortality worldwide: sources, methods and major patterns in GLOBOCAN 2012", *Int J Cancer*, Vol. 136/5, pp. E359-86, http://dx.doi.org/10.1002/ijc.29210. [31]

Graves, N. et al. (2010), "Estimating the cost of health care-associated infections: mind your p's and q's", *Clin Infect Dis*, Vol. 50/7, pp. 1017-1021, http://dx.doi.org/10.1086/651110. [19]

Jirka, T. et al. (2014), "Estimating the economic costs of antimicrobial resistance: Model and Results", https://www.rand.org/content/dam/rand/pubs/research_reports/RR900/RR911/RAND_RR911.pdf. [14]

Johns, B., R. Baltussen and R. Hutubessy (2003), "Programme costs in the economic evaluation of health interventions", *Cost Eff Resour Alloc*, Vol. 1/1, p. 1, https://www.ncbi.nlm.nih.gov/pubmed/12773220. [18]

KPMG (2014), *The global economic impact of anti-microbial resistance*, http://www.kpmg.co.uk (accessed on 07 September 2018). [12]

Laxminarayan, R. et al. (2016), "Access to effective antimicrobials: a worldwide challenge", *Lancet*, Vol. 387/10014, pp. 168-175, https://doi.org/10.1016/S0140-6736(15)00474-2. [2]

Leaper, D. et al. (2004), "Surgical site infection - a European perspective of incidence and economic burden", *International Wound Journal*, Vol. 1, pp. 247-273, http://dx.doi.org/10.1111/j.1742-4801.2004.00067.x. [27]

Luengo-Fernandez, R. et al. (2013), "Economic burden of cancer across the European Union: a population-based cost analysis", *The Lancet Oncology*, Vol. 14/12, pp. 1165-1174, https://doi.org/10.1016/S1470-2045(13)70442-X. [30]

O'Neill, J. (2016), *Tackling Drug-Resistant Infections Globally: Final Report and Recommendations*, HM Government, London, https://amr-review.org/sites/default/files/160525_Final%20paper_with%20cover.pdf (accessed on 24 July 2018). [13]

Pinkney, T. et al. (2013), "Impact of wound edge protection devices on surgical site infection after laparotomy: multicentre randomised controlled trial (ROSSINI Trial).", *BMJ (Clinical research ed.)*, Vol. 347, p. f4305, http://dx.doi.org/10.1136/bmj.f4305. [23]

Sipahi, O. (2008), "Economics of antibiotic resistance", *Expert Review of Anti-infective Therapy*, Vol. 6/4, pp. 523-539, http://dx.doi.org/10.1586/14787210.6.4.523. [4]

Smith, R. and J. Coast (2013), "The true cost of antimicrobial resistance", *BMJ*, Vol. 346, p. f1493, http://dx.doi.org/10.1136/bmj.f1493. [11]

Stewardson, A. et al. (2016), "The health and economic burden of bloodstream infections caused by antimicrobial-susceptible and non-susceptible Enterobacteriaceae and Staphylococcus aureus in European hospitals, 2010 and 2011: a multicentre retrospective cohort study", *Euro Surveillance*, Vol. 21/33, http://dx.doi.org/10.2807/1560-7917.ES.2016.21.33.30319. [8]

Tansarli, G. et al. (2013), "Impact of antimicrobial multidrug resistance on inpatient care cost: an evaluation of the evidence", *Expert Revue of Anti-infective Therapy*, Vol. 11/3, pp. 321-331, http://dx.doi.org/10.1586/eri.13.4. [5]

Teillant, A. et al. (2015), "Potential burden of antibiotic resistance on surgery and cancer chemotherapy antibiotic prophylaxis in the USA: a literature review and modelling study", *The Lancet*, Vol. 15/12, pp. 1429-1437, https://doi.org/10.1016/S1473-3099(15)00270-4. [9]

WHO (2003), *Making Choices in Health: WHO Guide to Cost-Effectiveness Analysis*, World Health Organization, http://apps.who.int/iris/bitstream/handle/10665/42699/9241546018.pdf?sequence=1. [17]

World Bank (2016), *Drug-Resistant Infections: A Threat to Our Economic Future (Discussion Draft)*, World Bank. [15]

Annex 4.A.

Annex Table 4.A.1. Characteristics of health economic models identified

Reference	ECDC 2009	RIVM 2011	KPMG 2014	RAND 2014	Teillant et al. 2015	Stewardson et al. 2016
Time perspective	2007	2007-2015	2012-2050	2011-2050	2010	2010-2011
Geographical scope	Europe	Europe	World	World	United States	Europe
Infections	MRSA, VRE, C3EC, C3KP, CRPA, PRSP	MRSA, C3EC	MRSA, C3EC, C3KP, HIV, TB, Malaria	MRSA, C3EC, C3KP HIV, TB, Malaria	MRSA, VRE, C3EC, C3KP, CRPA + other resistant bacteria s	3GCRE, 3GCSE, MRSA, MSSA
Infection site	Bloodstream, respiratory tract, urinary tract, skin/soft tissues	Bloodstream	Bloodstream, respiratory tract, urinary tract, skin/soft tissues	Not specified	Surgical site infections for 10 most common surgical procedures in the US	Bloodstream
Approach	prevalence-based attributable fraction	Prevalence-based attributable fraction	Prevalence-based attributable fraction	General equilibrium model	Prevalence-based attributable fraction	Cox regressions, Non-markov multi-stage model & micro-simulation
Scenarios	-	Linear trend / regression-derived	↑ 40% / 100% current resistance rates Doubling of current resistant rates & ↑ 40% / 100% of MRSA, C3EC. Pneumoniae, HIV, TB, Malaria	↑5% / 40% / 100% current resistance rates	↑10% / 30% / 70% / 100% current resistance rates	-
Outcomes	Infections, aLOS	Number of Infections, aLOS and extra deaths	Number of Infections, aLOS and extra deaths	Working age population loss	Number of Infections, aLOS and extra deaths	Number of Infections, aLOS and extra deaths
Cost inpatient/ outpatient	Both costs included	Only inpatient costs	Only inpatient costs	No cost included	No cost included	Only inpatient costs
Production losses	Included	Not included	Included	Included	Not included	Not included

Note: § The hospitals included in the analysis were located in Italy (3), Germany (2), UK (2), France (1), Spain (1), and Switzerland (1). HAIs: health care acquired infections; HIV: human immunodeficiency virus; TB: tuberculosis; MRSA: Methicillin-resistant *Staphylococcus aureus*; MSSA: Methicillin-susceptible *Staphylococcus aureus*; C3EC: *Escherichia coli* with resistance to third- generation cephalosporins; C3KP: *Klebsiella pneumoniae* with resistance to third-generation cephalosporins; PRSP:Penicillin-resistant *Streptococcus pneumonia*; ColRKP: *Klebsiella pneumoniae* with colistin resistance; CRKP: *Klebsiella pneumoniae* with carbapenem resistance ; CRPA: Carbapenem-resistant Pseudomonas *aeruginosa*; 3GCSE: third-generation cephalosporin susceptible *Enterobacteriaceae*, 3GCRE: third-generation cephalosporin-resistant *Enterobacteriaceae*, aLOS: average length of stay.

Chapter 5. Policies to combat antimicrobial resistance

Michele Cecchini, Stella Danek and Jennifer Deberardinis

During the last few years, there has been a growing interest in developing and implementing policies to combat the spread of antimicrobial resistance (AMR). This chapter provides an overview of the current status of OECD, Group of Twenty (G20) and European countries' action plans for tackling AMR and highlights the critical need for extensive international collaboration among all stakeholders. It looks at varied policy options to promote the prudent use of antimicrobials, stop the spread of infections, and prevent infections all together. Actions such as antimicrobial stewardship programmes, improved environmental hygiene, and vaccination use are examined and their effectiveness illustrated in a variety of contexts. The chapter describes some of the implementation decisions and challenges associated with these interventions, and where possible, addresses the degree to which these policies have been adopted globally.

The statistical data for Israel are supplied by and under the responsibility of the relevant Israeli authorities. The use of such data by the OECD is without prejudice to the status of the Golan Heights, East Jerusalem and Israeli settlements in the West Bank under the terms of international law.

Note by Turkey:

The information in this document with reference to "Cyprus" relates to the southern part of the Island. There is no single authority representing both Turkish and Greek Cypriot people on the Island. Turkey recognises the Turkish Republic of Northern Cyprus (TRNC). Until a lasting and equitable solution is found within the context of the United Nations, Turkey shall preserve its position concerning the "Cyprus issue".

Note by all the European Union Member States of the OECD and the European Union:

The Republic of Cyprus is recognised by all members of the United Nations with the exception of Turkey. The information in this document relates to the area under the effective control of the Government of the Republic of Cyprus.

Key findings

- There is widespread international recognition of the need to develop and implement policies to combat the spread of antimicrobial resistance (AMR), and most countries have now established action plans that address antimicrobial resistance in the health sector.
- In designing and implementing national action plans to combat AMR, countries have a broad arsenal of policy options from which to choose: key among them are policies related to promoting prudent use of antimicrobials, improving infection prevention and control, and increasing vaccinations.
- A growing body of evidence supports many of these interventions, especially those that reduce and/or rationalise the use of antimicrobials.
- Although some policies require major investments and involve complex implementation, a number of policies – such as hygiene interventions – can be effectively implemented in resource-constrained settings.
- The need for international coordination and the wide variety of stakeholders involved in AMR reduction renders policy making particularly challenging. In order to be effective, many policies will need to be coordinated among countries and address multiple types of stakeholders.
- Countries that have successfully addressed AMR tend to use a multi-pronged approach, with interventions targeting a variety of stakeholders and with different goals.

5.1. Introduction

There is widespread international recognition of the need to develop and implement policies to combat the spread of AMR. All OECD member countries have approved the World Health Organization's (WHO) 2015 global action plan, whose goal is to ensure the continuity of successful treatment and prevention of infectious diseases with effective and safe medicines that are quality-assured, used in a responsible way, and accessible to all who need them (WHO, 2015[1]). The plan hinges on five strategic objectives:

- improve awareness and understanding of AMR
- strengthen knowledge through surveillance and research
- reduce the incidence of infection
- optimise the use of antimicrobial agents
- develop the economic case for sustainable investment that takes account of the needs of all countries and increase investment in new medicines, diagnostic tools, vaccines and other interventions.

The Sixty-eighth World Health Assembly also urged all member states to develop and put in place, by 2017, national action plans on AMR that are aligned with the objectives of the global plan. The G20 health ministers reiterated this commitment in 2017, highlighting their focus on improving surveillance of AMR, raising awareness, improving infection prevention and control, promoting vaccination, and facilitating the prudent use of antimicrobials (G20, 2017[2]). In addition, the Food and Agriculture Organization of the United Nations (FAO) recently published its action plan on AMR in the food and the agricultural sector, which identified four key pillars: awareness, surveillance and monitoring, governance, and the promotion of good practices (FAO, 2016[3]).

As of 2011, fewer than half of all countries had implemented many of the basic policies needed to ensure appropriate use of antimicrobials, such as regular monitoring of use, regular updating of clinical guidelines, maintaining a medicine information centre for prescribers, and having therapeutics committees in most hospitals or regions (Holloway and van Dijk, 2011[4]). While there has been some progress in developing and implementing global action plans, only half of the 194 WHO Member States reported that they had a national action plan on AMR in place as of 2017 (WHO, FAO and OIE, 2018[5]). Another quarter reported to have such a plan under development. According to the same survey, 84% of OECD, G20, and remaining European Union (EU) countries had developed a national action plan, with the remaining countries undertaking the development of a plan at the time of the survey (Figure 5.1).

In designing and implementing national action plans to combat antimicrobial resistance, countries have a broad arsenal of policy options from which to choose and the opportunity to tailor each of these policies to their unique needs. Fortunately, a growing body of evidence supports many of these interventions, and a number of international success stories can help to guide their design and implementation. This chapter will provide an overview of a broad set of interventions aimed at decreasing AMR, describe some of the implementation decisions and challenges associated with these interventions, and where possible, address the degree to which these policies have been adopted globally.

While the information that follows focuses on policies in the human health sector, it is important to note that these represent just a portion of broader antimicrobial policies that governments are developing. As the agricultural sector accounts for a significant portion of resistance development, agricultural policy is also a critical part of the multi-sectoral one-health approach (Box 5.1).

Figure 5.1. National AMR action plans among OECD, G20, and other EU countries

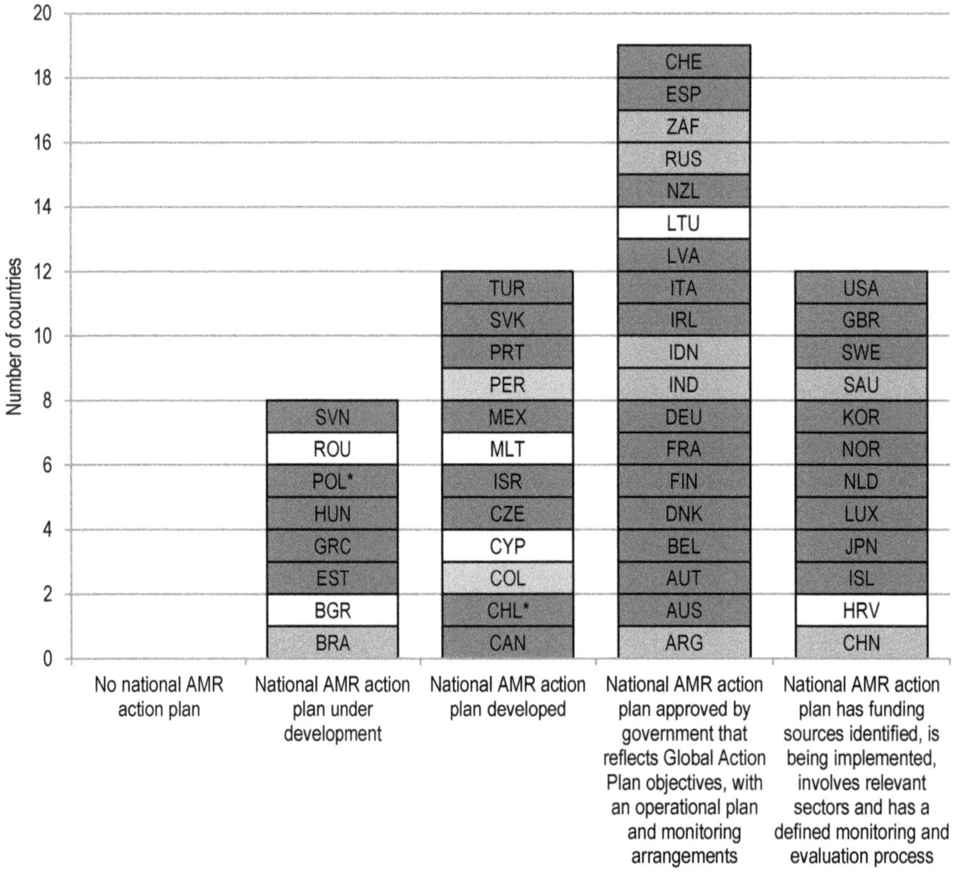

Note: countries in alphabetical order within each category. OECD countries in dark blue; other G20 non-OECD countries in light blue; other EU non-OECD countries in white; other countries partnering with the OECD in grey. Countries with * did not report in 2017 and 2016 data was used instead.
Source: OECD analysis on (WHO, FAO and OIE, 2018[6]).

StatLink http://dx.doi.org/10.1787/888933855010

Box 5.1. One Health approach and agricultural policies

The magnitude of antimicrobials in livestock production underscores the critical role of the agricultural sector in combatting AMR. In the United States, antimicrobial use in food animals has been estimated to account for approximately 80% of antimicrobial consumption in the country and is expected to increase by two-thirds by 2030 (Van Boeckel et al., 2015[7]). This widespread use of antimicrobials in agriculture is a major driver of the emergence and spread of antimicrobial resistant microbes in humans and the environment, and interventions reducing antimicrobial use in animals have been shown to affect resistance development in humans. A meta-analysis of nearly 200 studies evaluating the impact of interventions to reduce antimicrobial use in food-producing animals found not only a difference in resistance among animals but also a 24% lower incidence of resistance in human populations, particularly those with direct animal contact (Tang et al., 2017[8]).

Through the multisectoral One Health approach, WHO, the World Organisation for Animal Health (OIE), and the Food and Agriculture Organization of the United Nations (FAO) are tackling all causes of antimicrobial resistance and addressing its public health implications. Such a holistic view of resistance is critical given that resistant bacteria spread between humans, animals, and the environment, meaning that success in one sector requires success in others. The broad aims of the One Health approach are to (WHO, 2017[9]):

- ensure that antimicrobial agents continue to be effective and useful for curing diseases in humans and animals
- promote prudent and responsible use of antimicrobial agents
- ensure global access to medicines of good quality.

Specific policy measures that have been implemented in the agricultural sector include regulatory measures that limit the use of over-the-counter antimicrobials, wholesale bans of specific antimicrobials and growth promoters, manufacturing requirements and quality control, and surveillance and monitoring of agricultural use (Cogliani, Goossens and Greko, 2011[10]; Goutard, 2017[11]). Because of the use of antimicrobials to prevent and manage disease outbreaks among livestock populations, effective antimicrobial resistance policy within the agricultural sector will also need to involve interventions that improve animal health.

5.2. Effective antimicrobial policy requires global coordination

The ability of microbes and antimicrobial resistance to cross geographical borders presents a unique challenge for policy makers and underscores the importance of international collaboration to curb its spread. Even in the absence of direct collaboration, ensuring impact of many policies requires international harmonisation, such as intellectual property and regulatory policies that universally encourage companies to pursue innovation in vaccines, medicines and diagnostics.

WHO specifically calls for international collaboration to establish networks that can undertake surveillance, develop international inspection teams to monitor drug quality, encourage innovation within the pharmaceutical industry, and support research to contain AMR. Conducting surveillance in particular requires close international collaboration, given that consistent data collection is critical to understand national and international trends (Shah et al., 2017[12]). To that end, European countries have developed the ESAC-Net and the EARS-Net networks while, at the global level, WHO has launched a Global Antimicrobial Resistance Surveillance System (GLASS), which collects and reports resistance rates aggregated at a national level, to standardise surveillance of AMR.

Despite the critical role of international collaboration, national and local strategies need to be tailored to the specific area's culture, existing practices, and antimicrobial resistance profile in order to be most effective. Evaluations of several policy interventions aimed at curbing antimicrobial use suggest that certain policies are more effective in countries with higher or lower antimicrobial use. Across a sample of OECD countries, the frequency of non-prescription antimicrobial use varied between 3% and 44% (Morgan et al., 2011[13]), with countries in Northern and Western Europe, particularly Scandinavia, presenting lower frequency compared to countries in Southern and Eastern Europe as well as Mexico. The appropriateness of different interventions is also shaped by the legal environment of specific countries, such as whether antimicrobials are available over the counter, and typical health care practices, including in which settings antimicrobials are most often prescribed.

Box 5.2. Complex coordination of many stakeholders creates additional challenges for policy makers

Beyond the need for international collaboration, the required coordination of many different types of stakeholders, even at the local and regional levels, makes antimicrobial policy making particularly challenging. AMR is a clear case in which cooperation between national governments and agencies, professional societies, non-governmental organisations, and international agencies is needed to develop and implement successful strategies. Also key to successful implementation are local level stakeholders, such as hospitals, pharmacies, and other care facilities. For example, effective resistance surveillance requires individual physicians to collect cultures, hospitals to build laboratory capacity, and national health authorities to aggregate and disseminate data (DiazGranados, Cardo and McGowan, 2008[14]).

The WHO's global strategy specifically lays out policy recommendations for the general public, physicians, pharmacists, hospitals, national governments and health systems, and pharmaceutical companies (WHO, 2001[15]):

- **Patient** interventions include education about both the appropriate use of antimicrobials and infection transmission prevention, with the aim of aligning expectations with appropriate practice and avoiding self-medication
- **Prescriber and dispenser** interventions include education and training on appropriate antimicrobial use and infection control, prescription management such as auditing and guideline development, and regulatory requirements for professional registration. These strategies aim to combat lack of training and access to information as well as other factors that lead to poor antimicrobial and infection control practices, such as peer pressure, patient pressure, and perverse economic incentives

- **Hospital** interventions include establishing infection control programmes, antimicrobial use committees, and monitoring systems as well as bolstering diagnostic laboratory services. Hospitals are also key in implementing infection control measures (e.g., through cleaning practices) and promoting prudent antimicrobial use through audit feedback, formularies, and guidelines
- **National governments and health system** interventions may include creating task forces, allocating appropriate resources, establishing dispensation regulations, marketing authorisation and manufacturing, and safety/quality standards. Governments may also be responsible for developing guidelines for appropriate treatment practices, national drug lists, and immunisation as well as conducting national education programmes and maintaining surveillance systems

Studies have shown that those policy interventions that are most effective at addressing AMR tend to target multiple stakeholders simultaneously. For example, campaigns raising awareness about resistance seem to be more effective when they address both the general public and health care professionals, including physicians and nurses, than when focused on only one group (McNulty et al., 2010[16]). Despite historically focusing on physicians, many interventions are increasingly recognising the importance of other health care professionals (WHO-Europe, 2014[17]). In particular, pharmacists play a critical role as the interface between physicians and patients, with the potential to dramatically influence their behaviour by creating greater patient awareness on the importance of appropriate antimicrobial consumption while simultaneously guiding physician decision making. Achieving the buy-in of a wide variety of health care workers will be critical to implementing policies promoting better hygiene in the health care sector.

5.3. Strategies to reduce antimicrobial resistance address varied goals

Policies aimed at addressing AMR can be broadly categorised based on the goal of the intervention. The three major goals of policies concern avoiding the development of resistant infections (largely through controlling the use of antimicrobials), stopping the spread of resistant infections (typically involving improved hygiene practices), and promoting vaccination.

Other key differences among antimicrobial policies are whether such interventions are prescriptive (restrictive methods/requirements) or persuasive (suggestive). Prescriptive policies require or prevent a behaviour, such as hospital prescription controls that limit antimicrobial prescribing to particular specialists or patients (Pulcini, 2015[18]). Persuasive policies, on the other hand, tend to involve education, advice, and feedback in an attempt to change behaviour but not mandate it. A Cochrane review of over 50 studies assessing the impact of various interventions showed that restrictive methods tend to have a larger impact on reducing antimicrobial resistance than persuasive methods. However, this differential effect appeared to be short-lived; there were no significant differences at 12 or 24 months between restrictive and persuasive policies in terms of prescribing outcomes (Davey et al., 2013[19]).

In this chapter, we will characterise policies based on their goal: reducing the development of AMR, preventing its spread, and promoting immunisation, given that a comprehensive approach to antimicrobial policy involves all three types of interventions. The policies described herein were selected based on several key criteria involving their scope, goal, and current deployment. Selected policies that concern the human sector, rather than agricultural or environmental sectors, are consistent with the WHO Global Action Plan objectives of improving awareness and understanding of AMR, reducing incidence of infection, and optimising the use of antimicrobial products. To the extent possible, we focused on interventions whose effectiveness at reducing resistance has been evaluated in multiple studies.

5.4. Policies may target specific stakeholders, care settings, and microbes

Given the widespread potential for pathogen transmission and the development of resistance, policies targeting antimicrobial resistance are often broad in scope, rather than focused on particular sub-groups. However, accounting for the scale of the problem and limited resources, it may be effective to employ more targeted polices. Policies can be tailored to specific health care stakeholders, health care setting, and microbial targets.

Policies targeting specific stakeholders are most common. Policies may target specific patient populations at higher risk for developing microbial resistance, including pregnant women, children, people with chronic illnesses, and the elderly. Emigrants and travellers hospitalised in another country also tend to have high rates of antimicrobial resistance (Van der Bij and Pitout, 2012[20]). The most obvious target involves health care workers, who have the greatest exposure to microbes and may transmit resistant bacteria from patient to patient.

Polices may also target specific settings of care (e.g., community care vs. hospitals), where there is often significant disparity in terms of the severity of antimicrobial resistance and likelihood of pathogen transmission. Many interventions are targeted to the primary care setting, where antimicrobial prescribing tends to be the highest, accounting for about three-quarters of all human prescriptions globally, but where up to half of respiratory infections cannot be effectively treated with antimicrobials (Scott and Del Mar, 2017[21]). In addition, infections presenting in this setting tend to be self-limiting and less severe, which makes the setting particularly amenable to policies limiting antimicrobials or delaying the prescription of antimicrobials. Certain interventions may also work better in certain hospital settings than others, such as the intensive care unit vs. medical wards, based on the patient profiles, prescribing behaviour and nature of interactions that could potentially spread bacteria, among other differences.

Finally, specific microbial targets, such as those that are most susceptible to developing resistance and cause the most severe infections, may serve as policy targets. For example, overuse of several antimicrobials has been associated with increased risk of methicillin-resistant *Staphylococcus aureus* (MRSA) infections (Kinoshita et al., 2017[22]). Because of its high prevalence in both hospital and community settings, some policies have targeted MRSA specifically; the United Kingdom established an MRSA screening policy in 2010, mandating all patients in all health care facilities to be screened for MRSA when first admitted (Otter et al., 2013[23]). France, Germany, Belgium, and Italy have also implemented surveillance policies and national guidelines specifically targeted at MRSA infections (Kinoshita et al., 2017[22]).

Box 5.3. Policy design: Moving from an understanding of what to why

Traditionally, evaluations of policies have involved determining the impact of those policies on processes, outputs, and outcomes, such as prescribing, administration, patient outcomes, and resistance development. However, researchers have increasingly criticised these evaluations for failing to address *why* specific interventions are successful, thereby informing future policy development and implementation.

Increasingly, researchers are focusing on determinants of behaviours that influence the development of AMR in order to inform effective policy design. Behavioural science may also be used to explain large differences in the impact of similar policies implemented in different settings, such as the fact that effect of dissemination of educational materials has varied between 3.1% and 50.1% improvement (Hulscher and Prins, 2017[24]). Other prescribing interventions such as audit and feedback, educational outreach, specialist approval, and others have seen similar disparities in effect size.

A recent study demonstrated the time-dependent nature of antimicrobial prescribing, as physicians tend to prescribe more antimicrobials as they fatigue later in the day (Linder et al., 2014[25]). Another study found that physicians' senior colleagues tend to wield significant influence over their antimicrobial prescribing (Charani et al., 2011[26]). By identifying the types of interventions most likely to influence physician prescribing, these types of insights can help to guide the development of stewardship programmes, such as those involving engagement with senior colleagues who can influence more junior physicians and teams that oversee physician prescribing.

5.5. Specific interventions in toolkit: Prevent or reduce emergence of resistance

5.5.1. Stewardship programmes

Among the most widely deployed types of interventions, stewardship programmes involve the simultaneous implementation of regulations, guidelines, monitoring, and education and campaigns around the prescribing of antimicrobials, optimising the selection, dose, and duration. As such, these programmes help to determine whether a patient should be prescribed an antimicrobial, which antimicrobial should be prescribed, and for how long it should be taken. The Infectious Disease Society of America and Society for Healthcare Epidemiology of America describe the complexity of these types of interventions as "a multidisciplinary approach by a team consisting of infectious disease clinicians, pharmacists, microbiologists, hospital epidemiologists, and infection preventionists" (Goff et al., 2016[27]). Stewardship programmes can be either persuasive or prescriptive and often involve both types of interventions.

Stewardship programmes have been shown to be widely effective as a means to reduce antimicrobial prescribing and resistance, particularly when implemented together with infection control measures such as hand-hygiene interventions (Baur et al., 2017[28]). However, their impact tends to differ among clinical settings and existing prescribing landscapes. A large body of evidence supports the effectiveness of stewardship programmes in both hospital and community care settings. A Cochrane review showed that implementation of a stewardship programme in a hospital setting decreases both antimicrobial prescription rates (median change up to -40%) and AMR prevalence rates (median change between -24% to -68%, depending on the type of infective bacteria)

(Davey et al., 2013[19]). Specifically evaluating the inpatient setting, a more recent meta-analysis of stewardship programmes yielded similar results, showing that these programmes reduced the incidence of infections and colonisation with multidrug-resistant Gram-negative bacteria, extended-spectrum β-lactamase-producing Gram-negative bacteria, and methicillin-resistant *Staphylococcus aureus (S. aureus)*, and *Clostridium difficile* (*C. difficile*) infections by approx. 30-50% (Baur et al., 2017[28]).

The effects of stewardship programmes tend to be less dramatic in both areas and specific hospital settings that already have lower rates of antimicrobial prescribing. For example, programmes involving audit and feedback report insignificant effects in Scandinavian countries, where use of antimicrobials tends to be low (Ellegård, Dietrichson and Anell, 2017[29]). Another study showed a much higher effect in the critical care setting — deemed the "epicentre of resistance development"—than in medical wards (Brusselaers, Vogelaers and Blot, 2011[30]). However, there is limited evidence on effectiveness in long-term care settings, where inappropriate microbial prescribing can be particularly high (up to 50% of residents colonised with resistant organisms) (Morrill et al., 2016[31]).

While there is limited evidence on the impact of stewardship programmes at different types of hospitals, certain hospitals tend to more readily adopt antimicrobial stewardship programmes than others. In the United States, over half of hospitals with more than 50 beds were compliant with the Centre for Disease Control's (CDC) Hospital Antibiotic Stewardship Program, while only 26% of hospitals with 25 beds or less were compliant (Nebraska Medicine, 2017[32]). These findings suggest that successful antimicrobial stewardship policies may need to provide additional support, such as financial and educational support to particular types of institutions.

Despite significant evidence on the effectiveness of stewardship programmes in general, there is limited evidence on the specific types of interventions within such programmes that are most effective. Programmes evaluated have included pre-approval strategies for antimicrobials, audit and feedback, guidelines and formulary restrictions, and educational components—often employed simultaneously, making it challenging to assess the effect of particular interventions. However, there is some evidence that antimicrobial stewardship programmes in the hospital setting were more effective when implemented with infection control measures, particularly hand hygiene initiatives (Baur et al., 2017[28]).

While there is not a universal set of initiatives included as part of a stewardship programme, the CDC has outlined several core elements of stewardship programmes (CDC, 2017[33]):

- **Leadership Commitment:** Dedicating necessary human, financial and information technology resources
- **Accountability:** Appointing a single leader responsible for programme outcomes. Experience with successful programmes shows that a physician leader is effective
- **Drug Expertise:** Appointing a single pharmacist leader responsible for working to improve antimicrobial use
- **Action:** Implementing at least one recommended action, such as systemic evaluation of ongoing treatment need after a set period of initial treatment (i.e. "antimicrobial time out" after 48 hours)
- **Tracking:** Monitoring antimicrobial prescribing and resistance patterns

- **Reporting:** Regular reporting information on antimicrobial use and resistance to doctors, nurses and relevant staff
- **Education:** Educating clinicians about resistance and optimal prescribing.

Many countries have been successful in implementing stewardship programmes at both national and sub-national levels (Huttner, Harbarth and Nathwani, 2014[34]). Over 92% of OECD, G20, and other European countries had at least some national policy and/or regulations related to antimicrobial stewardship as of 2017 (Figure 5.2). While many stewardship programmes require significant financial investments, they have also been successful in resource-limited settings. A group of private hospitals in South Africa reported a 20% drop in antimicrobial consumption through implementation of a pharmacist-driven, prospective audit and feedback strategy for antimicrobial stewardship (Brink et al., 2016[35]). A review of 27 studies carried out in low and middle-income countries suggests that stewardship interventions have a positive effect on antimicrobial resistance reduction (Van Dijck, Vliegheb and Coxc, 2018[36]). However, successful implementation of interventions in these countries — as opposed to higher income countries — will need to take into account high levels of heterogeneity among health care centres in terms of resources, organisation, and prescribing practices (e.g., differences between urban and rural areas). It is also critical to identify easily measurable elements that can be used to track outcomes (e.g., infection with particular organisms), which may be different from those in countries with more substantial resources.

Given the highly variable nature of the interventions included in stewardship programmes, it is challenging to evaluate their economics. However, several studies have demonstrated significant cost savings associated with these programmes, both in terms of direct, antimicrobial costs themselves, and indirect costs, such as length of hospital stay and additional care required. Implementation of stewardship programmes was associated with a significant drop in antimicrobial costs by over a third, without including other potential decreases in health care expenditure such as reduced side effects and hospital length of stay (Karanika et al., 2016[37]).

Figure 5.2. Stewardship programmes among OECD, G20, and other EU countries

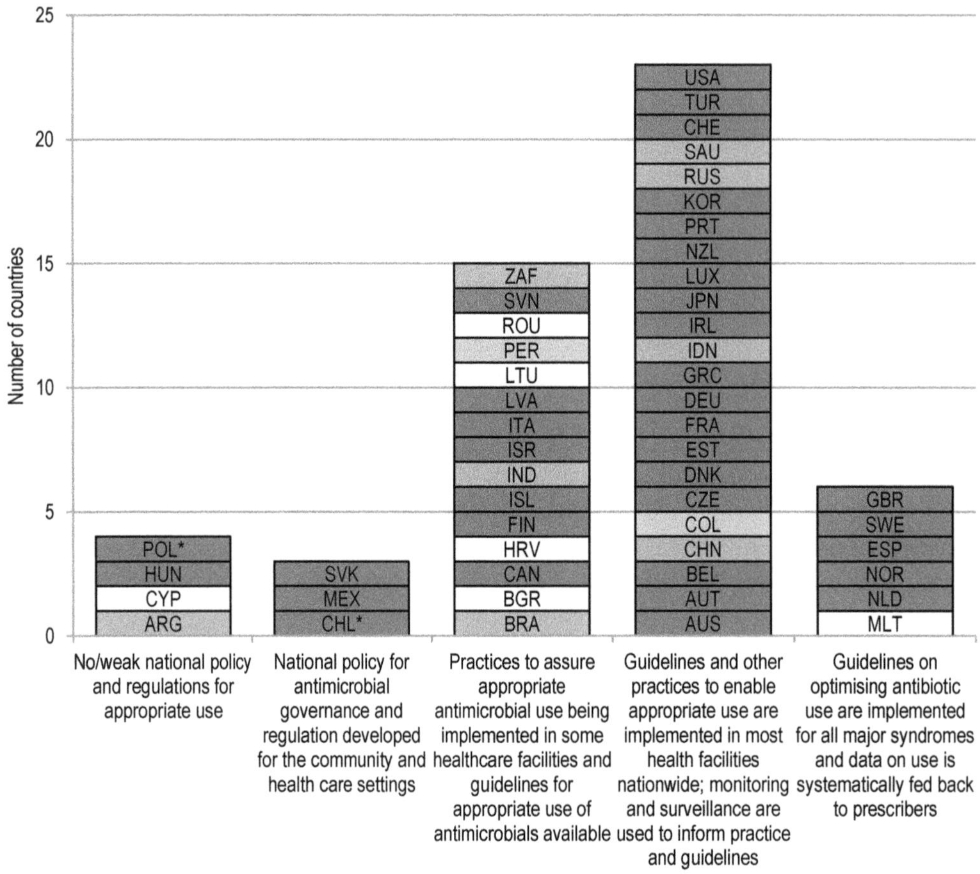

Note: countries in alphabetical order within each category. OECD countries in dark blue; other G20 non-OECD countries in light blue; other EU non-OECD countries in white; other countries partnering with the OECD in grey. Countries with * did not report in 2017 and 2016 data was used instead.
Source: OECD analysis on (WHO, FAO and OIE, 2018[6]).

StatLink http://dx.doi.org/10.1787/888933855029

Box 5.4. National stewardship programme in China

With the ability to purchase antimicrobials over the counter, high reliance on antimicrobials for treatment by both patients and physicians, and financial incentives associated with drug sales, China faces a relatively high prevalence of antimicrobial resistance compared with other countries (Xiao et al., 2013[38]). Over a 10-year period, Chinese health administration authorities established a suite of largely persuasive interventions, including issuing guidance on rational antimicrobial use, creating a national surveillance system, requiring hospitals to establish drug and therapeutics committees, creating continuing education programmes, and emphasising hand hygiene and cleaning measures. However, these policies did not appear to affect the resistance rate, largely due to poor implementation and insufficient enforcement (Xiao et al., 2013[38]).

In 2011, the Chinese Ministry of Health initiated a new strategy: a stewardship programme featuring mandatory management strategies with targets, taskforce organisation, and audit and inspection systems. The strategy required hospitals to have antimicrobial administrative groups, strict formulary restrictions, and prescribing rights given to different physicians. The strategy employed specific targets, including antimicrobials serving as less than specific portions of all drugs prescribed (60% for hospitalised patients and 20% for outpatients) and reducing prophylactic antimicrobial use and duration, among others. These targets would be linked to evaluations of hospitals and "allocation of medical resources". Hospitals that failed to meet targets would be downgraded to lower classifications by the Chinese Ministry of Health.

While these policies seemed to have early success, longer-term studies have shown a continuation of the increase in antimicrobial resistance. A 2013 study using IMS Research data found the percentage of drug sales for antimicrobials decreased from 25% in 2011 to 17% in 2012, corresponding to a reduction in the volume of antimicrobials sold (Xiao et al., 2013[38]). However, a study of 468 tertiary hospitals found that total antimicrobial consumption increased by 26% between 2011 and 2015, despite some success in isolated areas such as Shanghai, whose antimicrobial consumption decreased by 25% (Wushouer et al., 2017[39]).

These mixed results highlight the importance of multi-faceted policies that target a variety of factors influencing the use of antimicrobials. The stewardship programme did not address significant economic incentives for physicians to prescribe drugs that exist in China (mark-up policies) or patient education to reduce prescribing pressure on physicians (Wang et al., 2016[40]). Prescriptive policies aimed at physicians also need to be complimented by thorough educational programmes as part of formal and informal training (Xiao et al., 2013[38]).

Box 5.5. Regional antimicrobial stewardship programmes in Canada

Two western Canadian provinces, Alberta and British Columbia (BC), implemented regional education-based antimicrobial stewardship programmes ("Do Bugs Need Drugs?") in 2005 with the aim of promoting both improved hygiene and more prudent use of antimicrobials. Through a variety of programme components including multimedia tools, classroom materials, and social media, the effort focused on the importance of hand washing, the need to limit antimicrobial use, and the inability of antimicrobials to work against viruses (Carson and Patrick, 2015[41]). The programme targeted both clinicians (physicians, nurses, pharmacists) and the public (children, parents, teachers, employers, long-term care facilities).

As an example of key partnerships, the programme forms part of primary school Grade 2 curricula, delivered by medical and nursing students. By aligning the interests to both train future health care workers and educate young children about disease prevention and prudent antimicrobial use, the partnership contributes to the relatively low cost of the overall campaign (Carson and Patrick, 2015[41]).

A 2011 assessment of the programme confirmed significant improvement in health care professionals' clinical knowledge of appropriate treatment against upper respiratory tract infections (McKay et al., 2011[42]). Overall consumption of antimicrobials in BC, including fluoroquinolones and macrolides, decreased by 7.5% between programme implementation and 2013, with an even larger decrease in children aged under 14 (25%). In addition, the proportion of overall inappropriate use of antimicrobials in the treatment of respiratory tract infections, except acute bronchitis, also declined (BCCDC, 2014[43]).

Importantly, antimicrobial resistance against various clinically important antimicrobials declined or at least remained stable in a majority of pathogens after 2005. For example, resistance of MRSA to erythromycin declined from approximately 95% in 2007 to 82% in 2013 in BC (BCCDC, 2014[43]).

5.5.2. Delayed prescribing

The majority of respiratory infections are viral and self-limiting, meaning that symptoms are likely to resolve without any prescription treatment (Peters et al., 2011[44]). However, antimicrobials are often prescribed for these conditions, which account for much of the 30% of antimicrobials that are estimated to be prescribed inappropriately (Fleming-Dutra et al., 2016[45]). Delayed prescribing involves asking patients to wait up to 3 days or the worsening of their health status before filling a prescription for antimicrobials, with the aim of reducing antimicrobial use in those cases that will resolve themselves. Unlike not prescribing at all, delayed prescribing offers a perceived "safety net" for those few patients who may develop complications and is more amenable for patients than receiving no prescription at all. Delayed prescribing is mostly used in the community care (rather than hospital) setting, where patients' infections are likely to be less severe.

There is substantial evidence that delayed prescribing reduces antimicrobial prescription rates. A Cochrane review of patients with respiratory infections, including sore throat, middle ear infection, cough (bronchitis), and the common cold found that antimicrobial use was greatest in a group prescribed antimicrobials immediately (93%), followed by delayed antimicrobials (31%), and no antimicrobials (14%) (Spurling et al., 2017[46]). Studies have also consistently demonstrated that delayed prescribing is not associated with any negative impact on patient safety, including symptoms like fever, pain, feeling unwell, cough and runny nose (Little et al., 2017[47]). In addition, primary care practices that prescribe fewer antimicrobials for self-limiting respiratory tract infections encounter only a slightly higher incidence of a variety of infections. A study in the United Kingdom concluded that if an average-size general practice reduced the proportion of respiratory tract consultations with antibiotics prescribed by 10%, it would face only one additional case of pneumonia a year (Gulliford et al., 2016[48]).

Delayed prescribing can be implemented in a number of ways:

- with a post-dated prescription, the patient may obtain an antimicrobial treatment only at a later point in time, by the date indicated within the prescription
- re-contact a patient after an initial clinical visit for re-assessment or to instruct the patient to retrieve the prescription at a later appointment
- verbally instruct the patient to delay filling the prescription.

Physicians can also choose not to provide a prescription at the time of the initial consultation but wait for the patient to return if case symptoms do not resolve (Ryves et al., 2016[49]). While data comparing the effectiveness of these methods are limited, a clinical trial showed no differences in terms of severity or duration of symptoms, antimicrobial prescribing and patient satisfaction between different means of implementation (Little et al., 2014[50]).

Delayed prescribing may be implemented at the local, national, or international levels. In the United Kingdom, the National Institute for Health and Clinical Excellence (NICE) guidelines recommend delayed prescribing for patients with a number of conditions (NICE, 2008[51]). NICE guidelines also require physicians to provide patients with advice about the nature of their conditions (e.g. timing of symptom resolution). Like other interventions that target physician prescribing behaviour, delayed prescribing interventions may benefit from audit and feedback components, wherein prescribing is monitored and communicated back to physicians. Studies have shown that audit and feedback can help to improve physician adherence to prescribing guidelines (Høgli et al., 2016[52]) and may help to assuage physician concerns that less antimicrobial prescribing is associated with poorer patient outcomes. Physicians may also require guidance on addressing patient concerns and answering questions without prescribing antimicrobials in order to maintain positive relationships with patients (Ryves et al., 2016[49]).

5.5.3. Limiting use of antimicrobials without prescription and counterfeit and substandard antimicrobials

Limiting counterfeit and substandard antimicrobials and antimicrobial consumption without a prescription are another set of interventions aimed at reducing inappropriate antimicrobial use. Counterfeit drugs are a major issue in much of the world, potentially accounting for over 30% of all drugs in Africa, Asia, and the Middle East (though a likely less than 1% in the United States and Western Europe) (El-Jardali et al., 2015[53]). Containing a wrong active ingredient or no active ingredient at all, counterfeit drugs can result in improper concentrations of antimicrobials in the body and the unnecessary escalation to later line antimicrobials, ultimately promoting antimicrobial resistance (Blackstone, Fuhr and Pociask, 2014[54]). Efforts to limit counterfeit and substandard antimicrobials are extremely varied and can include drug regulatory measures and establishment of drug regulatory authorities, onsite inspection and surveillance systems, drug laws, legislation and decrees, product authentication technology, pharmacovigilance systems, public awareness and education, and recursive trust labelling (Fadlallah et al., 2016[55]).

While there are limited data on the scale of use of antimicrobials without a prescription, it has emerged as a challenge not only in countries lacking regulations on over-the-counter sales but also for regulated markets because of access to internet sales. A study in India found that antimicrobial drugs were obtained without a prescription from 174 of 261 (66.7%) pharmacies visited (Shet, Sundaresan and Forsberg, 2015[56]). A 2009 study found 138 unique online vendors selling and shipping antimicrobials without a prescription in the United States (Mainous et al., 2009[57]).

Though the sale of antibiotics without prescriptions is illegal in many markets, online pharmacies are often able to circumvent such regulations by allowing customers to purchase antimicrobial products and other drugs in other countries with poor regulation or enforcement (O'Neill, 2015[58]). The global nature of antimicrobial e-commerce underscores the need for international collaboration to address the availability of antimicrobials without a prescription: for example, the recent Operation Pangea X: a global cooperative effort led by INTERPOL meant to address the sale and distribution of illegal drugs on the internet (FDA, 2017[59]). From ten participating countries at its launch, the operation has now attracted 123 countries to participate in its week of action each year (INTERPOL, 2018[60]), and the 2017 effort saw the seizure of more than USD 51 million worth of medicines (INTERPOL, 2017[61]).

There is very limited evidence on the impact of interventions specifically targeted at counterfeit or substandard antimicrobials, but some data suggest that certain policies are effective at limiting counterfeit drugs more generally. A review of studies evaluating methods to control counterfeit drugs identified regulatory measures such as drug registration and WHO prequalification of drugs to effectively reduce the prevalence of counterfeit drugs (El-Jardali et al., 2015[53]). Despite more limited evidence, additional interventions such as deployment of handheld spectrometry technologies at various inspection points, an international cross-disciplinary model of collaboration, and public awareness campaigns on the danger of counterfeit medicine from illegal drug outlets may also be effective (El-Jardali et al., 2015[53]).

A review of studies examining various types of system-level interventions to combat counterfeit drugs identified a number of features of successfully implemented systems (Fadlallah et al., 2016[55]). Particularly critical are regulatory interventions, which involve the control of drug use by international agreement or national regulatory authorities (e.g., European Medicines Agency or US Food and Drug Administration). These interventions can address the online purchase of drugs, inclusion of public education campaigns, effective pharmacovigilance systems, and onsite surveillance and inspection systems. All policies need to promote communication among stakeholders across the supply chain, including manufacturers, wholesalers, providers, and regulatory bodies.

Policies that limit access to antimicrobials need to take into account the potential consequences of policies on the treatment landscape at large. For example, an unintended effect of over-the-counter antimicrobial sales restrictions in Mexico and Brazil occurred when users substituted antimicrobials with non-steroidal anti-inflammatory drugs and analgesics in both countries as well as cough and cold medicines in Mexico (Santa-Ana-Tellez et al., 2016[62]).

5.5.4. Mass media campaigns

As their name suggests, mass media campaigns are aimed at raising awareness about inappropriate antimicrobial prescribing and consumption. Campaigns are commonly used across OECD countries as a way to promote rational prescribing (Earnshaw et al., 2009[63]). As of 2017, over half of OECD, G20, and other European countries had national-level awareness campaigns in place to influence antimicrobial prescribing (Figure 5.3). Efforts can be targeted at a variety of stakeholders involved in pharmaceutical consumption but typically address patients and physicians. By illustrating the impact of rational or inappropriate antimicrobial use, campaigns aim to improve physician practice and better align patient expectations with good prescribing practice. Many campaigns have focused on antimicrobial prescribing for children, given that they comprise a very high percentage of antimicrobial prescriptions (Huttner, Harbarth and Nathwani, 2014[34]).

While the exact nature of campaigns varies widely, the basic form involves the development and dissemination of campaign materials through channels such as print, television, radio, internet, and social media. While campaigns are often broad in scope (i.e., do not focus on specific illnesses), some campaigns specifically highlight respiratory tract infections and the flu, for which antimicrobials are typically inappropriate.

Few studies have been able to draw conclusions on the effectiveness of mass media campaigns, but the available evidence suggests that campaigns affect patient attitudes toward antimicrobials and result in a modest decrease in antimicrobial prescriptions. A meta-analysis concluded that mass media campaigns have a small but statistically significant effect on the general population's satisfaction and knowledge toward appropriate antimicrobial use (Thoolen, de Ridder and van Lensvelt-Mulders, 2011[64]). Three studies assessing the effectiveness of mass media campaigns in England (Lambert, Masters and Brent, 2007[65]), Italy (Formoso et al., 2013[66]) and the United States (Gonzales et al., 2008[67]) concluded that implementation of a mass media campaign is responsible for a 4% to 9% decrease in antimicrobial prescriptions.

According to an international survey by WHO, less than half of campaigns involved any evaluation component, making it challenging to evaluate these programmes in practice (WHO, 2016[68]).

Box 5.6. Mass media campaigns in Belgium

The Belgian Antimicrobial Policy Coordination Committee (BAPCOC), a national committee established by the Ministry of Health to promote rational antimicrobial use and improved hygiene in both the health and agricultural sectors, undertook a multi-year public awareness campaign targeting improper antimicrobial use (Goossens et al., 2008[69]). While no specific targets were set, the public awareness campaign maintained general goals to improve the public's understanding of self-limiting infections, explain when antimicrobials are needed, and communicate the importance of antimicrobial resistance. The Belgian campaign ran over three consecutive winter seasons – when antibiotic consumption increases – and was broadcast through booklets, handouts, posters, prime-time television, radio spots, and websites.

The campaign involved fairly simple messaging and a multi-stakeholder approach. Messages included: "Use antimicrobials less frequently, but better", "Save antimicrobials, they may save your life", and "Talk to your doctor, talk to your pharmacist". During one winter season, the campaign focused on communicating that antimicrobials are ineffective for common viral diseases such as cold and flu. Beyond directly targeting the general public, physicians were sent personalised letters with campaign materials that they were asked to present to patients.

The fact that the broader BAPCOC suite of interventions, including publication of clinical practice guidelines, surveillance programmes, and campaigns to promote better hygiene, were implemented concurrently makes it challenging to isolate the specific impact of the prudent use public awareness campaign. However, studies of antimicrobial prescriptions and antimicrobial resistance suggest that the campaign at least contributed to major improvements. Outpatient antimicrobial use decreased by 36% from 1997 to 2007 in Belgium, including several broad-spectrum antimicrobials known to cause resistance. In an evaluation of actual outcomes, macrolide resistance in *Streptococcus pyogenes* decreased dramatically from 17% of strains in 2001 to 2% in 2007. The Belgian campaign also demonstrated that mass media campaigns can be executed with relatively modest investments. The Belgian campaign cost approximately EUR 400 000 per year (Zowawi et al., 2015[70]). On the other hand, a French antimicrobial awareness campaign from 2002 to 2007 was estimated to cost EUR 500 million over a six-year period[1] (Huttner and Harbarth, 2009[71]).

Figure 5.3. Awareness campaigns among OECD, G20, and other EU countries

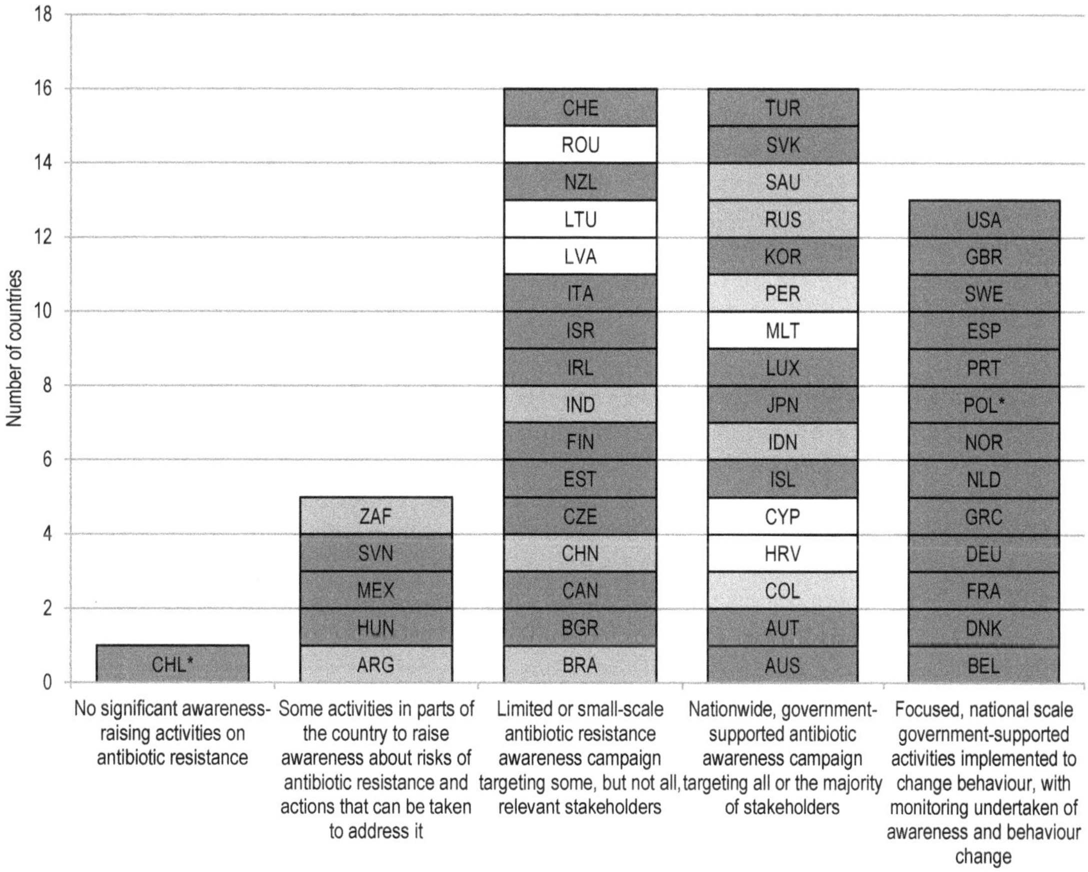

Note: countries in alphabetical order within each category. OECD countries in dark blue; other G20 non-OECD countries in light blue; other EU non-OECD countries in white; other countries partnering with the OECD in grey. Countries with * did not report in 2017 and 2016 data was used instead.
Source: OECD analysis on (WHO, FAO and OIE, 2018[6]).

StatLink http://dx.doi.org/10.1787/888933855048

5.5.5. Prescriber education

Prescriber education entails a wide range of informative activities to enhance physicians' knowledge of evidence-based medicine or to improve physicians' communication skills as they relate to antimicrobial prescribing. Like mass media campaigns, education can be delivered through a number of channels, including formal coursework, workshops, dissemination of educational material, and one-on-one coaching/feedback. They can also target various personnel involved in prescribing and dispensing antimicrobials, including physicians and nurses in community care, hospital, and long-term care settings. The scale on which educational programmes are implemented also varies considerably from country to country, as programmes may be offered locally through universities or employers or nationally through national health authorities. While most OECD, G20, and other European countries report that regular training is offered as part of professional curricula or continuing education, only 14% of countries had an integrated programme that systematically incorporates antimicrobial resistance into pre-medical service training for all relevant healthcare stakeholders as of 2017 (Figure 5.4).

Many studies have evaluated the impact of educational programmes on various outcomes related to prescribing, including adherence to guidelines, antimicrobials prescribed, attitude toward antimicrobial prescribing, and development of resistance. However, evidence on the degree to which prescriber education affects antimicrobial resistance is not as compelling as that associated with some other interventions, particularly in terms of overall antimicrobials prescribed. A recent Cochrane review determined that the quality of evidence associated with studies focused on physician education interventions was very low, preventing any conclusions about the impact of education in primary care (Tonkin-Crine et al., 2017[72]). Another review found that only 41% of studies evaluating the intervention found a decrease in total antimicrobials prescribed (Roque et al., 2014[73]).

Some evidence suggests that prescriber education can be most helpful at promoting more rational prescribing of particular antimicrobials, rather than reducing antimicrobial use overall. A study in Greece that included both prescriber and public education found no decrease in the overall volume of antimicrobials prescribed but that choice of antimicrobials changed to be more aligned with clinical guidelines, including decrease in broad-spectrum antimicrobials (Plachouras et al., 2014[74]). Similarly, a US study of paediatric prescribing found that prescriber education, along with audit and feedback, resulted in a 6.7% decrease in the portion of broad spectrum antimicrobials prescribed (Gerber, Prasad and Fiks, 2013[75]).

Interactive types of educational programmes tend to be the most effective. A review of evidence on these programmes found that interventions such as education outreach, workshops, small group-discussions, and other practice-based interventions were more effective than the dissemination of leaflets or other written materials (Roque et al., 2014[73]).

A well-known physician education programme, Choosing Wisely, combines physician education with guidelines as well as tools to help physicians communicate with patients. Started in 2012 by the American Board of Internal Medicine Foundation, the campaign has now expanded to over 20 countries and includes not only antimicrobials but also a host of treatments and procedures that are believed to be "overused" across specialities (Born and Levinson, 2017[76]). Two of the top ten international recommendations concern avoiding the use of antimicrobials for particular types of infections.

Figure 5.4. Education and training in human health among OECD, G20, and other EU countries

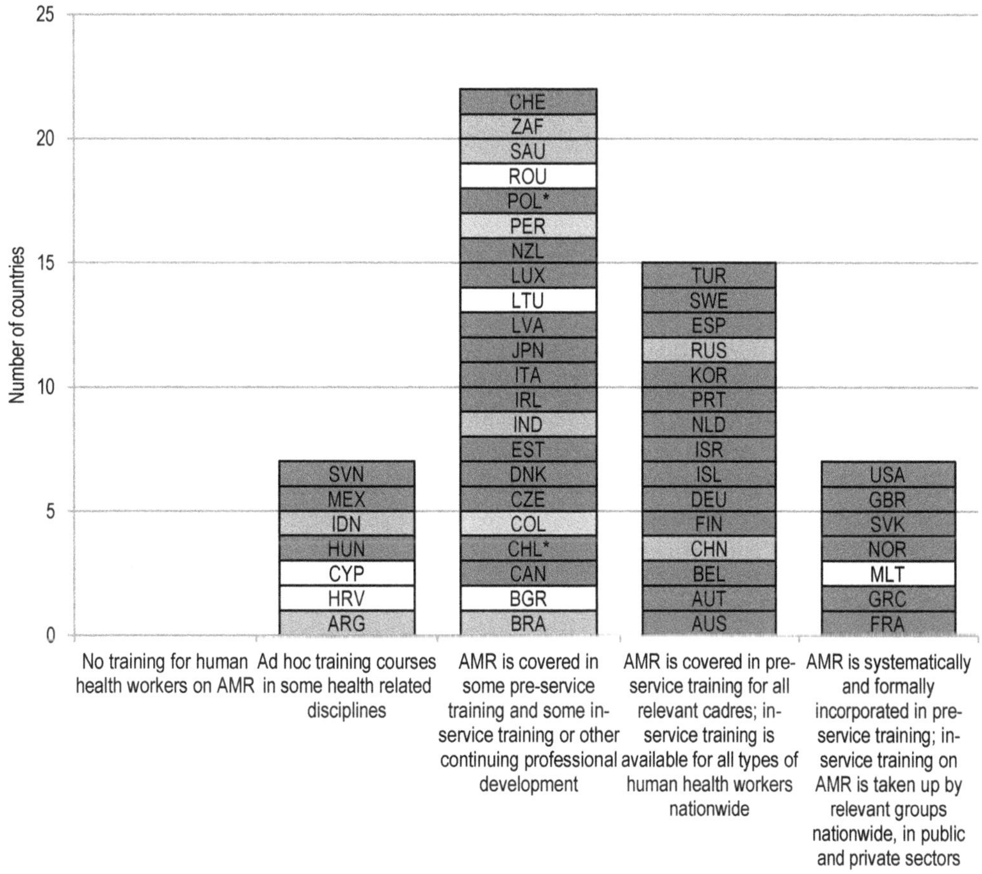

Note: countries in alphabetical order within each category. OECD countries in dark blue; other G20 non-OECD countries in light blue; other EU non-OECD countries in white; other countries partnering with the OECD in grey. Countries with * did not report in 2017 and 2016 data was used instead.
Source: OECD analysis on (WHO, FAO and OIE, 2018[6]).

StatLink http://dx.doi.org/10.1787/888933855067

5.5.6. Use of existing and new medical technologies such as rapid diagnostic tests

In determining whether to prescribe antimicrobials and which antimicrobials to prescribe, physicians have a number of diagnostic tools at their disposal. However, traditional diagnostic testing methods used to identify bacteria and evaluate antimicrobial susceptibility often require 48-72 hours, which limits their usefulness in guiding antimicrobial prescribing. New technology is allowing clinicians to rapidly acquire information that can guide treatment decisions, such as whether an infection is viral or bacterial, the specific type of bacterial infection, and whether the infection is susceptible to specific antimicrobials. As such, use of existing and new medical technologies such as rapid diagnostic tests (RDTs) can determine whether antimicrobials will be useful in treating an infection and in some cases, which specific antimicrobial will be most useful. By reducing the time to results to hours or minutes, these medical technologies have the potential to reduce unnecessary antimicrobial use, particularly the use of broad-spectrum antimicrobials, and improve patient outcomes. They can be used directly at all sites of care, including community care, outpatient, and emergency setting.

Among the most widely used RDTs are C-reactive protein (CRP) tests and rapid viral diagnostics. CRP testing, which measures inflammation, is used to rapidly detect the presence of bacteria. Rapid viral diagnostics can be conducted in 15-60 min and can detect the presence of certain viruses, such as influenza A and B and other common respiratory viruses, effectively ruling out the need for antimicrobials.

The use of a variety of medical technologies such as rapid diagnostic tests is growing globally. For example, an assay that can detect a bacterium that causes tuberculosis (TB) and resistance to an important antimicrobial (rifampicin) is now used in 122 of 145 developing countries with high TB burden (Sachdeva et al., 2015[77]), increasing the detection of multi-drug resistant TB by three to eight-fold (Albert et al., 2016[78]). Recent treatment guidelines have also supported the uptake of testing. In the United Kingdom, NICE recommends that physicians should consider carrying out rapid diagnostic tests that detect bacterial infection, CRP tests, for people presenting in primary care with symptoms of lower respiratory tract infection, if it is not clear whether antimicrobials should be prescribed (NICE, 2018[79]). The guidance goes on to recommend no antimicrobials or delayed antimicrobial prescribing for some patients based on the result.

The effectiveness of rapid diagnostic testing at reducing antimicrobial prescribing appears to vary among different technologies, and there have been limited comprehensive studies evaluating the impact of many types of rapid diagnostic tests. Because effectiveness has been widely demonstrated for CRP testing and the test can be widely used to distinguish bacterial from viral infections, the remainder of this section will focus on this particular test as a case study. However, it is important to acknowledge the heterogeneity among RDTs.

As reported in a Cochrane review, multiple trials have shown that CRP tests reduce antimicrobial prescribing, typically by approximately 25% in both primary and emergency care (Tonkin-Crine et al., 2017[72]). This effect appears to be sustained one month up to consultation (Aabenhus et al., 2014[80]; Huang et al., 2013[81]). While it reduces antibiotic prescribing, CRP testing does not affect symptom duration, patient satisfaction, or consultation. Importantly, studies have demonstrated the impact of CRP testing in both developed and developing countries. For example, CRP point-of-care testing reduced antimicrobial use for non-severe acute respiratory tract infection without compromising patients' recovery in primary health care in Vietnam (Do et al., 2016[82]).

Evidence supporting the impact of other types of RDT is sparser. A review of the impact of a number of RDTs identifying specific pathogens found a few studies suggesting they reduce antimicrobial prescribing, time to appropriate antimicrobial therapy, and hospital length of stay (Bauer et al., 2014[83]). The utilisation of rapid antigen-detection tests for Strep A has been associated with a lower prescribing of antimicrobials for patients with sore throat but showed no clear benefits over clinical scoring (Little et al., 2013[84]). An evaluation of several clinical trials showed no statistically significant evidence that rapid viral diagnostics have an impact on antimicrobial prescribing in emergency departments for paediatric patients (Doan et al., 2012[85]).

As tests vary considerably in their methodology, implementation of RDTs varies significantly depending on the test, including the need for investment in capital equipment and personnel needed to conduct testing (Frickmann, Masanta and Zautner, 2014[86]). CRP testing is generally simple to implement in routine practice given both the ease of conducting and interpreting the blood test. In clinical practice, large-scale implementation of RDTs could involve the need to refine workflow between the laboratory, physician, and other clinical staff (for example, discussion between laboratory technician and physician to ensure results are acted upon).

However, it can be more challenging to implement guidance for how to use the test results: i.e., which patients receive antimicrobials and for which patients delayed prescribing or no prescribing is more appropriate. Beyond building the testing infrastructure, successful implementation often requires an education and training component. Several studies involving the impact of RDTs have included training programmes that helped physicians explain the test results to patients and an additive effect was observed when CRP tests and training sessions in communication skills were combined (Aabenhus et al., 2014[80]).

Despite their promise, a combination of technical, social, regulatory, economic, and infrastructural barriers have hindered the more widespread uptake of RDTs (Miller and Sikes, 2015[87]). Clear regulatory pathways are necessary to ensure that tests used are sufficiently accurate and specific to yield confidence in their results. Integration of testing within standard clinical practice is also challenging. In low-resource countries, the widespread use of diagnostics is limited by low ability to pay for the diagnostics themselves and limited resources for training. Successful adoption across countries will also hinge upon sufficient quality assurance to ensure accurate results that can appropriately guide treatment decisions (Peeling and Boeras, 2016[88]).

Facilitating the development of new RDTs at the national and international level will be critical to drive their impact in reducing antimicrobial resistance. A report by the National Academies of Sciences advises health care systems to create financial incentives for test development. Specifically, the report recommends developing specific target product profiles to ensure companies develop the most appropriate test, create a rapid and inexpensive regulatory pathway to bring tests to market quickly, and establish pre-purchase agreements or sales guarantees with companies to offset a portion of the development cost (Mundaca-shah et al., 2017[89]). Future development of multiplex tests—those able to detect susceptibility among a wide variety of organisms—should decrease the implementation burden of rapid diagnostic testing that must currently be done as separate tests.

RDTs have the potential to save significant health care costs via reduced antimicrobial prescribing, need for follow-up visits, and length of stay (Doan et al., 2012[85]). When conducted by nurses, CRP testing has been shown to be cost effective (Hunter, 2015[90]). In its cost-effectiveness analysis, NICE estimated that a CRP test would cost GBP 12–15 in the United Kingdom, including the cost of reagents, equipment depreciation and staff time (Chaplin, 2015[91]; Hunter, 2015[90]). However, one time and recurring costs vary significantly depending on the specific test conducted (Frickmann, Masanta and Zautner, 2014[86]).

C-reactive testing for patients with lower respiratory tract infections has been implemented in a number of EU countries, including Sweden, Norway, the Netherlands, Germany, Switzerland, the Czech Republic and Estonia (Huddy et al., 2016[92]). In 2014, the UK's NICE included CRP thresholds, which specify the CRP levels at which antimicrobials should be prescribed, in antibiotic prescribing guidelines. A qualitative assessment of the success factors of CRP implementation within the EU identified the inclusion of testing in guidelines and treatment algorithms, central laboratory capacity, effective quality control, and management of potential work flow impacts as key success factors (Huddy et al., 2016[92]). However, because of the significant efforts required, the process from initial adoption to large-scale national implementation of new testing technologies can vary from 2-7 years.

Box 5.7. Policies to increase use of RDTs in Slovenia

Measures restricting the use of antimicrobials and strongly incentivising the use of RDTs significantly decreased antimicrobial consumption in Slovenia. Implemented in 2000, these efforts were part of a broader antimicrobial stewardship policy to tackle the substantial increase in antimicrobial consumption and resistance within the country. The policy includes restrictive prescription criteria for amoxicillin and clavulanic acid (co-amoxiclav), fluoroquinolones, third-generation cephalosporins, and macrolides in community care and hospital settings (Cizman et al., 2015[93]). For example, fluoroquinolones can only be prescribed for urinary tract infections as a second-line treatment (i.e. when the first-line treatment does not produce any positive clinical effect) or when microbial susceptibility is demonstrated by diagnostic test results. Similar measures were implemented for antimicrobials at high risk of inappropriate use.

While introduction of this policy did not make use of RDTs compulsory, it strongly incentivised their increased use. The concurrent introduction of educational interventions for professionals also supports higher use of RDTs in clinical practice.

The policy resulted in a significant increase in the use of RDTs and positive effects on antimicrobial use and AMR. Between 1999 (the year before the new policy was introduced) and 2003, the use of two common RDTs (C-reactive protein testing and streptococcal antigen detection test) in primary care settings increased by 220% (Cizman et al., 2005[94]). Following more widespread use of RDTs, overall antimicrobial consumption decreased by 20.3%, and consumption of restricted antimicrobials also decreased by 27.7% between 2000 and 2007. Penicillin resistance among invasive pneumococci also decreased (Cizman, 2008[95]).

5.5.7. Economic incentives

Economic incentives refer to a host of policies that encourage appropriate antimicrobial behaviour via financial bonuses and/or penalties. Such incentives are widely applied in the health sector to foster specific behaviours—such as reduced consumption of various health care resources—and have more recently been applied specifically to antimicrobial prescribing and consumption to promote more rational use (Schaffer, Sussex and Feng, 2015[96]). While policies are most often targeted at physicians, they may also be used to promote specific behaviours among patients.

Studies that have evaluated specific pay-for-performance programmes have shown that these incentives do influence physician prescribing, but the magnitude of their impact is variable. A large-scale antimicrobial prescription pay-for-performance scheme targeting general practitioners was established in Sweden between 2006 and 2013 with the goal of converting some antimicrobial prescribing from broad to narrow spectrum antimicrobials for respiratory infections. The financial incentives, which accounted for between 0.05% and 1.2% of physicians' total reimbursement, depending on geographical area, were tied to the share of narrow spectrum penicillin prescriptions of total respiratory tract antimicrobials. The programme led to a 3% reduction in narrow-spectrum penicillin V share (Ellegård, Dietrichson and Anell, 2017[29]). A study in the United Kingdom found similar outcomes in the hospital setting (McDonald et al., 2015[97]), and a study of the primary care setting in China also showed a reduction in antimicrobial prescribing associated with a change from fee-for-service to capitated payments (Yip et al., 2014[98]).

However, all of these studies have key methodological weaknesses, limiting the ability to draw definitive conclusions on the impact of economic incentives.

The impact of employing financial incentives to alter antimicrobial prescribing for physicians is consistent with the impact of such incentives on changing physician behaviour in general. A Cochrane review including 32 studies found that financial incentives are effective at changing a variety of health care professionals' practice, including prescribing, referrals and admissions, and guideline compliance. While the review does not distinguish between bonuses and penalties (Flodgren et al., 2011[99]), whether incentive payments involve incentives or penalties creates major consequences for the difficulty of achieving the buy-in of providers. Because penalties typically require significantly more negotiation between payers and providers, administrative cost considerations tend to favour the establishment of bonus payments to influence antimicrobial prescribing (Cashin et al., 2014[100]).

Economic incentives targeting patients are less widespread and their impact less studied than physician-targeted economic incentives. Patient incentives most often take the form of higher cost-sharing on antimicrobials, with the aim of limiting use in situations where they are unnecessary. A classic study of the impact of cost-sharing on medical care in general, conducted in six US cities across 2 000 households, demonstrated that an increase in co-payment was associated with a significant reduction in antimicrobial use (Newhouse and the insurance experiment group, 1993[101]). However, more recent studies have demonstrated that higher patient cost-sharing is linked to antimicrobial resistance. By incentivising patients to seek medical care from less well-regulated private providers, a 10% increase in the expenditures that were out-of-pocket was associated with a 3.2% increase in resistant isolates across 47 low and middle-income countries (Alsan et al., 2015[102]). Higher cost-sharing in the public sector led patients to seek medical care in the private sector, wherein antimicrobial prescribing was less tightly controlled (Alsan et al., 2015[102]).

While economic incentives have proven to be successful in the past, their design can be challenging, requiring the determination of appropriate outcomes and size of the financial incentive. Importantly, however, evidence suggests that incentives do not need to involve significant financial stakes for physicians to be effective. Physicians have been consistently responsive to very nominal bonuses, suggesting that the mechanism behind successful pay-for-performance schemes is "lowering physicians' psychological barriers to changing prescription routines" (Celhay et al., 2015[103]).

While there is no universal formula for the development of successful economic incentive programmes, incentive design needs to consider a number of factors (Kondo et al., 2016[104]):

- focus on measures targeting process-of-care or clinical outcomes that are transparently evidence-based and viewed as clinically important
- incentive structure needs to consider several factors, including incentive size, frequency, and target group.
- programmes need to be able to change over time based on measurement and physician input
- target areas of poor performance and consider de-emphasising areas that have achieved high performance.

In designing effective economic incentive policies, it is also key to keep in mind unintended economic consequences that can create perverse incentives for physicians and patients. For example, after the reduction of China's 15% mark-up policy, which incentivised physicians to overprescribe because drug administration made up a significant portion of their revenue, some hospitals provided additional inpatient care services as well as increased use of intravenous prescriptions (Wang et al., 2016[40]). In health care systems with both public and private channels, changes in patient cost-sharing likely only have the potential to be effective if implemented across both.

Box 5.8. Reimbursement of antimicrobials in Japan

Since 1996, Japan's health care system has employed a reimbursement-based fee schedule for medical services and prescription medicine. The schedule contains embedded economic incentives in the form of bonuses to promote prudent use of medical resources, including the use of antimicrobials, in hospitals (Federal Ministry of Health, 2015[105]). The most recent national action plan on AMR includes a set of policies to enhance capacity building and training on adaptation of diagnostic and treatment technologies, clinical and public health expertise on infectious diseases, and rapid response to AMR emergence. In fulfilling the level of activities dedicated to reducing inappropriate antimicrobial consumption, the programme sets out specific performance indicators, such as the number of antimicrobial stewardship seminars carried out each year and the number of cases of antimicrobial-resistant infections at each medical institution. Upon meeting specific targets, hospitals are rewarded reimbursement credits that can eventually be recovered as hospital revenues (AMR Special Group, 2016[106]).

Conversely, health care providers can only be fully reimbursed by the insurer for the costs of prescribed antimicrobials when required stewardship precautions are demonstrated and the treatment of choice is judged prudent. Under the Health Insurance Act and the Act on Assurance of Medical Care for Elderly People, physicians are required to not prescribe medicines beyond necessity (Japan Ministry of Health, 2016[107]).

At the community level, additional economic incentives are in place to facilitate regional co-operation of hospitals regarding infection control through mutual audit and feedback. A support network of specialists in the community aims to increase awareness and provide adequate expertise and consultation to facilitate aspects of AMR prevention.

Box 5.9. Role of business stakeholders in promoting prudent use of antimicrobials

While many interventions are targeted at physicians and the patients taking antimicrobials, stakeholders who benefit commercially from the sale and dispensation of antimicrobials, such as pharmaceutical manufacturers and private pharmacies, also have a significant role to play in promoting rational use of antimicrobials.

Numerous pharmaceutical companies, which can be involved in interventions from reducing counterfeit products to ensuring sales and marketing practices are transparent, have publicly committed to tackling AMR, with many signing the Davos Declaration in 2016 (IFPMA, 2016[108]). This Declaration was followed by the publication, by a core group of manufacturers, of an "Industry Roadmap for Progress on Combating Antimicrobial Resistance" (IFPMA, 2016[109]). The Access to Medicines Foundation developed an evaluation metric for pharmaceutical companies to assess their impact on AMR, with a focus on:

- ensuring affordability and limiting shortages
- registering products
- ensuring manufacturing quality
- supporting/engaging in antimicrobial stewardship
- supporting/engaging in surveillance systems
- adapting packaging to enable rational use
- supporting efforts to limit uncontrolled use
- employing ethical sales and marketing practices

The Foundation found that a number of pharmaceutical manufacturers have made progress in promoting the prudent use of antibiotics, such as AMR surveillance and promotional activities (Foundation, 2018[110]). Almost half of companies that market antimicrobials have undertaken surveillance across 147 countries. Only four companies, however, are working to reduce overuse of antimicrobials by modifying sales incentives to be separate from the volume of antibiotics sold, thereby disincentivising the sale of unnecessarily high volumes.

Private pharmacies not only influence antimicrobial use by educating patients on appropriate antimicrobial use but also in how they dispense antimicrobials. Even in markets where antimicrobials are prescription-only, some pharmacy outlets—both online and more traditional brick-and-mortar facilities—dispense them without a prescription. In a 2017 World Bank study, antimicrobials were dispensed without a prescription derived from appropriate clinical diagnosis in more than 60% of pharmacy visits in Botswana, Georgia, Ghana, Nicaragua, and Peru (World Bank, 2016[111]). A recent survey of 20 online pharmacies that deliver to the United Kingdom found that 45% of them did not require a prescription prior to purchase. Even among those requiring a prescription, nearly all of the pharmacies allowed customers to select the specific antimicrobial they wanted, along with the dose and treatment duration (Boyd et al., 2017[112]). Importantly, it was unclear whether most of the pharmacies surveyed were actually operating in the United Kingdom, highlighting the critical importance of international collaboration in pharmacy regulatory policy.

Some private pharmacies are actively working to promote rational prescribing. For example, one pharmacy chain conducted an antimicrobial resistance audit across the home care facilities it supported to ultimately improve antimicrobial dispensation (PharmacyMagazine, 2017[113]). However, significantly more work is needed in order for pharmacies to curtail the inappropriate acquisition of antimicrobials by patients.

5.6. Specific interventions in toolkit: Prevent spread or transmission of resistance in health care settings

5.6.1. Improved environmental hygiene in health care settings

Environmental hygiene in health care settings encompasses the decontamination, disinfection, cleaning and sterilisation of the environment and equipment as well as proper disposal of items that have potentially come into contact with infected individuals. Because many organisms are able to live in the health care environment for days, proper hygiene is critical to preventing the spread of resistant bacteria. Studies have shown that only 50% of surfaces in hospital rooms are sufficiently cleaned between patient stays, meaning rooms previously occupied by patients with multidrug-resistant organisms are at an increased risk of subsequent infection or colonisation with these organisms (Anderson et al., 2017[114]).

Cleaning practices are extremely variable in terms of frequency, method, equipment, benchmarks, monitoring, and standards (Dancer, 2014[115]). While the types of interventions applied to improve these cleaning practices differ widely, they can be clustered into three broad categories (Donskey, 2013[116]).

- **Disinfectant substitution** involves a change from detergent to disinfectant, or to a different disinfectant assumed to have higher effectiveness against certain pathogens.
- **No-touch cleaning** involves the use of an automated cleaning device, emitting hydrogen peroxide vapour or ultraviolet (UV) radiation, to disinfect rooms after routine cleaning. UV and hydrogen peroxide attack the molecular bonds in DNA and other essential cell components, thereby destroying the microorganisms (Weber, Kanamori and Rutala, 2016[117]).
- **Interventions to improve effectiveness of cleaning** may include additional cleaning time through the employment of new staff; audit, monitoring and feedback regarding cleaning practices and thoroughness (Curtis, 2008[118]); staff education as well as novel techniques of applying products, such as using disposable wipes or colour-coded cloths.

Several studies have found that improved cleaning practices have decreased contamination with antimicrobial resistant bacteria, both on humans and within the health care environment. A recent clinical trial investigated the effect of three enhanced strategies for terminal room cleaning on the acquisition of several types of antimicrobial-resistant organisms at eight hospitals in the United States. The three strategies tested comprised the use of bleach and ultraviolet-C decontamination as well as a combination of both compared to standard cleaning with quaternary ammonium. On all target organisms, UV-C cleaning alone was the most effective and resulted in a significant 30% decrease in pathogen transmission (Anderson et al., 2017[114]).

A number of studies have also demonstrated the impact of improved hygiene practices on contamination and infections more generally. A study of four US hospitals found that a change in gown and glove donning and removal technique resulted in a significant reduction in skin and clothing contamination that was sustained for up to three months (Tomas et al., 2015[119]). Other studies have identified various cleaning methods that reduce contamination of hospital rooms. For example, one study identified that a solution used to disinfect pieces of equipment in intensive care units significantly reduced catheter-related infections (Chopra and Saint, 2015[120]).

Though it may seem straightforward, implementation of improved cleaning practices involves both process improvements (e.g., skin disinfection or use of UV lights) as well as education and training, with an eye to key "socioadaptive" considerations (Chopra and Saint, 2015[120]). Medical personnel need to be not only trained but also effectively encouraged and incentivised to adhere to hygiene practices (Chopra and Saint, 2015[120]). Most hygiene programmes evaluated include both educational and evaluative components, with training, proficiency monitoring, and feedback (Doll and Bearman, 2015[121]; Tomas et al., 2015[119]). Particularly effective programmes have included immediate visual feedback on contaminated surfaces to allow health care workers to improve their practices.

However, interventions also need to address some of the broader challenges surrounding medical facility cleaning in general, such as poor compensation of staff, which can undermine proper hygiene. In community settings, proper sanitation infrastructure and education of the public on the importance of environmental hygiene are essential to prevent contamination with resistant pathogens (Cecchini, Langer and Slawomirski, 2015[122]). In 2015 in India, the National Health Mission launched the Kayakalp (clean hospital initiative) Award Scheme, which aims to promote infection control practices in health care facilities (Swaminathan et al., 2017[123]). Under the scheme, health facilities are incentivised to achieve certain cleanliness, hygiene, waste management, and infection control practices with monetary rewards (MoHFW, 2016[124]). Funds provided through the scheme may be used for cleaning equipment, improved cleaning practices, and staff training. Introduced to district hospitals in 2016 and 2017, the programme is now being rolled out to community health centres and other health care facilities.

Studies in the United Kingdom and Canada have shown that enhanced environmental hygiene can lead to substantial cost-savings ranging from GBP 31 600 to CAD 500 000 per year (Conlon-Bingham et al., 2016[125]; Dancer et al., 2009[126]; Semret et al., 2016[127]). If resources are limited, targeted approaches could be considered such as enhanced cleaning for patients deemed to be at higher risk of infection (e.g., those in exposed rooms or those undergoing critical care) (Siegel et al., 2017[128]).

5.6.2. Improved hand hygiene

Transmission via hand contact, in particular through health care workers' hands, is deemed the most important vector for spreading healthcare-associated pathogens. Since microorganisms can survive on the skin for several minutes, pathogens can be readily spread from patient to patient (Allegranzi and Pittet, 2009[129]; Sroka, Gastmeier and Meyer, 2010[130]). The ease with which infections can spread on the hands highlights the critical importance of hand hygiene as a mechanism to control infections. Often, however, hand hygiene is extremely inadequate: a global review of hand hygiene compliance found that compliance with hand hygiene guidelines was just 40% on average (Erasmus et al., 2010[131]).

The WHO World Alliance for Patient Safety campaign, launched in 2005, initiated a series of international and national efforts to improve hand hygiene. The campaign strategy featured five key components: system change, training and education, observation and feedback, reminders in the hospital, and a hospital safety climate. Since then, a number of countries have established hand hygiene guidelines and national policies. Many of the most recent guideline updates recommend hand cleaning after removal of gloves (Wilson et al., 2016[132]), such as the UK's NICE guidelines (NICE, 2012[133]).

There is some evidence suggesting that specific hand hygiene measures can reduce the spread of infections; however, many of these studies have significant limitations, including inadequate sample sizes, inappropriate analyses and failure to compare the efficacy of different types of interventions (Fätkenheuer, Hirschel and Harbarth, 2015[134]). Despite these drawbacks, a European study demonstrated that increased use of alcohol-based handrubs was associated with reduced MRSA rates (Fätkenheuer, Hirschel and Harbarth, 2015[134]). In a study focused on rural hospitals in New Hampshire, a hospital-wide hygiene initiative targeting both nurses and physicians was associated with a reduction in the incidence of hospital-associated infections (Kirkland et al., 2012[135]).

The most successful hand hygiene interventions tend to be the most comprehensive, such as those that include accountability, feedback, education and training, marketing and communication, in addition to simply making cleaning products available (Bauer-Savage et al., 2013[136]; Kirkland et al., 2012[135]). The multi-faceted WHO-5 intervention, which includes goal setting, reward incentives, and accountability also appears to improve health care worker compliance (Luangasanatip et al., 2015[137]). While such comprehensive solutions are useful in specific settings, simple changes can also drive improvements in resource-limited settings. More straightforward solutions such as WHO-recommended locally-produced handrubs have been rolled out in many countries, eliminating the need for resource-constrained health care facilities to purchase cleaning products (Bauer-Savage et al., 2013[136]).

Key regulatory actions are also important in improving hand hygiene, particularly in ensuring that products used for cleaning are appropriate and effective. In light of no evidence supporting the effectiveness of 19 chemicals used in soap products, the US Food and Drug Administration (FDA) banned the use of 19 different chemicals in consumer hand soap in 2016 (Food and Drug Adminnistration, HHS, 2016[138]). Before the ban, about 40% of soaps – including liquid hand soap and bar soap – contained the chemicals.

Box 5.10. National Hand Hygiene Initiative in Australia

Introduced in 2006, Australia's National Hand Hygiene Initiative, commissioned by the Australian Commission on Quality and Safety in Health Care, has achieved significant reductions in infection rates of resistant bacteria. The programme aims to improve both surveillance and hand hygiene practice, including improvements in hand hygiene compliance rates, reducing rates of healthcare-associated infections, as well as accurately measure rates of staphylococcal disease and an effective education and credentialing system to improve knowledge about hand hygiene (Hand Hygiene Australia, 2018[139]). The hand hygiene strategy hinges upon the "5 Moments" when hand hygiene should be performed: before touching a patient, before a procedure, after a procedure or body fluid exposure, after touching a patient, and after touching a patient's surroundings.

While the initiative initially focused on acute care public hospitals, it now includes a variety of both public and private health care facilities, and it tracks compliance rates across the country, with breakdowns by specific moment in patient journey, health care worker type, hospital wards, and types of hospitals. As of 2017, the national compliance rate (84.8%) has exceeded the 80% benchmark established by the Australian Health Ministers' Advisory Council (Hand Hygiene Australia, 2017[140]).

Two evaluations of the Initiative found it yielded both improved health outcomes and cost savings. A study of 38 hospitals across eight states and territories found that the initiative was associated with infection rate reductions from 8% per year in South Australia to 28% in the Australian Capital Territory (Barnett et al., 2014[141]). A cost-effectiveness analysis including 50 hospitals determined the cost effectiveness ratio of AUD 29 700 per life year gained, with total implementation costs of the programme amounting to AUD 2.85 million (Graves et al., 2016[142]).

5.6.3. Screening and isolation of infected patients

Aimed at reducing the transmission of infections from patient to patient, screening and isolation involves the quarantining of specific patients to separate areas of a health care facility (most typically a hospital). The intervention can be broad or targeted, involving patients colonised with epidemiologically important bacteria (such as MRSA and vancomycin-resistant *Enterococci*) after screening or pre-emptive isolation of high-risk patients. Isolation itself can range from contact precautions (e.g., gloves and gowns for contact with patients) to patient cohorting (groups of patients in one area) or single-room isolation (Worby et al., 2013[143]).

Evidence evaluating the effectiveness of policies to screen and isolate infected patients in reducing antimicrobial resistance is limited. A number of observational studies have suggested that isolation of patients, when included as part of a bundle of interventions, can reduce the spread of MRSA (Fätkenheuer, Hirschel and Harbarth, 2015[134]). However, these studies tend to be low quality and often couple isolation with other actions such as decolonisation, thus making it challenging to disentangle the impact of one intervention from the another (Worby et al., 2013[143]). For example, a screening and isolation policy in the Netherlands was successful at controlling a large MRSA outbreak (Vos, Ott and Verbrugh, 2005[144]). Following an outbreak of MRSA, in a university hospital, the proportion of a particular strain of MRSA rose from 3% to 33%. An intensive "search-and-destroy" policy on patients and health care workers lowered the portion of that strain to 5% over several years. National guidelines for the more sensitive detection of strains with low-level resistance were also implemented across laboratories nationally.

While isolation of infected patients may seem straightforward, there are major open questions related to the implementation of screening and isolation policies. A first issue concerns where and under what circumstances patients should be isolated (Tacconelli, 2009[145]). Because screening tests can often require 24-72 hours to yield results, a period during which patients could spread infections, there is a significant trade-off between isolating patients pre-emptively as opposed to isolating them after receiving screening results. There is also a lack of consensus surrounding which patients should be screened; some evidence suggests that screening and isolation may be most effective and best implemented in intensive care units rather than other wards of the hospital. Finally, some investigators have expressed concern that isolation may decrease overall quality of care for isolated patients because of the more limited time health care professionals spend with them (Fätkenheuer, Hirschel and Harbarth, 2015[134]).

Despite very limited evidence on the impact of screening and isolation on infection control, at least on a theoretical basis, the intervention could be both clinically sound and cost effective. As screening would reduce expensive nosocomial infections, such as MRSA, the intervention might result in significant cost savings. A few studies have shown savings from USD 100-150 000 annually in individual hospitals: the result of both fewer infections and reduced use of antimicrobials (Tacconelli, 2009[145]). However, the need for single rooms in many cases makes this intervention particularly resource-intensive. Most guidelines recommend the use of a single room along with contact precautions for patients infected with multi-drug resistant bacteria, which can be virtually impossible to provide in countries with a limited supply of rooms (Otter et al., 2015[146]).

Box 5.11. Hospital screening to combat rising resistance in Hong Kong

In Hong Kong, the authority managing the city's public hospitals and other health care facilities has recently established more stringent screening guidelines for hospitalised patients in an attempt to address rising rates of antimicrobial resistance. High resistance rates and spread largely result from historically high antimicrobial use and a significant population of international visitors (Tsang et al., 2012[147]). A recent study showed that antimicrobials cephalexin, amoxicillin, ofloxacin and erythromycin were ubiquitous in seawater throughout Victoria Harbour as a result of continuous discharge into the environment (Cheng et al., 2015[148]). Hong Kong faces particular concerns about the spread of carbapenem-resistant *Enterobacteriaceae* (CRE): a so-called "super bug" because it is resistant to nearly all antimicrobial products.

In recent years, Hong Kong established a hospital surveillance system that involves routine screening of high risk patients, including those who were hospitalised overseas within six months or had received a surgical operation outside Hong Kong within 12 months of admission (Cheng et al., 2015[148]). In many cases, patients hospitalised for 14 days or more are also screened.

If screened patients are found to harbour certain types of resistant bacteria, an infection control team carries out a bedside assessment and establishes strict contact precautions, including isolation of the patient to a single room. In addition, all of their hospital contacts are tracked for potential secondary cases and immediately screened. If those patients have been discharged from the hospital into secondary care facilities, they are screened at those facilities. For patients who have been discharged to home, the hospital computer system records their status, and they are screened upon readmission (Cheng et al., 2015[148]).

However, with a major increase in CRE cases between 2016 and 2017 (340 cases to 473), Hong Kong has announced multiple changes to the screening programme. Public hospitals will now conduct screening on site within hospitals, and criteria for screening may also be expanded to include more patients, given an increasing number of cases of CRE reported in patients who were not hospitalised outside of Hong Kong (van Dongen, 2018[149]).

Screening is just one component of Hong Kong's comprehensive national action plan, which includes efforts to optimise the use of antimicrobials in both humans and animals, reduce the incidence of infection, improve surveillance, grow awareness about resistance, and promote relevant research and development (The Government of the Hong Kong Special Administrative Region, 2017[150]).

5.6.4. Decolonisation

Colonisation of body surfaces with drug-resistant pathogens, in particular patient skin, serves as a key vector for transmission and is linked to an increased risk of infection. Approaches to decolonisation can be highly variable. Decolonisation may target individuals with a specific infection or a broad set of infections; it can occur pre-emptively (before admission) or following screening, and may target health care workers or specific patients, such as those undergoing surgery or treatment in the intensive care unit. Decolonisation can also be carried out using one of several methods:

- nasal decolonisation involving topical antimicrobials and usually targeting a specific pathogen
- selective decontamination involving prophylactic application of antimicrobials in the stomach
- skin decolonisation with topical antiseptics involving use of an antiseptic and can thus be used for a variety of drug-resistant bacteria.

Because decolonisation may involve the use of antimicrobials, there is a risk not only of additional resistance development but also other adverse events such as allergic skin reactions. Resistance to a topical antimicrobial product has been reported in some studies of MRSA decolonisation (Edgeworth, 2011[151]; Robicsek et al., 2009[152]), making decolonisation relatively controversial among hygiene interventions (Edgeworth, 2011[151]; Worby et al., 2013[143]).

Despite its risks, however, decolonisation has been proven to be effective in reducing infections in high-risk patient groups, such as those with surgical site infections and wound complications. The pooled effects of 17 studies showed that decolonisation had a significantly protective effect against surgical site infection associated with *S. aureus* both when all patients and only *S. aureus* patients underwent decolonisation (Schweizer et al., 2013[153]). A review of 19 studies showed a reduction in surgical site infections (effect ranging from 13% to 200%) by instituting an *S. aureus* screening and decolonisation protocol in elective orthopaedic (total joints, spine, and sports) and trauma patients. The screening and decolonisation protocol also saved costs in orthopaedic patients (Chen, Wessel and Rao, 2013[154]).

Because decolonisation runs the risk of actually increasing antimicrobial resistance, effective implementation typically involves specific patient populations that are likely to yield the most benefit. For example, decolonisation may be used for patients increased risk of developing an MRSA infection during a specific period, such as patients admitted to inpatient care units and those undergoing cardiothoracic surgery (Clarke, 2014[155]). UK guidance suggests screening only patients at high risk for organisms such as MRSA and carbapenemase-producing *Enterobacteriaceae* and decolonising only select MRSA patients (Public Health England, 2017[156]).

Box 5.12. Role of business stakeholders in promoting hygiene in the natural environment

While hygiene within health care facilities falls to the facilities themselves, business stakeholders have a profound responsibility in promoting broader environmental hygiene in order to combat antimicrobial resistance. Antimicrobial manufacturing, which is largely concentrated in India and China, releases antimicrobials into the environment and has been cited as a major source of antimicrobial resistance. A 2009 study showed antimicrobial concentrations in rivers around Hyderabad higher than in the bloodstream of a patient undergoing antimicrobial treatment (Rotthier and Gharabaghi, 2015[157]). A 2016 study recommended that regulators not only set targets on maximum levels of antimicrobial discharge but also that pharmaceutical companies improve monitoring of their manufacturing and that of their suppliers (Milmo, 2017[158]). The lack of environmental regulation and enforcement in some countries underscores the need for pharmaceutical manufacturers to adhere to the most rigorous environmental hygiene practices.

Beyond prudent antimicrobial use, the Access to Medicines Foundation also evaluates pharmaceutical manufacturers on their environmental risk management efforts. Currently, only 8 of 19 companies are reducing antimicrobial release into the environment through limits on antimicrobial wastewater discharge and none of them publishes discharge levels (Foundation, 2018[110]). In 2016, a group of companies within the International Federation of Pharmaceutical Manufacturers & Associations (IFPMA) published a roadmap that includes specifying steps they would undertake to control the release of antimicrobials from pharmaceutical plants (IFPMA, 2016[159]). The companies agreed to review their manufacturing and supply chains, build a common framework for assessing and mitigating antimicrobial discharge, and begin to apply the framework to their own practices in 2018. They have also worked with external experts and have developed targets for antimicrobial discharge concentrations (AMR Industry Alliance, 2018[160]).

5.7. Specific interventions in toolkit: Vaccination

Vaccination is a key intervention that can reduce antimicrobial resistance by lowering the incidence of diseases that are treated with antimicrobials, particularly those bacteria that tend to develop resistant strains. Vaccines essentially train the immune system to recognise pathogens and mount an immune response, thereby reducing the severity of infection or preventing its establishment all together (Jansen, Knirsch and Anderson, 2018[161]). Vaccines also protect unvaccinated individuals through herd immunity by reducing the likelihood of transmission. While vaccination is one of a suite of infection prevention measures, such as better nutrition, clean water, and hygiene, vaccination can be easier to implement and produces significant results (Ginsburg and Klugman, 2017[162]).

Vaccination, particularly for *Streptococcus pneumoniae* (*S. pneumoniae*) and *Haemophilus influenzae* type b (Hib), can help to combat antimicrobial resistance by both reducing the incidence of resistant strains of bacteria as well as allowing for differential diagnoses that allow narrower spectrum antimicrobials to be used when vaccinated patients become ill. For the most part, vaccines do not specifically target resistant strains of bacteria but address all strains of a particular type of bacteria. One notable exception is pneumococcal conjugate vaccines (PCVs), which address specific serotypes of *pneumoniae* that have a high resistance frequency. Highlighting the potential impact of vaccination in curbing antimicrobial use, universal coverage by a PCV could yield a 47% reduction in the amount of antimicrobials used for pneumonia cases caused by *S. pneumoniae* (Laxminarayan et al., 2016[163]).

Vaccination has been shown to be extremely effective in reducing the incidence of many clinical diseases, including those pathogens with high rates of resistance. In the United States, after the introduction of the PCV into the routine childhood immunisation programme, incidence of penicillin non-susceptible invasive pneumococcal disease decreased by 81% in children under the age of two (Kyaw, 2006[164]). Within four years of the introduction of the PCV in children under two years of age in South Africa, reductions of greater than 80% were recorded in the incidence of invasive pneumococcal disease caused by penicillin, ceftriaxone, and multidrug non-susceptible serotypes (von Gottberg et al., 2014[165]).

Although they do not target bacterial pathogens, influenza vaccines also help to reduce AMR by both preventing secondary bacterial infections, which occur as a result of viral infections, and preventing inappropriate antibiotic use for patients with viral infections (Jansen, Knirsch and Anderson, 2018[161]). The impact of influenza vaccination on inappropriate antimicrobial use is particularly profound in light of the fact that in the United States, approximately one-third of antimicrobial prescriptions are unnecessary, with the majority of these prescriptions written for respiratory illnesses caused by viruses (CDC, 2016[166]). A study in Canada showed that following the introduction of a universal influenza vaccination in Ontario, influenza-associated antibiotics were prescribed 64% less often than prior to the implementation of the vaccination policy (Kwong et al., 2009[167]).

Despite its demonstrated effectiveness at not only reducing disease burden but also decreased antimicrobial resistance, implementation of more widespread vaccination faces ideological, logistical, and financial hurdles. Global vaccination rates—the portion of children who receive vaccinations—have recently levelled out at approximately 86%, with certain diseases such as pneumococcal diseases achieving much lower rates (42%) (WHO, 2018[168]). Though developed countries tend to have high vaccination rates, global coverage rates for the Hib and PCVs are, respectively, only 45% and 19% (Greenwood, 2014[169]).

Several key factors need to be addressed to bolster vaccination coverage in low and middle-income countries, including simultaneous licensure in developed and developing countries, faster rollout of vaccines, logistics improvements to grow vaccination rates in remote areas, increasing funding, and reducing public resistance. In 2017, the Ministers of Health from 194 countries endorsed a resolution to improve efforts to achieve the goals of the Global Vaccine Action Plan, which aims to achieve more equitable access to vaccines by 2020. The resolution includes efforts to bolster national immunisation programmes as well as monitoring systems, mobilise financing, and expand immunisations to adolescents and adults (WHO, 2018[168]).

Although vaccination rates are fairly high across OECD and G20 countries (Figure 5.5), coverage falls short of the WHO's 95% target for each vaccine in the routine vaccination schedule by the age of two (Williams et al., 2011[170]). It is therefore critical to not only focus on the need to promote vaccine uptake in low-income countries but also on continuing to improve vaccination rates in higher income countries. A review of strategies to improve vaccination rates in preschool children identified successful interventions targeting both parents and providers (Williams et al., 2011[170]). Parental reminders increased immunisation rates by 34%, while physician-targeted reminders, educational programmes, and feedback programmes increased rates by 7%, 8%, and 19% respectively.

While these efforts can improve utilisation of current vaccines, realising the full potential impact of vaccination on AMR will also require the development of novel vaccines. There are no licensed vaccines for any bacterial species that address bacteria considered "critical" or "high" on the WHO Priority Pathogens List (WHO, 2017[171]). In addition, only 4% of research and development spending on products to prevent infections specifically related to AMR is spent on diagnostics, vaccines, or other technologies, with 95% on antimicrobials (OECD et al., 2017[172]). This suggests that sustaining viable markets and supporting new vaccine research, in addition to supporting uptake of current vaccines, will be critical to combatting the spread of AMR. Pipeline vaccines such as those to prevent *C. difficile* or *S. aureus* infection, PCVs with extended serotype coverage, and vaccines to prevent infections with Gram-negative bacteria offer the promise of significantly reduced infection and antimicrobial prescribing (Jansen, Knirsch and Anderson, 2018[161]).

Figure 5.5. Vaccination rates among OECD, G20, and other EU countries

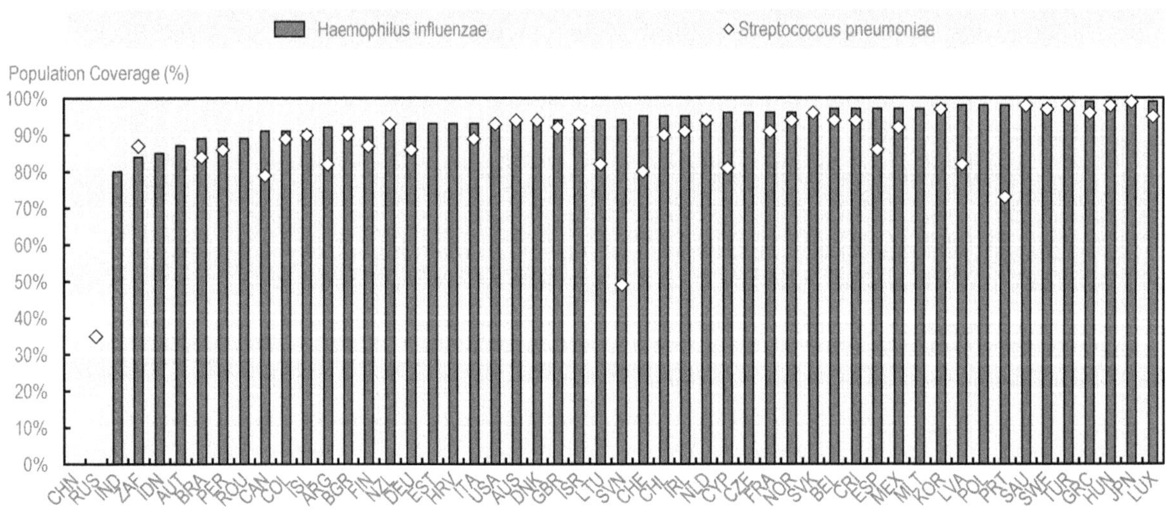

Note: cross-country discrepancies exist on the population for which data is reported. For example, certain countries may report data only for certain age groups or for population sub-groups.
Source: OECD analysis on (WHO, 2018[173]; WHO, 2017[174]).

StatLink http://dx.doi.org/10.1787/888933855086

Conclusions

In developing policies to combat antimicrobial resistance, policy makers have a lengthy menu of interventions from which to choose. Interventions aimed at promoting more rational use of antimicrobials, improving environmental hygiene in the health care setting, and bolstering vaccination rates have all been shown to lower the burden of antimicrobial resistance. Additionally, many of these policies have been effectively used in a variety of health care settings and across geographies, demonstrating the potential of policies to be successfully tailored to meet local needs. The fact that many of these efforts have been studied and work in consort, rather than separately, underscores the need to implement a wide variety of policies rather than attempt to identify and select the most effective one. In addition, given the global nature of microbes and antimicrobial resistance, successfully reducing resistance development will also require global surveillance, co-operation, and coordination for the impact of antimicrobial policies to be fully realised.

Note

[1] While this cost seems much higher than the cost of the mass media campaign in Belgium, it is noteworthy that the authors report that the reduction in antibiotic costs was higher than the cost to implement the mass media campaign. A significant share of the total budget was devoted to buying television broadcast time.

References

Aabenhus, R. et al. (2014), "Biomarkers as point-of-care tests to guide prescription of antibiotics in patients with acute respiratory infections in primary care (Review)" 11, https://www.cochranelibrary.com/cdsr/doi/10.1002/14651858.CD010130.pub2. [80]

Albert, H. et al. (2016), "Development, roll-out and impact of Xpert MTB/RIF for tuberculosis: What lessons have we learnt and how can we do better?", *European Respiratory Journal*, Vol. 48/2, pp. 516-525, http://dx.doi.org/10.1183/13993003.00543-2016. [78]

Allegranzi, B. and D. Pittet (2009), "Role of hand hygiene in healthcare-associated infection prevention", *Journal of Hospital Infection*, Vol. 73/4, pp. 305-315, https://doi.org/10.1016/j.jhin.2009.04.019. [129]

Alsan, M. et al. (2015), "Out-of-pocket health expenditures and antimicrobial resistance in low- and middle-income countries", *Lancet Infectious Diseases*, Vol. 15/10, pp. 1203–1210, https://doi.org/10.1016/S1473-3099(15)00149-8. [102]

AMR Industry Alliance (2018), *AMR Industry Alliance Antibiotic Discharge Targets*, https://www.amrindustryalliance.org/wp-content/uploads/2018/09/AMR_Industry_Alliance_List-of-Predicted-No-Effect-Concentrations-PNECs.pdf (accessed on 08 October 2018). [160]

AMR Special Group (2016), *National Action Plan on Antimicrobial Resistance*, The Government of Japan, https://www.mhlw.go.jp/file/06-Seisakujouhou-10900000-Kenkoukyoku/0000138942.pdf (accessed on 3 October 2018). [106]

Anderson, D. et al. (2017), "Enhanced terminal room disinfection and acquisition and infection caused by multidrug-resistant organisms and Clostridium difficile (the Benefits of Enhanced Terminal Room Disinfection study): a cluster-randomised, multicentre, crossover study", *The Lancet*, Vol. 389/10071, pp. 805-814, https://doi.org/10.1016/S0140-6736(16)31588-4. [114]

Barnett, A. et al. (2014), "Changes in Healthcare-Associated Staphylococcus aureus Bloodstream Infections after the Introduction of a National Hand Hygiene Initiative", *Infection Control and Hospital Epidemiology*, Vol. 35/8, pp. 1-10, http://dx.doi.org/10.1086/677160. [141]

Bauer, K. et al. (2014), "Review of rapid diagnostic tests used by antimicrobial stewardship programs", *Clinical infectious diseases : an official publication of the Infectious Diseases Society of America*, Vol. 59/March, pp. S134-S145, http://dx.doi.org/10.1093/cid/ciu547. [83]

Bauer-Savage, J. et al. (2013), "Local production of WHO-recommended alcohol-based handrubs: feasibility, advantages, barriers and costs.", *Bulletin of the World Health Organization*, Vol. 91/September, pp. 963-9, http://dx.doi.org/10.2471/BLT.12.117085. [136]

Baur, D. et al. (2017), "Effect of antibiotic stewardship on the incidence of infection and colonisation with antibiotic-resistant bacteria and Clostridium difficile infection: a systematic review and meta-analysis", *The Lancet Infectious Diseases*, Vol. 17/9, pp. 990-1001, https://doi.org/10.1016/S1473-3099(17)30325-0. [28]

BCCDC (2014), *Do Bugs Need Drugs? Annual Evaluation Report*, http://www.bccdc.ca/health-professionals/data-reports/antimicrobial-resistance/do-bugs-need-drugs-evaluation-reports (accessed on 1 October 2018). [43]

Blackstone, E., J. Fuhr and S. Pociask (2014), "The health and economic effects of counterfeit drugs.", *American health & drug benefits*, Vol. 7/4, pp. 216-24, https://www.ncbi.nlm.nih.gov/pubmed/25126373 (accessed on 1 October 2018). [54]

Born, K. and W. Levinson (2017), "Choosing Wisely: An International Campaign to Combat Overuse", *To the Point (The Commonwealth Fund)*, https://www.commonwealthfund.org/blog/2017/choosing-wisely-international-campaign-combat-overuse (accessed on 2 October 2018). [76]

Boyd, S. et al. (2017), "Obtaining antibiotics online from within the UK: a cross-sectional study", *Journal of Antimicrobial Chemotherapy*, Vol. 72/5, pp. 1521-28, http://dx.doi.org/10.1093/jac/dkx003. [112]

Brink, A. et al. (2016), "Antimicrobial stewardship across 47 South African hospitals: an implementation study", *The Lancet Infectious Diseases*, Vol. 16/9, pp. 1017-1025, https://doi.org/10.1016/S1473-3099(16)30012-3. [35]

Brusselaers, N., D. Vogelaers and S. Blot (2011), "The rising problem of antimicrobial resistance in the intensive care unit", *Annals of Intensive Care*, Vol. 1/1, p. 47, http://dx.doi.org/10.1186/2110-5820-1-47. [30]

Carson, M. and D. Patrick (2015), "Do Bugs Need Drugs?" A community education program for the wise use of antibiotics", *Canada Communicable Disease Report*, Vol. 41/S4, pp. 5-8, https://doi.org/10.14745/ccdr.v41is4a02. [41]

Cashin, C. et al. (eds.) (2014), *Paying for Performance in Health Care: Implications for health system performance and accountability*, European Observatory on Health Systems and Policies Series, http://www.euro.who.int/__data/assets/pdf_file/0020/271073/Paying-for-Performance-in-Health-Care.pdf (accessed on 2 October 2018). [100]

CDC (2017), *Core Elements of Hospital Antibiotic Stewardship Programs*, https://www.cdc.gov/antibiotic-use/healthcare/pdfs/core-elements.pdf (accessed on 2 October 2018). [33]

CDC (2016), "CDC: 1 in 3 antibiotic prescriptions unnecessary", *CDC Newsroom*, CDC Newsroom Releases, https://www.cdc.gov/media/releases/2016/p0503-unnecessary-prescriptions.html (accessed on 2 October 2018). [166]

Cecchini, M., J. Langer and L. Slawomirski (2015), *Antimicrobial Resistance in G7 Countries and Beyond : Economic Issues, Policies and Options for Action*, OECD, Paris, http://www.oecd.org/els/health-systems/Antimicrobial-Resistance-in-G7-Countries-and-Beyond.pdf (accessed on 19 January 2018). [122]

Celhay, P. et al. (2015), "Long Run Effects of Temporary Incentives on Medical Care Productivity", *Nber Working Paper Series*, Vol. 21361, pp. 1-60, http://dx.doi.org/10.3386/w21361. [103]

Chaplin, S. (2015), "CRP testing could reduce antibiotic prescribing", *Prescriber*, Vol. 26/18, pp. 29-30, http://dx.doi.org/10.1002/psb.1387. [91]

Charani, E. et al. (2011), "Behavior change strategies to influence antimicrobial prescribing in acute care: A systematic review", *Clinical Infectious Diseases*, Vol. 53/7, pp. 651-662, http://dx.doi.org/10.1093/cid/cir445. [26]

Chen, A., C. Wessel and N. Rao (2013), "Staphylococcus aureus screening and decolonization in orthopaedic surgery and reduction of surgical site infections infection", *Clinical Orthopaedics and Related Research*, Vol. 471/7, pp. 2383-2399, http://dx.doi.org/10.1007/s11999-013-2875-0. [154]

Cheng, V. et al. (2015), "Strategic measures for the control of surging antimicrobial resistance in Hong Kong and mainland of China", *Emerging Microbes and Infections*, Vol. 4/2, p. 0, http://dx.doi.org/10.1038/emi.2015.8. [148]

Chopra, V. and S. Saint (2015), "Vascular catheter infections: Time to get technical", *The Lancet*, Vol. 386/10008, pp. 2034-2036, https://doi.org/10.1016/S0140-6736(15)00245-7. [120]

Cizman, M. (2008), "Experiences in Prevention and Control of Antibiotic Resistance in Slovenia", *Eurosurveillance*, Vol. 13/46, https://www.eurosurveillance.org/content/10.2807/ese.13.46.19038-en (accessed on 2 October 2018). [95]

Cizman, M. et al. (2015), "The long-term effects of restrictive interventions on consumption and costs of antibiotics", *Journal of Global Antimicrobial Resistance*, Vol. 3/1, pp. 31-35, https://doi.org/10.1016/j.jgar.2014.11.004. [93]

Cizman, M. et al. (2005), "Analysis of the causes and consequences of decreased antibiotic consumption over the last 5 years in Slovenia", *Journal of Antimicrobial Chemotherapy*, Vol. 55/5, pp. 758-763, http://dx.doi.org/10.1093/jac/dki098. [94]

Clarke, K. (2014), "When Should You Decolonize Methicillin-Resistant Staphylococcus aureus (MRSA) in Hospitalized Patients?", *The Hospitalist*, Vol. 11, https://www.the-hospitalist.org/hospitalist/article/122734/antimicrobial-resistant-infections/when-should-you-decolonize-methicillin (accessed on 2 October 2018). [155]

Cogliani, C., H. Goossens and C. Greko (2011), "Restricting Antimicrobial Use in in Food Animals : Lessons from Europe", *Microbe Magazine*, Vol. 6/6, pp. 274-279, http://dx.doi.org/10.1128/microbe.6.274.1. [10]

Conlon-Bingham, G. et al. (2016), "Reduction in the incidence of hospital-acquired MRSA following the introduction of a chlorine dioxide 275 ppm based disinfecting agent in a district general hospital", *European Journal of Hospital Pharmacy*, Vol. 23/1, pp. 28-32, http://dx.doi.org/10.1136/ejhpharm-2014-000608. [125]

Curtis, L. (2008), "Prevention of hospital-acquired infections: review of non-pharmacological interventions", *Journal of Hospital Infection*, Vol. 69/3, pp. 204-219, https://doi.org/10.1016/j.jhin.2008.03.018. [118]

Dancer, S. (2014), "Controlling hospital-acquired infection: Focus on the role of the environment and new technologies for decontamination", *Clinical Microbiology Reviews*, Vol. 27/4, pp. 665-690, http://dx.doi.org/10.1128/CMR.00020-14. [115]

Dancer, S. et al. (2009), "Measuring the effect of enhanced cleaning in a UK hospital: a prospective cross-over study", *BMC MEDICINE*, Vol. 7, http://dx.doi.org/10.1186/1741-7015-7-28. [126]

Davey, P. et al. (2013), "Interventions to improve antibiotic prescribing practices for hospital inpatients", *The Cochrane database of systematic reviews*, Vol. 4/4, p. CD003543, http://dx.doi.org/10.1002/14651858.CD003543.pub3. [19]

DiazGranados, C., D. Cardo and J. McGowan (2008), "Antimicrobial resistance: international control strategies, with a focus on limited-resource settings", *International Journal of Antimicrobial Agents*, Vol. 32/1, pp. 1-9, http://dx.doi.org/10.1016/j.ijantimicag.2008.03.002. [14]

Doan, Q. et al. (2012), "Rapid viral diagnosis for acute febrile respiratory illness in children in the Emergency Department", *Cochrane Database of Systematic Reviews* 9, pp. 4-6, http://dx.doi.org/10.1002/14651858.CD006452.pub3. [85]

Doll, M. and G. Bearman (2015), "The Increasing Visibility of the Threat of Health Care Worker Self-contamination.", *JAMA internal medicine*, Vol. 175/12, pp. 1911-1912, http://dx.doi.org/10.1001/jamainternmed.2015.5457. [121]

Donskey, C. (2013), "Does improving surface cleaning and disinfection reduce health care-associated infections?", *American Journal of Infection Control*, Vol. 41/5 SUPPL., pp. S12-S19, http://dx.doi.org/10.1016/j.ajic.2012.12.010. [116]

Do, N. et al. (2016), "Point-of-care C-reactive protein testing to reduce inappropriate use of antibiotics for non-severe acute respiratory infections in Vietnamese primary health care: a randomised controlled trial", *The Lancet Global Health*, Vol. 4/9, pp. e633-e641, https://doi.org/10.1016/S2214-109X(16)30142-5. [82]

Earnshaw, S. et al. (2009), "European Antibiotic Awarness Day 2008", *Eurosurveillance*, Vol. 14/30, https://doi.org/10.2807/ese.14.30.19280-en. [63]

Edgeworth, J. (2011), "Has decolonization played a central role in the decline in UK methicillin-resistant Staphylococcus aureus transmission? A focus on evidence from intensive care", *Journal of Antimicrobial Chemotherapy*, Vol. 66/SUPPL. 2, pp. 41-47, http://dx.doi.org/10.1093/jac/dkq325. [151]

El-Jardali, F. et al. (2015), "Interventions to combat or prevent drug counterfeiting: A systematic review", *BMJ Open*, Vol. 5/3, pp. 1-11, http://dx.doi.org/10.1136/bmjopen-2014-006290. [53]

Ellegård, L., J. Dietrichson and A. Anell (2017), "Can pay-for-performance to primary care providers stimulate appropriate use of antibiotics?", *Health Economics*, Vol. 27/1, pp. e39-e54, http://dx.doi.org/10.1002/hec.3535. [29]

Erasmus, V. et al. (2010), "Systematic Review of Studies on Compliance with Hand Hygiene Guidelines in Hospital Care", *Infection Control & Hospital Epidemiology*, Vol. 31/03, pp. 283-294, http://dx.doi.org/10.1086/650451. [131]

Fadlallah, R. et al. (2016), "Strategies and Systems-Level Interventions to Combat or Prevent Drug Counterfeiting: A Systematic Review of Evidence Beyond Effectiveness", *Pharmaceutical Medicine*, Vol. 30/5, pp. 263-276, http://dx.doi.org/10.1007/s40290-016-0156-4. [55]

FAO (2016), *The FAO Action Plan on Antimicrobial Resistance 2016-2020*, http://www.fao.org/3/a-i5996e.pdf (accessed on 2 October 2018). [3]

Fätkenheuer, G., B. Hirschel and S. Harbarth (2015), "Screening and isolation to control meticillin-resistant Staphylococcus aureus: sense, nonsense, and evidence", *The Lancet*, Vol. 385/9973, pp. 1146-1149, https://doi.org/10.1016/S0140-6736(14)60660-7. [134]

FDA (2017), *FDA conducts major global operation to protect consumers from potentially dangerous prescription drugs sold online*, FDA News Release, https://www.fda.gov/NewsEvents/Newsroom/PressAnnouncements/ucm577178.htm (accessed on 2 October 2018). [59]

Federal Ministry of Health (2015), *Combating Antimicrobial Resistance: Examples of Best-Practices of the G7 Countries*, Federal Ministry of Health, Germany, https://www.bundesgesundheitsministerium.de/fileadmin/Dateien/3_Downloads/G/G7/Best-Practices-Broschuere_G7.pdf (accessed on 2 October 2018). [105]

Fleming-Dutra, K. et al. (2016), "Prevalence of inappropriate antibiotic prescriptions among us ambulatory care visits, 2010-2011", *JAMA - Journal of the American Medical Association*, Vol. 315/17, pp. 1864-1873, http://dx.doi.org/10.1001/jama.2016.4151. [45]

Flodgren, G. et al. (2011), "An overview of reviews evaluating the effectiveness of financial incentives in changing healthcare professional behaviours and patient outcomes", *Cochrane Database of Systematic Reviews* 7, http://dx.doi.org/10.1002/14651858.CD009255. [99]

Food and Drug Adminnistration, HHS (2016), "Safety and Effectiveness of Consumer Antiseptics; Topical Antimicrobial Drug Products for Over-the-Counter Human Use. Final rule", *Federal register*, Vol. 81/172, pp. 61106-61130, https://www.federalregister.gov/documents/2016/09/06/2016-21337/safety-and-effectiveness-of-consumer-antiseptics-topical-antimicrobial-drug-products-for (accessed on 2 October 2018). [138]

Formoso, G. et al. (2013), "Feasibility and effectiveness of a low cost campaign on antibiotic prescribing in Italy: Community level, controlled, non-randomised trial", *BMJ (Online)*, Vol. 347/7926, pp. 1-10, http://dx.doi.org/10.1136/bmj.f5391. [66]

Foundation, A. (2018), *Antimicrobial Resistance Benchmark 2018*, Access to Medicine Foundation, https://amrbenchmark.org/wp-content/uploads/2018/04/Antimicrobial-Resistance-Benchmark-2018.pdf. [110]

Frickmann, H., W. Masanta and A. Zautner (2014), "Emerging rapid resistance testing methods for clinical microbiology laboratories and their potential impact on patient management", *Biomed Res Int*, Vol. 2014, p. 375681, http://dx.doi.org/10.1155/2014/375681 [doi]. [86]

G20 (2017), "Berlin Declaration of the G20 Health Ministers" May, pp. 1-7., https://www.bundesgesundheitsministerium.de/fileadmin/Dateien/3_Downloads/G/G20-Gesundheitsministertreffen/G20_Health_Ministers_Declaration_engl.pdf (accessed on 2 October 2018). [2]

Gerber, J., P. Prasad and A. Fiks (2013), "Effect of an Outpatient Antimicrobial Stewardship Intervention on Broad-Spectrum Antibiotic Prescribing by Primary Care PediatriciansA Randomized Trial", *JAMA - Journal of the American Medical Association*, Vol. 309/22, pp. 2345–2352, http://dx.doi.org/10.1001/jama.2013.6287. [75]

Ginsburg, A. and K. Klugman (2017), "Vaccination to reduce antimicrobial resistance", *The Lancet Global Health*, Vol. 5/12, https://doi.org/10.1016/S2214-109X(17)30364-9. [162]

Goff, D. et al. (2016), "A global call from five countries to collaborate in antibiotic stewardship: united we succeed, divided we might fail.", *The Lancet. Infectious diseases*, Vol. 3099/16, pp. 1-8, https://doi.org/10.1016/S1473-3099(16)30386-3. [27]

Gonzales, R. et al. (2008), ""Get Smart Colorado": Impact of a Mass Media Campaign to Improve Community Antibiotic Use", *Medical Care*, Vol. 46/6, pp. 597-605, http://dx.doi.org/10.1097/MLR.0b013e3181653d2e. [67]

Goossens, H. et al. (2008), "Achievements of the Belgian Antibiotic Policy Coordination Committee (BAPCOC)", *Eurosurveillance*, Vol. 13/46, pp. 6-9, https://doi.org/10.2807/ese.13.46.19036-en. [69]

Goutard, F. (2017), "Antimicrobial policy interventions in food animal production in South East Asia", *The BMJ*, Vol. 358/September 2016, http://dx.doi.org/10.1136/bmj.j3544. [11]

Graves, N. et al. (2016), "Cost-Effectiveness of a national initiative to improve hand hygiene compliance using the outcome of healthcare associated staphylococcus aureus bacteraemia", *PLoS ONE*, Vol. 11/2, pp. 1-17, http://dx.doi.org/10.1371/journal.pone.0148190. [142]

Greenwood, B. (2014), "The contribution of vaccination to global health: past, present and future", *Philosophical Transactions of the Royal Society B: Biological Sciences*, Vol. 369/1645, pp. 20130433-20130433, http://dx.doi.org/10.1098/rstb.2013.0433. [169]

Gulliford, M. et al. (2016), "Safety of reduced antibiotic prescribing for self limiting respiratory tract infections in primary care: cohort study using electronic health records", *BMJ*, Vol. 354354, pp. 1-10, http://dx.doi.org/10.1136/bmj.i3410. [48]

Hand Hygiene Australia (2018), *Hand Hygiene Australia*, https://www.hha.org.au/hand-hygiene/hha (accessed on 2 October 2018). [139]

Hand Hygiene Australia (2017), *National Data Period Three 2017*, https://www.hha.org.au/audits/national-data/2017 (accessed on 2 October 2018). [140]

Høgli, J. et al. (2016), "An audit and feedback intervention study increased adherence to antibiotic prescribing guidelines at a Norwegian hospital", *BMC Infectious Diseases*, Vol. 16/1, pp. 1-11, http://dx.doi.org/10.1186/s12879-016-1426-1. [52]

Holloway, K. and L. van Dijk (2011), *The World Medicines Situation 2011: Rational Use of Medicines*, World Health Organization, http://www.who.int/medicines/areas/policy/world_medicines_situation/WMS_ch14_wRational.pdf (accessed on 2 October 2018). [4]

Huang, Y. et al. (2013), "Association between point-of-care CRP testing and antibiotic prescribing in respiratory tract infections: A systematic review and meta-analysis of primary care studies", *British Journal of General Practice*, Vol. 63/616, pp. 787-794, http://dx.doi.org/10.3399/bjgp13X674477. [81]

Huddy, J. et al. (2016), "Point-of-care C reactive protein for the diagnosis of lower respiratory tract infection in NHS primary care : a qualitative study of barriers and facilitators to adoption", *BMJ Open*, Vol. 6/3, pp. 1-9, http://dx.doi.org/10.1136/bmjopen-2015-009959. [92]

Hulscher, M. and J. Prins (2017), "Antibiotic stewardship: does it work in hospital practice? A review of the evidence base", *Clinical Microbiology and Infection*, Vol. 23/11, pp. 799-805, https://doi.org/10.1016/j.cmi.2017.07.017. [24]

Hunter, R. (2015), "Cost-Effectiveness of Point-of-Care C-Reactive Protein Tests for Respiratory Tract Infection in Primary Care in England", *Advances in Therapy*, Vol. 32/1, pp. 69-85, http://dx.doi.org/10.1007/s12325-015-0180-x. [90]

Huttner, B. and S. Harbarth (2009), "Antibiotics Are Not Automatic Anymore—The French National Campaign To Cut Antibiotic Overuse", *PLoS Medicine*, Vol. 6/6, https://www.ncbi.nlm.nih.gov/pmc/articles/PMC2683568/pdf/pmed.1000080.pdf (accessed on 2 October 2018). [71]

Huttner, B., S. Harbarth and D. Nathwani (2014), "Success stories of implementation of antimicrobial stewardship: A narrative review", *Clinical Microbiology and Infection*, Vol. 20/10, pp. 954-962, http://dx.doi.org/10.1111/1469-0691.12803. [34]

IFPMA (2016), "Declaration by the Pharmaceutical, Biotecnology, and Diagnostics Industries on Combatting Antimicrobial Resistance" January, https://www.ifpma.org/resource-centre/declaration-by-the-pharmaceutical-biotechnology-and-diagnostics-industries-on-combating-antimicrobial-resistance/ (accessed on 2 October 2018). [108]

IFPMA (2016), "Global Biopharmaceutical Industry Takes Action to Combat Antimicrobial Resistance (AMR)", https://www.ifpma.org/resource-centre/global-biopharmaceutical-industry-takes-action-to-combat-antimicrobial-resistance-amr/ (accessed on 2 October 2018). [109]

IFPMA (2016), "Industry Roadmap for Progress on Combating Antimicrobial Resistance – September 2016", https://www.ifpma.org/wp-content/uploads/2018/06/Roadmap-for-Progress-on-AMR-FINAL.pdf (accessed on 2 October 2018). [159]

INTERPOL (2018), *Pharmaceutical-crime - Operations*, https://www.interpol.int/Crime-areas/Pharmaceutical-crime/Operations/Operation-Pangea (accessed on 2 October 2018). [60]

INTERPOL (2017), *Millions of medicines seized in largest INTERPOL operation against illicit online pharmacies*, INTERPOL News Release, https://www.interpol.int/News-and-media/News/2017/N2017-119. [61]

Jansen, K., C. Knirsch and A. Anderson (2018), "The role of vaccines in preventing bacterial antimicrobial resistance", *Nature Medicine*, Vol. 24/1, pp. 10-20, http://dx.doi.org/10.1038/nm.4465. [161]

Japan Ministry of Health (2016), "About the Handling of Procedures Relating to Facility Standards and the Notification of Basic Medical Care Fee (Japanese)", https://www.mhlw.go.jp/file/06-Seisakujouhou-12400000-Hokenkyoku/0000114881.pdf (accessed on 3 October 2018). [107]

Karanika, S. et al. (2016), "Systematic review and meta-analysis of clinical and economic outcomes from the implementation of hospital-based antimicrobial stewardship programs", *Antimicrobial Agents and Chemotherapy*, Vol. 60/8, pp. 4840-4852, http://dx.doi.org/10.1128/AAC.00825-16. [37]

Kinoshita, T. et al. (2017), "Policy implementation for methicillin-resistant <i>Staphylococcus aureus</i> in seven European countries: a comparative analysis from 1999 to 2015", *Journal of Market Access & Health Policy*, Vol. 5/1, p. 1351293, http://dx.doi.org/10.1080/20016689.2017.1351293. [22]

Kirkland, K. et al. (2012), "Impact of a hospital-wide hand hygiene initiative on healthcare-associated infections: Results of an interrupted time series", *BMJ Quality and Safety*, Vol. 21/12, pp. 1019-1026, http://dx.doi.org/10.1136/bmjqs-2012-000800. [135]

Kondo, K. et al. (2016), "Implementation Processes and Pay for Performance in Healthcare: A Systematic Review", *Journal of General Internal Medicine*, Vol. 31, pp. 61-69, http://dx.doi.org/10.1007/s11606-015-3567-0. [104]

Kwong, J. et al. (2009), "The Effect of Universal Influenza Immunization on Antibiotic Prescriptions: An Ecological Study", *Clinical Infectious Diseases*, Vol. 49/5, pp. 750-756, http://dx.doi.org/10.1086/605087. [167]

Kyaw, M. (2006), "Effect of introduction of the pneumococcal conjugate vaccine on drug-resistant Streptococcus pneumoniae", *New England Journal of Medicine*, Vol. 354, pp. 1455-1463, http://dx.doi.org/10.1056/NEJMoa051642. [164]

Lambert, M., G. Masters and S. Brent (2007), "Can mass media campaigns change antimicrobial prescribing? A regional evaluation study", *Journal of Antimicrobial Chemotherapy*, Vol. 59/3, pp. 537-543, http://dx.doi.org/10.1093/jac/dkl511. [65]

Laxminarayan, R. et al. (2016), "Access to effective antimicrobials: a worldwide challenge", *The Lancet*, Vol. 387/10014, pp. 168-175, https://doi.org/10.1016/S0140-6736(15)00474-2. [163]

Linder, J. et al. (2014), "Time of Day and the Decision to Prescribe Antibiotics", *JAMA Internal Medicine*, Vol. 174/12, pp. 2029–2031, http://dx.doi.org/10.1001/jamainternmed.2014.5225. [25]

Little, P. et al. (2014), "Delayed antibiotic prescribing strategies for respiratory tract infections in primary care: Pragmatic, factorial, randomised controlled trial", *BMJ (Online)*, Vol. 348/March, pp. 1-8, http://dx.doi.org/10.1136/bmj.g1606. [50]

Little, P. et al. (2013), "Clinical score and rapid antigen detection test to guide antibiotic use for sore throats: Randomised controlled trial of PRISM (primary care streptococcal management)", *BMJ (Online)*, Vol. 347/7930, pp. 1-10, http://dx.doi.org/10.1136/bmj.f5806. [84]

Little, P. et al. (2017), "Antibiotic prescription strategies and adverse outcome for uncomplicated lower respiratory tract infections: Prospective cough complication cohort (3C) study", *BMJ (Online)*, Vol. 357, http://dx.doi.org/10.1136/bmj.j2148. [47]

Luangasanatip, N. et al. (2015), "Comparative efficacy of interventions to promote hand hygiene in hospital: systematic review and network meta-analysis", *BMJ*, Vol. 351, p. h3728, http://dx.doi.org/10.1136/bmj.h3728. [137]

Mainous, A. et al. (2009), "Availability of antibiotics for purchase without a prescription on the internet", *Annals of Family Medicine*, Vol. 7/5, pp. 431-435, http://dx.doi.org/10.1370/afm.999. [57]

McDonald, R. et al. (2015), "A qualitative and quantitative evaluation of the Advancing Quality pay-for-performance programme in the NHS North West", *Health Services and Delivery Research*, Vol. 3/23, pp. 1-104, http://dx.doi.org/10.3310/hsdr03230. [97]

McKay, R. et al. (2011), "Evaluation of the Do Bugs need Drugs? Program in British Columbia: Can we curb antibiotic prescribing?", *Canadian Journal of Infectious Diseases and Medical Microbiology*, Vol. 22/1, pp. 19-24, http://dx.doi.org/10.1155/2011/745090. [42]

McNulty, C. et al. (2010), "The English antibiotic awareness campaigns: Did they change the public's knowledge of and attitudes to antibiotic use?", *Journal of Antimicrobial Chemotherapy*, Vol. 65/7, pp. 1526-1533, http://dx.doi.org/10.1093/jac/dkq126. [16]

Miller, E. and H. Sikes (2015), "Addressing Barriers to the Development and Adoption of Rapid Diagnostic Tests in Global Health", https://doi.org/10.5772%2F61114. [87]

Milmo, S. (2017), "Pharmaceutical Environmental Pollution and Antimicrobial Resistance", *Pharmaceutical Technology*, Vol. 41/10, http://www.pharmtech.com/pharmaceutical-environmental-pollution-and-antimicrobial-resistance (accessed on 3 October 2018). [158]

MoHFW (2016), *Operational Guidelines: Swachh Swasth Sarvtra*, Ministry of Health and Family Welfare, India, http://kayakalpraj.org/assets/Guideline/Swachh_swasth_sarvtra_Guidelines_-_for_ODF_CHC.pdf (accessed on 2 October 2018). [124]

Morgan, D. et al. (2011), "Non-prescription antimicrobial use worldwide: a systematic review.", *The Lancet. Infectious diseases*, Vol. 11/9, pp. 692-701, https://doi.org/10.1016/S1473-3099(11)70054-8. [13]

Morrill, H. et al. (2016), "Antimicrobial Stewardship in Long-Term Care Facilities: A Call to Action", *Journal of the American Medical Directors Association*, Vol. 17/2, pp. 183.e1-183.e16, http://dx.doi.org/10.1016/j.jamda.2015.11.013. [31]

Mundaca-shah, C. et al. (2017), *Combating Antimicrobial Resistance: A One Health Approach to a Global Threat*, National Academy of Sciences, http://dx.doi.org/10.17226/24914. [89]

Nebraska Medicine (2017), *Establishing Antimicrobial Stewardship Programs in Small and Critical Access Hospitals*, https://asap.nebraskamed.com/establishing-antimicrobial-stewardship-programs-small-critical-access-hospitals/ (accessed on 1 October 2018). [32]

Newhouse, J. and the insurance experiment group (1993), *Free for all? Lesson from the Rand Health Insurance experiment*, Harvard University Press. [101]

NICE (2018), *NICE Pathways: Pneumonia*, NICE Pathways, https://pathways.nice.org.uk/pathways/pneumonia. [79]

NICE (2012), "Healthcare-associated infections: prevention and control in primary and community care", *NICE Guideline* March, https://www.nice.org.uk/Guidance/CG139 (accessed on 2 October 2018). [133]

NICE (2008), *Respiratory tract infections (self-limiting): prescribing antibiotics*, https://www.nice.org.uk/Guidance/CG69 (accessed on 2 October 2018). [51]

OECD et al. (2017), *Tackling Antimicrobial Resistance Ensuring Sustainable R&D*, http://www.oecd.org/els/health-systems/G20-AMR-Final-Paper-2017.pdf (accessed on 08 May 2018). [172]

O'Neill, J. (2015), *Safe, Secure and Controlled: Managing the Supply Chain of Antimicrobials*, Review on Microbial Resistance, https://amr-review.org/sites/default/files/Safe,%20secure%20and%20controlled%20-%20Managing%20the%20supply%20chain%20of%20antimicrobials.pdf (accessed on 2 October 2018). [58]

Otter, J. et al. (2013), "Low prevalence of meticillin-resistant Staphylococcus aureus carriage at hospital admission: Implications for risk-factor-based vs universal screening", *Journal of Hospital Infection*, Vol. 83/2, pp. 114-121, http://dx.doi.org/10.1016/j.jhin.2012.10.008. [23]

Otter, J. et al. (2015), "Controversies in guidelines for the control of multidrug-resistant Gram-negative bacteria in EU countries", *Clinical Microbiology and Infection*, Vol. 21/12, pp. 1057-1066, http://dx.doi.org/10.1016/j.cmi.2015.09.021. [146]

Peeling, R. and D. Boeras (2016), *Diagnostic Innovation for Antimicrobial Resistance*, AMR Control, http://resistancecontrol.info/2016/diagnostics/diagnostic-innovation-for-antimicrobial-resistance/ (accessed on 2 October 2018). [88]

Peters, S. et al. (2011), "Managing self-limiting respiratory tract infections :", *British Journal of General Practice* March, pp. 579-589, https://doi.org/10.3399%2Fbjgp11X593866. [44]

PharmacyMagazine (2017), *Boots supports World Antibiotic Awareness Week*, https://www.pharmacymagazine.co.uk/boots-supports-world-antibiotic-awareness-week. [113]

Plachouras, D. et al. (2014), "Promoting prudent use of antibiotics: the experience from a multifaceted regional campaign in Greece.", *BMC public health*, Vol. 14/1, p. 866, http://dx.doi.org/10.1186/1471-2458-14-866. [74]

Public Health England (2017), *Guidance: Health matters: preventing infections and reducing antimicrobial resistance*, GOV.UK, https://www.gov.uk/government/publications/health-matters-preventing-infections-and-reducing-amr/health-matters-preventing-infections-and-reducing-antimicrobial-resistance (accessed on 2 October 2018). [156]

Pulcini, C. (2015), "Tackling Antimicrobial Resistance through Prescription Control in Human Health", *AMR Control* 12, pp. 62-66, http://www.globalhealthdynamics.co.uk/wp-content/uploads/2015/06/AMR2015-June-3.pdf (accessed on 2 October 2018). [18]

Robicsek, A. et al. (2009), "Topical Therapy for Methicillin-Resistant Staphylococcus aureus Colonization Impact on Infection Risk", *Infection Control & Hospital Epidemiology*, Vol. 30/07, pp. 623-632, http://dx.doi.org/10.1086/597550. [152]

Roque, F. et al. (2014), "Educational interventions to improve prescription and dispensing of antibiotics: a systematic review.", *BMC public health*, Vol. 14/1, p. 1276, http://dx.doi.org/10.1186/1471-2458-14-1276. [73]

Rotthier, K. and M. Gharabaghi (2015), "How the pharmaceutical industry is contributing to antimicrobial resistance", *The Pharmaceutical Journal*, https://www.pharmaceutical-journal.com/opinion/comment/how-the-pharmaceutical-industry-is-contributing-to-antimicrobial-resistance/20068073.fullarticle?firstPass=false (accessed on 2 October 2018). [157]

Ryves, R. et al. (2016), "Understanding the delayed prescribing of antibiotics for respiratory tract infection in primary care: A qualitative analysis", *BMJ Open*, Vol. 6/11, pp. 1-12, http://dx.doi.org/10.1136/bmjopen-2016-011882. [49]

Sachdeva, K. et al. (2015), "The potential impact of up-front drug sensitivity testing on India's epidemic of multi-drug resistant tuberculosis", *PLoS ONE*, Vol. 10/7, pp. 1-15, http://dx.doi.org/10.1371/journal.pone.0131438. [77]

Santa-Ana-Tellez, Y. et al. (2016), "Effects of over the counter sales restriction of antibiotics on substitution with medicines for symptoms relief of cold in Mexico and Brazil: Time series analysis", *Health Policy and Planning*, Vol. 31/9, pp. 1291-1296, http://dx.doi.org/10.1093/heapol/czw066. [62]

Schaffer, S., J. Sussex and Y. Feng (2015), "Incentives to follow Best Practice in Health Care", *OHE Briefing* 55 February, https://www.ohe.org/publications/incentives-follow-best-practice-health-care (accessed on 2 October 2018). [96]

Schweizer, M. et al. (2013), "Effectiveness of a bundled intervention of decolonization and prophylaxis to decrease Gram positive surgical site infections after cardiac or orthopedic surgery: Systematic review and meta-analysis", *BMJ (Online)*, Vol. 346/7912, pp. 1-13, http://dx.doi.org/10.1136/bmj.f2743. [153]

Scott, A. and C. Del Mar (2017), "Controlling antibiotic prescribing for lower respiratory tract infections", *Bmj*, Vol. 2398, p. j2398, http://dx.doi.org/10.1136/bmj.j2398. [21]

Semret, M. et al. (2016), "Cleaning the grey zones of hospitals: A prospective, crossover, interventional study", *American Journal of Infection Control*, Vol. 44/12, pp. 1582-1588, http://dx.doi.org/10.1016/j.ajic.2016.04.234. [127]

Shah, A. et al. (2017), "Strengthening laboratory surveillance of antimicrobial resistance in South East Asia.", *BMJ (Clinical research ed.)*, Vol. 358, p. j3474, http://dx.doi.org/10.1136/BMJ.J3474. [12]

Shet, A., S. Sundaresan and B. Forsberg (2015), "Pharmacy-based dispensing of antimicrobial agents without prescription in India: Appropriateness and cost burden in the private sector", *Antimicrobial Resistance and Infection Control*, Vol. 4/1, pp. 1-7, http://dx.doi.org/10.1186/s13756-015-0098-8. [56]

Siegel, J. et al. (2017), "Management of Multidrug - Resistant Organisms In Healthcare Settings, 2006", pp. 1-74, https://www.cdc.gov/infectioncontrol/pdf/guidelines/mdro-guidelines.pdf (accessed on 2 October 2018). [128]

Spurling, G. et al. (2017), "Delayed antibiotic prescriptions for respiratory infections", *Cochrane Database of Systematic Reviews*, Vol. 2017/9, http://dx.doi.org/10.1002/14651858.CD004417.pub5. [46]

Sroka, S., P. Gastmeier and E. Meyer (2010), "Impact of alcohol hand-rub use on meticillin-resistant Staphylococcus aureus: an analysis of the literature", *Journal of Hospital Infection*, Vol. 74/3, pp. 204-211, http://dx.doi.org/10.1016/j.jhin.2009.08.023. [130]

Swaminathan, S. et al. (2017), "Strengthening infection prevention and control and systematic surveillance of healthcare associated infections in India", *BMJ (Online)*, Vol. 358, pp. 59-62, http://dx.doi.org/10.1136/bmj.j3768. [123]

Tacconelli, E. (2009), "Screening and isolation for infection control", *Journal of Hospital Infection*, Vol. 73/4, pp. 371-377, http://dx.doi.org/10.1016/j.jhin.2009.05.002. [145]

Tang, K. et al. (2017), "Restricting the use of antibiotics in food-producing animals and its associations with antibiotic resistance in food-producing animals and human beings: a systematic review and meta-analysis", *The Lancet Planetary Health*, Vol. 1/8, pp. e316-e327, https://doi.org/10.1016/S2542-5196(17)30141-9. [8]

The Government of the Hong Kong Special Administrative Region (2017), "National Action Plan on Antimicrobial Resistance (2017-2022)", p. 57, https://www.chp.gov.hk/files/pdf/amr_action_plan_eng.pdf (accessed on 2 October 2018). [150]

Thoolen, B., D. de Ridder and G. van Lensvelt-Mulders (2011), "Patient-oriented interventions to improve antibiotic prescribing practices in respiratory tract infections: a meta-analysis", *Health Psychology Review*, Vol. 6/1, pp. 92-112, http://dx.doi.org/10.1080/17437199.2011.552061. [64]

Tomas, M. et al. (2015), "Contamination of Health Care Personnel During Removal of Personal Protective Equipment", *JAMA Internal Medicine*, Vol. 44106, pp. 1-7, http://dx.doi.org/10.1001/jamainternmed.2015.4535. [119]

Tonkin-Crine, S. et al. (2017), "Clinician-targeted interventions to influence antibiotic prescribing behaviour for acute respiratory infections in primary care: an overview of systematic reviews", *Cochrane Database of Systematic Reviews* 9, http://dx.doi.org/10.1002/14651858.CD012252.pub2. [72]

Tsang, K. et al. (2012), "Hong Kong experiences the 'ultimate superbug': NDM-1 Enterobacteriaceae", *Hong Kong Medical Journal*, Vol. 18/5, pp. 439-441, http://www.hkmj.org/system/files/hkm1210p439.pdf (accessed on 2 October 2018). [147]

Van Boeckel, T. et al. (2015), "Global trends in antimicrobial use in food animals", *Proceedings of the National Academy of Sciences*, Vol. 112/18, pp. 5649-5654, http://dx.doi.org/10.1073/pnas.1503141112. [7]

Van der Bij, A. and J. Pitout (2012), "The role of international travel in the worldwide spread of multiresistant enterobacteriaceae", *Journal of Antimicrobial Chemotherapy*, Vol. 67/9, pp. 2090-2100, http://dx.doi.org/10.1093/jac/dks214. [20]

Van Dijck, C., E. Vliegheb and J. Coxc (2018), "Antibiotic stewardship interventions in hospitals in low- and middle-income countries : a systematic review", *Systematic Reviews (World Health Organization)* January, pp. 266-280, http://dx.doi.org/10.2471/BLT.17.203448. [36]

van Dongen, M. (2018), *Full screening superbug begins as Hong Kong hospitals battle rising numbers*, AMR Insights, https://www.amr-insights.eu/en/full-screening-for-superbug-begins-as-hong-kong-hospitals-battle-rising-number-cases/ (accessed on 2 October 2018). [149]

von Gottberg, A. et al. (2014), "Effects of Vaccination on Invasive Pneumococcal Disease in South Africa", *New England Journal of Medicine*, Vol. 371/20, pp. 1889-1899, http://dx.doi.org/10.1056/NEJMoa1401914. [165]

Vos, M., A. Ott and H. Verbrugh (2005), "Successful Search-and-Destroy Policy for Methicillin-Resistant Staphylococcus aureus in The Netherlands", *Journal of Clinical Microbiology*, Vol. 43/4, pp. 2034-2035, https://dx.doi.org/10.1128%2FJCM.43.4.2034-2035.2005. [144]

Wang, L. et al. (2016), "Addressing antimicrobial resistance in China: policy implementation in a complex context", *Globalization and Health*, Vol. 12/1, p. 30, http://dx.doi.org/10.1186/s12992-016-0167-7. [40]

Weber, D., H. Kanamori and W. Rutala (2016), "'No touch' technologies for environmental decontamination: Focus on ultraviolet devices and hydrogen peroxide systems", *Current Opinion in Infectious Diseases*, Vol. 29/4, pp. 424-431, http://dx.doi.org/10.1097/QCO.0000000000000284. [117]

WHO (2018), *Global Health Observatory data repository - Immunization*, World Health Organization, http://apps.who.int/gho/data/node.main.A824?lang=en (accessed on 25 September 2018). [173]

WHO (2018), "Immunization coverage: Key Facts", http://www.who.int/en/news-room/fact-sheets/detail/immunization-coverage (accessed on 2 October 2018). [168]

WHO (2017), *Global Priority List of Antibiotic-resistant Bacteria to Guide Research, Discovery, and Development of New Antibiotics*, World Health Organization, http://www.who.int/medicines/publications/WHO-PPL-Short_Summary_25Feb-ET_NM_WHO.pdf (accessed on 2 October 2018). [171]

WHO (2017), "Immunization, Vaccines and Biologicals: WHO/UNICEF Joint Reporting Process", http://www.who.int/immunization/monitoring_surveillance/routine/reporting/en/ (accessed on 25 September 2018). [174]

WHO (2017), *One Health*, World Health Organization, http://www.who.int/features/qa/one-health/en/ (accessed on 09 May 2018). [9]

WHO (2016), *Evaluation of antibiotic awareness campaigns*, WHO Collaborating Centre on Patient Safety, Geneva, http://www.who.int/selection_medicines/committees/expert/21/applications/s6_antibiotic_awareness_campaigns.pdf?ua=1 (accessed on 2 October 2018). [68]

WHO (2015), *Global Action Plan on Antimicrobial Resistance*, World Health Organization, Geneva, http://apps.who.int/iris/bitstream/10665/193736/1/9789241509763_eng.pdf?ua=1 (accessed on 13 July 2017). [1]

WHO (2001), *WHO Global Strategy for Containment of Antimicrobial Resistance*, World Health Organization, http://www.who.int/drugresistance/WHO_Global_Strategy_English.pdf (accessed on 2 October 2018). [15]

WHO-Europe (2014), *The role of pharmacist in encouraging prudent use of antibiotics and averting antimicrobial resistance: a review of policy and experience*, World Health Organization - Europe, http://www.euro.who.int/__data/assets/pdf_file/0006/262815/The-role-of-pharmacist-in-encouraging-prudent-use-of-antibiotics-and-averting-antimicrobial-resistance-a-review-of-policy-and-experience-Eng.pdf (accessed on 2 October 2018). [17]

WHO, FAO and OIE (2018), *Global Database for AMRCSAT Country Self-Assessment Test*, https://extranet.who.int/sree/Reports?op=vs&path=%2FWHO_HQ_Reports/G45/PROD/EXT/amrcsat_AnswersForPublic (accessed on 18 May 2018). [5]

WHO, FAO and OIE (2018), *Global Database for Antimicrobial Resistance Country Self Assessment*, http://amrcountryprogress.org/ (accessed on 20 July 2018). [6]

Williams, N. et al. (2011), "Primary care strategies to improve childhood immunisation uptake in developed countries: systematic review", *JRSM Short Reports*, Vol. 2/10, pp. 1-21, http://dx.doi.org/10.1258/shorts.2011.011112. [170]

Wilson, A. et al. (2016), "Prevention and control of multi-drug-resistant Gram-negative bacteria: recommendations from a Joint Working Party", *Journal of Hospital Infection*, Vol. 92/1, pp. S1-S44, http://dx.doi.org/10.1016/j.jhin.2015.08.007. [132]

Worby, C. et al. (2013), "Estimating the effectiveness of isolation and decolonization measures in reducing transmission of methicillin-resistant staphylococcus aureus in hospital general wards", *American Journal of Epidemiology*, Vol. 177/11, pp. 1306-1313, http://dx.doi.org/10.1093/aje/kws380. [143]

World Bank (2016), "Drug-resistant infections: A Threat to Our Economic Future", *World Bank Report* September, pp. 1-132, http://documents.worldbank.org/curated/en/323311493396993758/final-report (accessed on 2 October 2018). [111]

Wushouer, H. et al. (2017), "Trends and patterns of antibiotic consumption in China's tertiary hospitals: Based on a 5 year surveillance with sales records, 2011-2015.", *PloS one*, Vol. 12/12, p. e0190314, http://dx.doi.org/10.1371/journal.pone.0190314. [39]

Xiao, Y. et al. (2013), "Changes in Chinese Policies to Promote the Rational Use of Antibiotics", *PLoS Medicine*, Vol. 10/11, pp. 1-4, http://dx.doi.org/10.1371/journal.pmed.1001556. [38]

Yip, W. et al. (2014), "Capitation combined with pay-for-performance improves antibiotic prescribing practices in Rural China", *Health Affairs*, Vol. 33/3, pp. 502-510, http://dx.doi.org/10.1377/hlthaff.2013.0702. [98]

Zowawi, H. et al. (2015), "The potential role of social media platforms in community awareness of antibiotic use in the gulf cooperation council states: Luxury or necessity?", *Journal of Medical Internet Research*, Vol. 17/10, http://dx.doi.org/10.2196/jmir.3891. [70]

Chapter 6. Cost-effectiveness of antimicrobial resistance control policies

Driss Ait Ouakrim, Michele Cecchini, Michael Padget and Tiago Cravo Oliveira

The impact of antimicrobial resistance (AMR) on health and health systems expenditure is substantial and set to increase dramatically if no action is taken to curb current trends. Existing AMR control policies have the potential to significantly influence the burden of AMR through first reducing the risk of transmission of infections or by reducing the inappropriate prescription and use of antimicrobials. This chapter reports the findings of a cost-effectiveness model developed to assess and compare the health and economic impact of a number of AMR control policies relative to a business-as-usual scenario in which there are no interventions. The OECD SPHeP-AMR model was used to assess performances of six selected policies – stewardship programmes, improved hand hygiene, enhanced environmental hygiene, rapid diagnostic tests, delayed prescriptions and mass media campaigns – if they were scaled up to national levels in 33 countries. The effects of each AMR control policy on health outcomes and health care expenditure for the 33 countries included in the microsimulation are presented, along with the possible impact of combining different policies. Finally, the strengths and weaknesses of the findings and sensitivity analysis of the main outcomes are discussed.

Note by Turkey:

The information in this document with reference to "Cyprus" relates to the southern part of the Island. There is no single authority representing both Turkish and Greek Cypriot people on the Island. Turkey recognises the Turkish Republic of Northern Cyprus (TRNC). Until a lasting and equitable solution is found within the context of the United Nations, Turkey shall preserve its position concerning the "Cyprus issue".

Note by all the European Union Member States of the OECD and the European Union:

The Republic of Cyprus is recognised by all members of the United Nations with the exception of Turkey. The information in this document relates to the area under the effective control of the Government of the Republic of Cyprus.

Key findings

- The majority of antimicrobial resistance (AMR) deaths can be prevented. Upscaling stewardship programmes, improved hand hygiene and enhanced environmental hygiene policies to national levels would reduce the annual AMR mortality by on average 54% to 58%.
- Hospital-based AMR control policies can result in up to 2 000 disability-adjusted life years (DALYs) gained per 100 000 persons per year across the included countries
- The health gains associated with the six control policies tested in the model appear almost immediately following their implementation.
- Control policies would substantially reduce the number of hospital days due to AMR – up to 800-1 000 hospital days avoided per 100 000 persons, per year for countries with the highest incidence of AMR.
- For most AMP control policies, implementation costs are largely offset by the savings generated, including for relatively expensive strategies, such as enhanced environmental hygiene, stewardship programmes and rapid diagnostic tests.
- Improved hand hygiene represents a particularly good investment as its average annual implementation across the countries considered is around USD PPP 8 500 per 100 000 persons for a net return of around USD PPP 140 000.
- Across all countries, the AMR control policies included in the model deliver high value for money, and for a number of them, represent "best buys" as they generate savings for the health care system.
- Combining multiple AMR control policies in a broader policy package would generate overall effects (in terms of disease burden and healthcare expenditure) close to the sum of the effects of the individual component policies.
- A policy package including all three hospital-based policies would save on average USD PPP 1.2 million per 100 000 persons, per year.
- A community-based policy package and a mixed policy package, would result, respectively, in average reductions in health care expenditure of approximately USD PPP 275 000 and USD PPP 920 000, per year.

6.1. Determining the opportunity cost due AMR

The potential impact of AMR on population morbidity and mortality, health care expenditure and the broader economy is a major cause of concern for health agencies, governments and a variety of policy makers and stakeholders worldwide. The number of recent initiatives and analyses that have attempted to assess the long-term effects of resistance illustrates an increased level of awareness, at the global economic and institutional level, of the threats of AMR. The O'Neil review and the World Bank report on drug-resistant infections, discussed in Chapter 4, are the most recent examples of a series of high-profile government-commissioned publications investigating the potential health and economic burden of AMR. This type of analytical work – which includes the OECD model presented in Chapter 4 – is primarily descriptive. As such, it is fundamental as it provides baseline information that can guide AMR policy and on which further analyses can be developed. In economic terms, however, such evaluations can be considered as partial because they do not provide a complete picture of the potential impact of AMR. More specifically, they fail to estimate the "opportunity cost" associated with AMR – which represents what society is missing out on by committing resources (treatment cost, productivity, life years, etc.) to dealing with the consequences of AMR and not allocating resources to something else. That opportunity cost can only be estimated through the comparison of alternative courses of action or events in terms of both their costs and consequences.

This chapter reports the findings of a cost-effectiveness model (see Box 6.1) developed to assess and compare the health and economic impact of a number of AMR control policies relative to a business-as-usual scenario in which there are no interventions. The objective of the model is to evaluate if the implementation of the selected policies, scaled up to national levels, can reduce the health and economic burden of AMR, the extent of that reduction, if any, and whether those policies would represent efficient investments for governments. The effects of each AMR control policy on health outcomes and health care expenditure for the 33 countries included in the microsimulation are presented, along with the possible impact of combining different policies. Finally, the strengths and weaknesses of the findings and sensitivity analysis of the main outcomes are discussed.

Box 6.1. Modelling the cost-effectiveness of AMR control policies

The cost-effectiveness analysis is based on the microsimulation and model parameters described in Chapter 4. The model relies on three main components:

- A demographic module, which allows the model to account for population demographic evolution (births and deaths). This approach enables the model to reproduce the population dynamics of the included countries.
- A risk factor module, which includes the exposures of interest. These are the incidence rates of the antibiotic-bacterium combinations included in the study, and the variations of those rates for specific interventions.
- An outcome module, which produces results from the two first modules and their interactions.

The model described in Chapter 4 constitutes the business-as-usual scenario and its estimates and projections of country-specific outcomes (i.e. AMR mortality, DALYs, health expenditure, and hospital days) were used as the base-case values to which the effects of the selected AMR control policies were compared. The analysis was performed under the assumption that no policies are implemented beyond the policies already in place, and that any potential effects of existing national AMR policies – in terms of reduction in the number of resistant infections – are fully reflected in the AMR incidence data implemented in the model. Figure 6.1 summarises the general approach of the model.

The cost-effectiveness of six AMR control policies and three packages of policies was determined, with specific models for each one of the 33 countries considered, based on the incremental cost-effectiveness ratio (ICER) associated with each policy or package of policies. Outcomes were calculated over the microsimulation period (2015-2050) and a 3% discount rate was applied to future estimates. For all countries, each policy scenario was run 20 000 times in Monte Carlo analyses, to determine 95% uncertainty intervals (UIs) and probabilities of cost-effectiveness.

Figure 6.1. Modelling approach

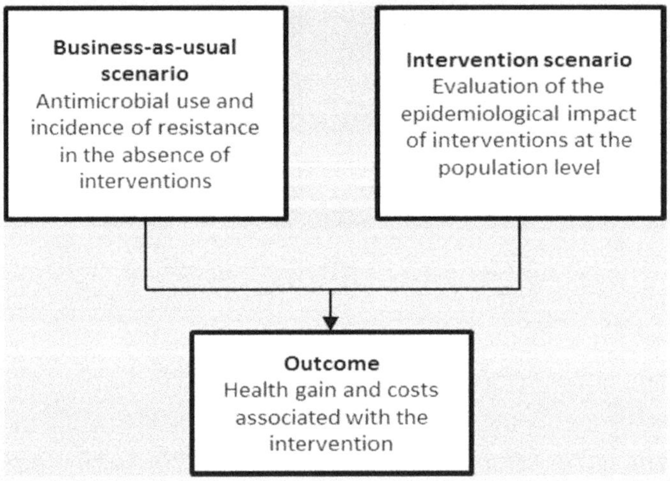

The cost-effectiveness status of the policies was determined in two steps:

1. The value of their ICERs was calculated – as the difference in costs between an intervention and the base-case scenario, divided by the difference in effects between an intervention and the base case. The ratio obtained represents the cost per unit of health outcome (i.e. DALY) (Weinstein and Stason, 1977[1]);
2. The probability of cost-effectiveness of each policy was then calculated against the standard threshold of USD 50 000 per health outcome threshold used to determine the cost-effectiveness of health interventions in industrialised economies – i.e. policy makers' willingness to pay.

Based on these probabilities, the modelled AMR control policies were categorised as either:

- Cost-saving (leading to an increase in health and net cost-savings),
- Cost-effective (ICER ≤ USD 50 000 per DALY averted),
- Non cost-effective (ICER > USD 50 000 per DALY averted),
- Inferior (i.e. achieving less health benefits and being more costly that the business-as-usual scenario).

This approach (i.e. presenting the probability of cost-effectiveness, instead of the usual display of the ICER associated with each strategy) was preferred as it allows a more informative evaluation and description of the performance of the policies modelled – particularly those with a cost-saving effect.

Country-specific resource needs and implementation costs of the policies were calculated according to the WHO-CHOICE approach. Costs are divided into two main components:

- Costs incurred at the point of delivery level (most often corresponding to the patient level)
- Costs incurred at the programme level (corresponding to central costs).

Patient-level costs involve face-to-face delivery by a provider (broadly defined but often corresponding to a health provider) to a recipient - e.g. medicines, outpatient visits, inpatient stays and individual health education messages. Programme-level costs include all resources required to establish and maintain an intervention - administration, publicity, training, delivery of supplies. Interventions like delivery of health education messages on mass media largely involve the latter, while treatment at health centres largely involves the former. A standardised ingredients approach is used, requiring information on the quantities of physical inputs needed and their unit cost (i.e. total costs are quantities of inputs multiplied by their unit costs) (Johns, Baltussen and Hutubessy, 2003[2]) (Johns, Adam and Evans, 2006[3]).

For patient-level costs, quantities are taken from a variety of sources. Where effectiveness estimates were available from published studies, the resources necessary to ensure the observed level of effectiveness are identified. In other cases, the resources implied by the activities outlined in WHO treatment practice guidelines were estimated (WHO, 2003[4]).

Unit costs for each input were derived from an extensive search of published and unpublished literature and databases along with consultation with costing experts.

6.2. How to tackle AMR

As discussed in Chapter 5, the multiple reports of increasing rates of AMR have pushed many stakeholders (governments, health agencies, individual hospitals etc.) to design and implement policies to control the progression of drug-resistance or prevent its occurrence in the first place. These policies can be broadly categorised into two groups:

1. Education interventions promoting effective use of antimicrobials – excessive and/or unnecessary use of antimicrobials is a key driver of AMR. The rationalisation of antimicrobial prescriptions would prevent and reduce the emergence of new resistant strains.
2. Interventions to prevent the spread of infections – by improving hygiene and reducing the contaminating potential of infected patients.

A variety of AMR control interventions and policies falling in one of these two categories have been described in the literature (Cecchini, Langer and Slawomirski, 2015[5]). However, not all of the exiting approaches to tackle AMR are currently suitable for inclusion in a quantitative modelling framework. The analysis presented here focuses on a subset of policy options for which a strong body of evidence of effectiveness is available. The selection of policies is the result of extended consultations with OECD member countries and relevant stakeholders, primarily members of the OECD Expert Group on the Economics of Public Health. The policies included in the cost-effectiveness model are presented in Table 6.1.

Table 6.1. Policy actions to tackle AMR included in the model

Objective	Healthcare-based interventions	Community-based interventions
Category of the intervention	Stewardship programmes	Delayed prescribing
	Improved hand hygiene	Mass media campaigns
	Enhanced environmental hygiene	Rapid diagnostic tests

Estimates of the effectiveness of the included policies at the population level (i.e. the scaling up of the intervention to the national level) were identified in the literature and modelled along three main dimensions. The first dimension is the effect of the intervention at the micro-level. For example, a campaign to improve hand-washing practices in hospitals produced a 48% decrease in AMR rates (Kirkland et al., 2012[6]). The second dimension is the potential coverage of the intervention, once it is scaled up. Even if an intervention is implemented nationally, it is likely that some hospitals will not apply it. A common assumption is that between 50% and 70% of health care structures will implement a policy, depending on the income of the country. The third dimension is the time to steady state (i.e. time for the intervention to produce an effect at the population level). Available evidence shows that interventions to tackle AMR require less than one year to reach the steady state (Cecchini and Lee, 2017[7]).

6.3. Healthcare-based interventions

6.3.1. Improved hand hygiene

Insufficient hand hygiene is unanimously recognised as the most important modifiable cause of hospital-acquired infections. Currently, hand-hygiene compliance rates are well below 50% in many OECD countries (Pittet et al., 2004[8]). The implementation of multimodal strategies has been shown very effective in increasing adherence to hand-washing guidelines (Kirkland et al., 2012[6]). The WHO-5 campaign is an example of a strategy promoting hand washing through system change, training and education, observation and feedback, reminders in the hospital, and a hospital safety climate (Kilpatrick, Allegranzi and Pittet, 2011[9]).

Few studies have investigated the effect of hand hygiene on AMR rates. Stone and colleagues calculated a 48% decline in methicillin-resistant *Staphylococcus aureus* (MRSA) bacteraemia rates following the implementation of the Clean-your-hands campaign (Stone et al., 2012[10]). Similarly, Grayson et al. (2008[11]) and Johnson et al. (2005[12]) concluded that the number of MRSA isolates would decrease by 53% and 40%, respectively. Positive effects were also demonstrated on resistant infections from *Escherichia coli* (*E. coli*) and *Klebsiella pneumoniae* (*K. pneumoniae*).

The effectiveness of this intervention was modelled by averaging the effectiveness reported by the three studies mentioned above (i.e. -48% of AMR for hospital-acquired infections). The intervention is assumed to be implemented by 70% of the health care structure in a country, affecting all health care-acquired infections (independently of whether they are susceptible or resistant) and its effectiveness is maintained constant over time. The intervention is assumed not to affect the incidence of community-acquired infections.

The intervention is designed as a hand hygiene culture-change programme with the objective to mimic, as much as possible, the WHO-5 campaign. More specifically, the intervention entails some structural changes to ensure that cleaning facilities are available at the point of care (e.g. alcohol-based handrub, soap and water, etc.), combined with training for health care personnel and regular hand-hygiene audits and feedback. Training for personnel and provision of material promoting hygiene is also an important part of the programme.

The cost of the intervention has been estimated at between USD 0.9 and USD 2.5 per capita per year, depending on the country. The calculation of the implementation costs was based on a recent systematic review, which has concluded that the median cost of delivering this type of intervention is around USD 1 per hospital bed per day (Luangasanatip et al., 2015[13]). In addition to the cost at the hospital level, our calculation also includes some costs towards strategic planning at the national level and coordination at the local level (e.g. hospital audit, monitoring, etc.).

6.3.2. Stewardship programmes

Antibiotic stewardship programmes represent a broad category of interventions that usually entail simultaneous implementation of multiple elements, including regulations, guidelines, monitoring, education and campaigns. These actions aim to increase awareness and to rationalise antimicrobial prescription practices among health care personnel. Stewardship programmes are designed and conducted by multidisciplinary teams including specialised physicians (e.g. experts in infectious diseases or microbiologists) and pharmacists.

A large body of evidence supports the effectiveness of stewardship programmes in both hospital and community care settings. A Cochrane review (Davey et al., 2017[14]) showed that implementation of a stewardship programme in a hospital setting decreases both antimicrobial prescription rates (median change up to -40%) and AMR prevalence rates (median change between -24% to -68%, depending on the type of infective bacteria). A more recent systematic review and meta-analysis concluded that stewardship programmes decrease antimicrobial consumption by 19% on average, AMR by 1.7% to 10.4%, and length of hospital stay by 9% (Karanika et al., 2016[15]).

The intervention is modelled on the effectiveness reported by Davey and colleagues (Davey et al., 2017[14]), under the assumption that the average stewardship programme is upscaled to the national level and that uptake from the hospital sector is at around 70% in all the countries included in the analyses. The programme only affects antibiotic-resistant infections acquired in health care settings and its effectiveness is assumed to remain constant over time. Susceptible infections in the hospital setting and susceptible and resistant infections acquired in the community are assumed not to be affected by this intervention.

The implementation of a stewardship programme entails the setting up of a multidisciplinary team including a specialist in infectious diseases, a microbiologist and a pharmacist. The team would review prescription patterns, provide consultation to the other doctors on which antibiotics to prescribe and develop guidelines for antibiotic prophylaxis and treatment aligned with national and international antibiotic guidelines. The team would also deliver specific courses, for example as part of an ongoing medical education programme, to train hospital personnel. As part of the intervention, brochures would be distributed to medical staff and hospital personnel.

The cost of implementing such a programme has been estimated between USD 2.5 and USD 12 per capita per year, depending on the country. The most expensive cost component is the salary of the stewardship team, which accounts for more than 90% of the total costs across countries. Remaining costs cover planning at the central and local level and material for the training of health care personnel in hospitals. The implementation costs vary quite substantially across countries. Wages of health care personnel as well as the number of health care facilities in the country are the most important drivers of such a difference.

6.3.3. Enhanced environmental hygiene

Hospital environments are a reservoir for drug-resistant organisms as pathogens can survive for up to seven months on inanimate surfaces (Donskey, 2013[16]) (Otter et al., 2013[17]). It is estimated that cross-transmission from the environment causes up to 20% of nosocomial infections (Weber, Anderson and Rutala, 2013[18]). Resistant bacteria contaminate objects when they are shed from the skin scales of colonised or infected individuals. These contaminated environmental surfaces and portable equipment such as stethoscopes or pagers can consequently transmit pathogens to susceptible individuals via direct or indirect contact (Blazejewski et al., 2015[19]).

Risk of AMR transmission from contaminated environments depends on the density of resistant pathogens, cleaning practices, patient comorbidities, and the intensity of medical care. Several studies have shown that the risk of acquiring multi-drug resistant organisms

(MDROs) is increased if a room has previously been occupied or used by a person colonised or infected by a resistant bacterium (Drees et al., 2008[20]). Systematic cleaning of equipment and the environment is therefore essential for reducing microbial contamination and the subsequent risk of transmission, in particular after discharging an infected individual. Enhanced environmental hygiene can therefore represent a key transmission prevention strategy. This encompasses the decontamination, disinfection, cleaning and sterilisation of the immediate environment and equipment. It further comprises the disposal of items which may have come into contact with infected individuals.

A systematic review was conducted to identify studies evaluating the effectiveness of enhanced environmental hygiene in reducing the transmission of AMR. Thirteen studies met the inclusion criteria and a meta-analysis was performed to calculate pooled estimates of their results. Based on this analysis, enhanced environmental hygiene interventions, depending on the MDRO considered, were estimated to reduce AMR rates by 26% to 49%.

An intervention enhancing environmental hygiene entails any of the following three actions (Donskey, 2013[16]):

- Disinfectant substitution: This involves a change from detergent to disinfectant, or to a different disinfectant assumed to have higher effectiveness against certain pathogens. The associated cost is estimated at USD PPP 14.2 per person per year.
- No-touch cleaning: This involves the use of an automated cleaning device, emitting hydrogen peroxide vapour or ultraviolet radiation, to disinfect rooms after routine cleaning. The associated cost is estimated at USD PPP 65 per person per year.
- Improving effectiveness of cleaning. This may include: additional cleaning time through the employment of new staff; audit, monitoring and feedback regarding cleaning practices and thoroughness; staff education as well as novel techniques of applying products, such as using disposable wipes or colour-coded cloths. The associated cost is estimated at USD PPP 12.6 per person per year.

The average cost of enhanced environmental hygiene interventions was estimated at USD PPP 30.6 per person per year, based on the components of the different types of interventions falling in one of the three categories above.

6.4. Community-based interventions

6.4.1. Delayed antimicrobial prescription

Delayed antimicrobial prescribing avoids unnecessary consumption of antimicrobials in outpatient and primary care settings. Patients are asked to wait up to three days or for a deterioration in their health status before collecting a medical prescription. This strategy both reduces antimicrobial consumption and educates patients that antimicrobials are not always necessary, especially for self-limiting illnesses. Meanwhile, having a prescription provides a sense of safety for both the patient and the clinician if the illness deteriorates (Spurling et al., 2013[21]).

Several reviews and meta-analyses demonstrate that delayed prescriptions reduce antimicrobial prescription rates. Based on the results of clinical trials spanning several OECD countries, Ranji et al. (2008[22]) found the intervention is most effective if patients have to return to the clinic to obtain a prescription if the symptoms do not resolve (Arroll, Kenealy and Kerse, 2003[23]; Spurling et al., 2013[21]).

The effectiveness estimates reported by Ranji and colleagues were used for the analysis. The authors reported that delayed prescriptions could lead to a 50% decrease in the consumption of antimicrobials in the community. A perfectly elastic relationship between consumption of antimicrobials and AMR rates was assumed in the model. This assumption is likely to be conservative as, for many antimicrobials, the relationship is found to be more than elastic (Kaier, 2011[24]). This intervention is also assumed to be implemented by 70% of drug prescribers, affect all the infections developed in the community and its effectiveness remains constant over time. The intervention is assumed not to affect the incidence of infections acquired in hospital settings or of susceptible infections acquired in the community.

The intervention is divided into two components. A first component entails setting up training programmes for general practitioners. General practitioners are given general information about AMR, are explained how to implement the intervention in their practice – the intervention requires the patient to return to the practice three days later if symptoms worsen – and how to respond to potential questions by the patient. A second component is the provision of brochures and posters for general practices. The informative material targets patients and provides information about AMR and the need to decrease antimicrobial consumption. Planning of the intervention is carried out at the national level but its implementation is managed locally.

The cost of the intervention has been estimated at between USD 0.30 and USD 1.30 per person per year. The majority of the resources are devoted to training, followed by the printing and the provision for the information to be handed out to patients. Our analysis does not take into account any economic impact caused by a decrease in the sales of antimicrobials or the extra time needed for doctors to provide a prescription during the second visit, under the assumption that the prescription would be prepared during the first visit.

6.4.2. Mass media campaigns

Raising public awareness about the dangers associated with inappropriate antimicrobial prescription is commonly used across OECD countries as a way to promote rational prescribing. Campaigns are usually delivered during the winter season through mass media, including TV, radio and billboards as well as new forms of media. In some cases, messages are reinforced at the health care service level (mainly in general practices) by providing brochures or leaflets. In many cases campaigns are designed and managed by national health authorities, but sometime the pharmaceutical industry contributes to their development (Huttner et al., 2010[25]).

Few studies have carried out formal quantitative assessments of the potential effectiveness of mass media campaigns. A meta-analysis by Thoolen et al. (2012[26])concluded that mass media campaigns have a small but statistically significant effect on the general population's attitudes and knowledge towards inappropriate antimicrobial use. By reviewing studies from Italy, the United Kingdom and the United States, Cecchini and Lee (2017[7]) concluded that mass media campaigns may be responsible for a 4% to 9% decrease in antimicrobial prescriptions. Based on these results, mass media campaign interventions were estimated to decrease antibiotic consumption by 6.5%. This was assumed to result in a 6.5% decrease in AMR rates for community-based infections, based on an assumption of perfect elasticity (Kaier,

2011[24]). The intervention is assumed not to affect the incidence of infections acquired in hospital settings or of susceptible infections acquired in the community.

Mass media campaigns are usually delivered over multiple channels, including national TV, radio and newspapers, billboards in major cities and flyers available in general practices and health care structures. Campaigns are modelled in yearly waves, with the media campaign to be reached during the winter season when infections (bacterial or viral) are more likely. A campaign would typically last for the rest of the year but at lower intensity (about half of the advertising coverage compared to the winter period). The cost of such an intervention ranges between USD 1.3 and USD 2.7 per capita per year, depending on the country. The majority of costs are incurred in buying advertising space on the media, followed by the costs of devising and planning the campaign.

6.4.3. Rapid Diagnostic Tests (C-reactive protein tests)

Traditional diagnostic testing methods used to identify bacteria and determine antibiotic susceptibility often require 48-72 hours, limiting their usefulness in guiding antibiotic prescribing and use. New rapid diagnostic tests (RDTs) can produce results within hours that allow clinicians to distinguish viral infections from bacterial infections, identify specific bacterial infections, and determine whether an antimicrobial treatment should be initiated and which drug should be used, based on the identified organism and its susceptibility profile. RDT technologies vary from standard assays to whole genome sequencing approaches and can be used in both hospital and primary care settings. By substantially reducing the time to results, RDTs have the potential to reduce unnecessary antibiotic use (particularly the use of broad-spectrum antibiotics) and improve patient outcomes. Their use is increasing globally.

To derive effectiveness and cost parameters for the RDT intervention in the microsimulation model, we focused on C-reactive protein tests, given the strong evidence in support of this technology and the fact that it can be used for many types of infections – as it effectively distinguishes bacterial from viral infections.

A recent Cochrane review including 9 trials conducted in emergency and primary care setting, reported that that C-reactive protein tests reduce antibiotic prescribing by approximately 25% (Tonkin-Crine et al., 2017[27]). Another review limited to trials conducted in the primary setting reported that use of C-reactive protein tests was associated with a 22% (95% confidence interval: 8% to 44%) reduction in antibiotic prescription. Based on these estimates, RDT interventions were estimated to reduce AMR by 22% in the microsimulation. The intervention was assumed not to affect the incidence of infections acquired in hospital settings or of susceptible infections acquired in the community.

The cost of C-reactive protein tests has been estimated at EUR 11.27 (95% confidence interval: 1.87-24.41 per patient) per patient (Oppong et al., 2013[28]). A study conducted by The National Institute for Health and Care Excellence (NICE) estimated the cost per patient at GBP 12-15 in the United Kingdom (Chaplin, 2015[29]; Hunter, 2015[30]), including the cost of reagents, equipment depreciation and staff time.

6.5. The impact of interventions on AMR

Each of the policies tested in the model seeks to reduce the burden of AMR by affecting one or more factors influencing AMR infections. Figure 6.2 illustrates these factors as well as the specific areas targeted by interventions tested in the model. Target 1 focuses on the selection pressure for AMR created by use of antimicrobials among humans in the community, Target 2 focuses on the selection pressure created by use of antimicrobials in hospital settings, and Target 3 focuses on the impact on bacterial infection rates created by substandard hygiene and living conditions.

Figure 6.2. Factors influencing resistant infections including targets for selected AMR control policies

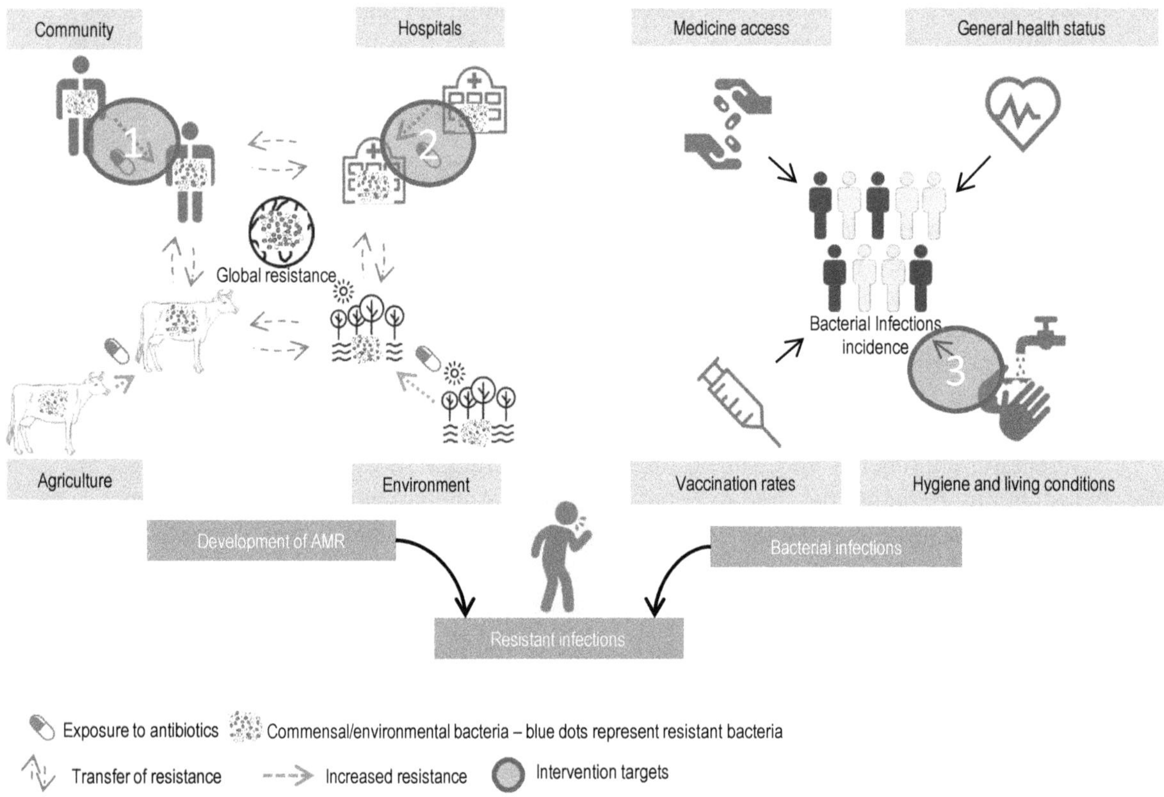

Several of the control policies included in the models seek to reduce resistant infections by focusing on Target 1. These policies include delayed prescribing strategies, mass media campaigns, and use of rapid diagnostic tests. The aim of these strategies is to reduce the selection pressure for resistance development and spread among humans in the community by reducing antibiotic consumption in this sector through various means. Lowered selection pressure will then ideally lead to a smaller proportion of resistant bacteria in the community, less transmission of resistance to other sectors, and less global resistance. Ultimately, this decrease in the proportion of pathogens that are resistant will in turn lower the proportion of all bacterial infections that are resistant to antibiotics leading to fewer resistant infections.

Interventions designed to modify Target 2 are based on the same principles as those designed for Target 1 but with a special focus on the hospital setting. As in the community, reducing antibiotic consumption in hospitals will reduce the selection pressure in these environments leading to fewer resistant bacteria and ultimately fewer resistant infections. Interventions focused on this target include stewardship programmes and mass media campaigns.

Lastly, two of the interventions tested, including enhanced environmental hygiene and improved hand hygiene, focus on Target 3. Unlike interventions focused on Targets 1 and 2, these interventions seek to reduce resistance infections by lowering the overall infection rate of both susceptible and resistant infections. This is achieved by reducing the spread of pathogenic bacteria through improved hygiene measures. By targeting all bacteria, these strategies aim to reduce the number but not necessarily the proportion of infections due to resistant bacteria. Interventions targeting bacterial infections may also indirectly affect Targets 1 and 2 by lowering the need for antibiotics in both the community and hospital settings through reduced infections rates.

6.6. The majority of deaths due to AMR can be prevented

All strategies tested in the model lead to reductions in AMR mortality and their effect was consistent across countries. Figure 6.3 shows the estimates per 100 000 persons, for each country, of the annual AMR mortality reductions associated with the six policies tested in the model. The overall preventive effect of the different policies is consistent across all the countries with the improved hand hygiene intervention being the most effective approach. The scale of effect, however, varies significantly between countries. The estimates of the improved hand hygiene policy, for example, range from ten AMR deaths prevented per 100 000 persons annually in Italy, to less than one AMR death per 100 000 persons prevented in the Netherlands or Norway. The differences in scale and magnitude of reductions reflect the heterogeneous epidemiological situation of the included countries, particularly in terms of baseline resistance proportions of infections and rates of change across countries – as discussed in Chapter 3.

Hospital-based policies have the largest impact on AMR mortality. Upscaling the improved hand hygiene, stewardship programmes, and enhanced environmental hygiene policies to national levels would reduce the total annual number of AMR deaths in the included countries by on average 58% (n=37 836), 54% (n=35 270), and 53% (34 931), respectively. These sharp reductions reflect current estimates from studies that have evaluated the included interventions in the clinical context. They are also consistent with the fact that all three interventions have a preventive effect on both resistant and susceptible infections as their impact is based on a reduction of the risk of transmission of all infections, regardless of their resistance status.

Community-based policies are also effective in preventing AMR deaths, albeit to a lesser extent than hospital-based policies. The average annual reduction in AMR mortality associated with the implementation of mass media campaigns, delayed prescription, and RDT is estimated at around 9% (n=5 872), 16% (n=10 214), and 25%, respectively, across the included countries. The lower preventive effect of community interventions on AMR mortality is due to the fact that their implementation would have an impact on resistant infections only. The three community-based policies do not decrease the total probability of acquiring an infection. Their primary effect is a reduction in antimicrobial consumption, which in turn results in a decrease of the probability that an acquired infection is resistant to antimicrobials. This shift, from resistant to susceptible infections, results in a net decrease in total mortality as the probability of dying from a susceptible infection is lower than that of dying from a resistant infection. On the other hand, two out of the three healthcare-based policies (i.e. improved hand hygiene and enhanced environmental hygiene), have an impact on both resistant and susceptible infections, by reducing risk of transmission, and therefore mortality from both types of infections. The stewardship programmes policy – which also affects the level of resistance through reduction in antimicrobial consumption – has a stronger effect on mortality than the community-based intervention because it reduces the probability of resistance of infections acquired in hospital, which are deadlier than those acquired in the community.

Figure 6.3. Number of deaths prevented per year, 2015-2050

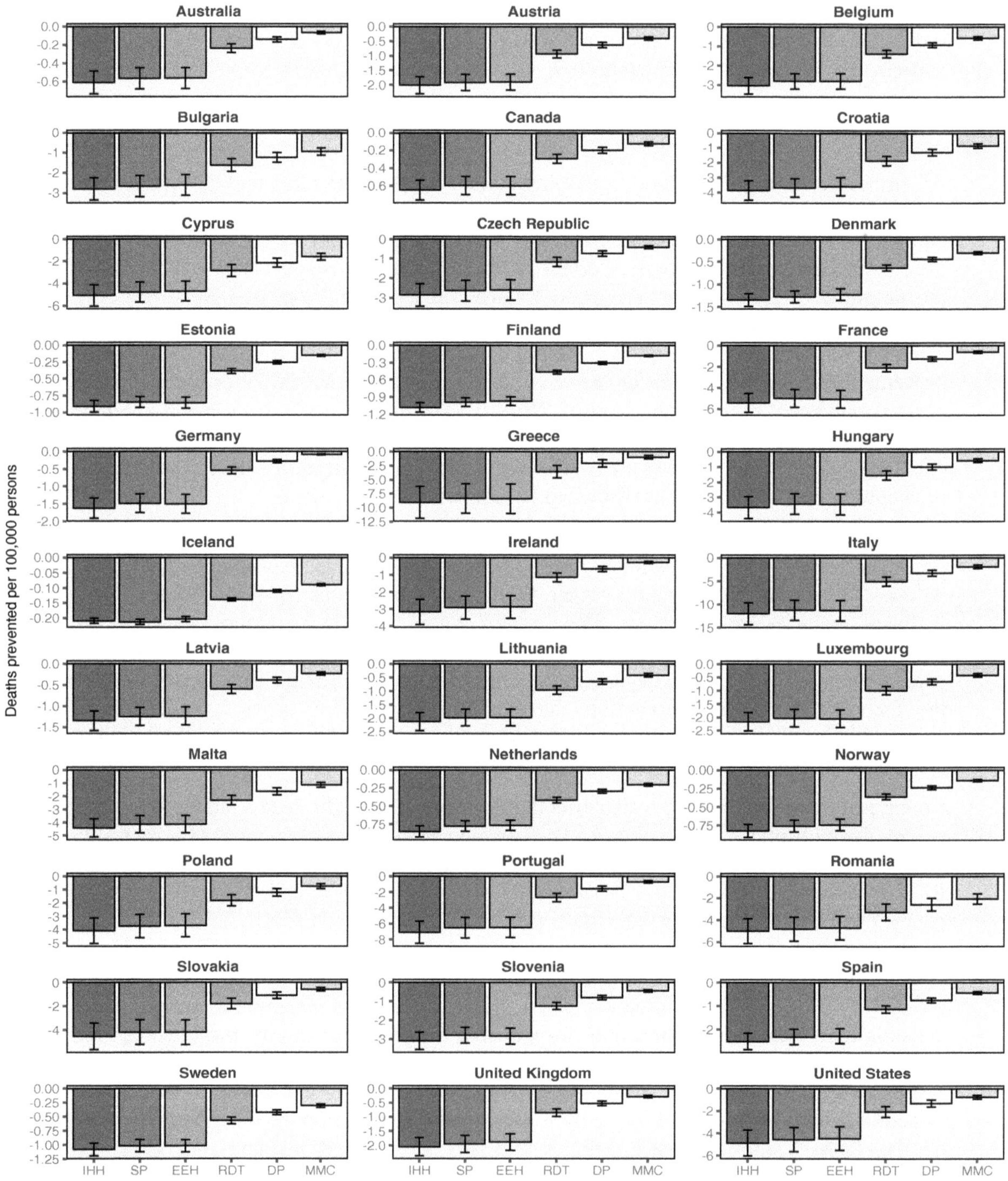

Note: IHH: improved hand hygiene, SP: stewardship programmes, EHH: enhanced environmental hygiene, RDT: rapid diagnostic tests. DP: delayed prescription, MMC: mass media campaigns.

Source: OECD analysis based on the OECD SPHeP-AMR model.

StatLink http://dx.doi.org/10.1787/888933855124

6.7. AMR control can deliver substantial health gains

The impact of the interventions in terms of health gains (i.e. DALYs) is consistent with their preventive effect on AMR mortality. Here too, the three healthcare-based interventions considered in the model have the potential of delivering the largest health gains – on average 1 500 to 2 000 DALYs gained per 100 000 persons per year across the included countries. The community-based interventions would generate smaller but meaningful gains at the population level with an average total across countries of 300 to 800 DALYs gained per 100 000 persons per year.

Figure 6.4 shows the evolution of DALYs gained associated with each policy for individual countries. For most countries, the progression tends to be more rapid in the initial phase for healthcare-based policies, while community-based policies gain momentum after five to ten years but deliver substantially less DALYs over time. Again, important heterogeneity exists between countries in terms of scale of the potential health gains, which reflect the baseline epidemiological differences mentioned above. The trends, however, are consistent across all countries, with the improved hand hygiene policy resulting in the highest number of DALYs gained over-time – followed closely by the stewardship programmes and enhanced environmental hygiene policies.

Importantly, the model's projections show that the potential health returns of AMR control policies would appear rapidly following their implementation. This means that putting in place any of the policies evaluated in the model would deliver virtually immediate health benefits to the population, as shown for all countries in Figure 6.4. This is in stark contrast with most existing population-based prevention policies – such as cancer screening programmes (Hanley, 2011[31]) and other chronic disease prevention initiatives (Cecchini et al., 2010[32]) – which are usually characterised by several years and sometimes decades (in the case of cancer screening for example) of long lead-time before any substantive public health benefit can be observed.

Box 6.2. Effect of AMR control policies on employment and productivity

An important aspect of the potential health gains that might result from the implementation at the national level of AMR control policies is the impact on employment and productivity. In the last few years, several evaluations of the potential impact of AMR on the global economy have been published. A report published in 2017 by the World Bank estimated that by 2050, the effects of AMR on labour supply and productivity in the livestock sector could result in a decline in the annual global gross domestic product (GDP) of 1.1% to 3.8%. The shortfall associated with such a contraction was projected to reach USD 1 trillion to USD 3.8 trillion per year after 2030. Increased mortality and its effects on the population size of countries were identified as the largest driver of the decrease in GDP. A detailed evaluation of the macro-economic effects of AMR and AMR control was beyond the scope of the model presented in this report. However, comparing the World Bank estimates to the potential health gains shown in Figure 6.3 and Figure 6.4 sheds light on the capacity of a large-scale implementation of AMR control policies to substantially mitigate any long-term negative effects of AMR in terms of labour supply, productivity, and the global economy.

Figure 6.4. DALYs averted by each AMR control policy over time – 2015-2050

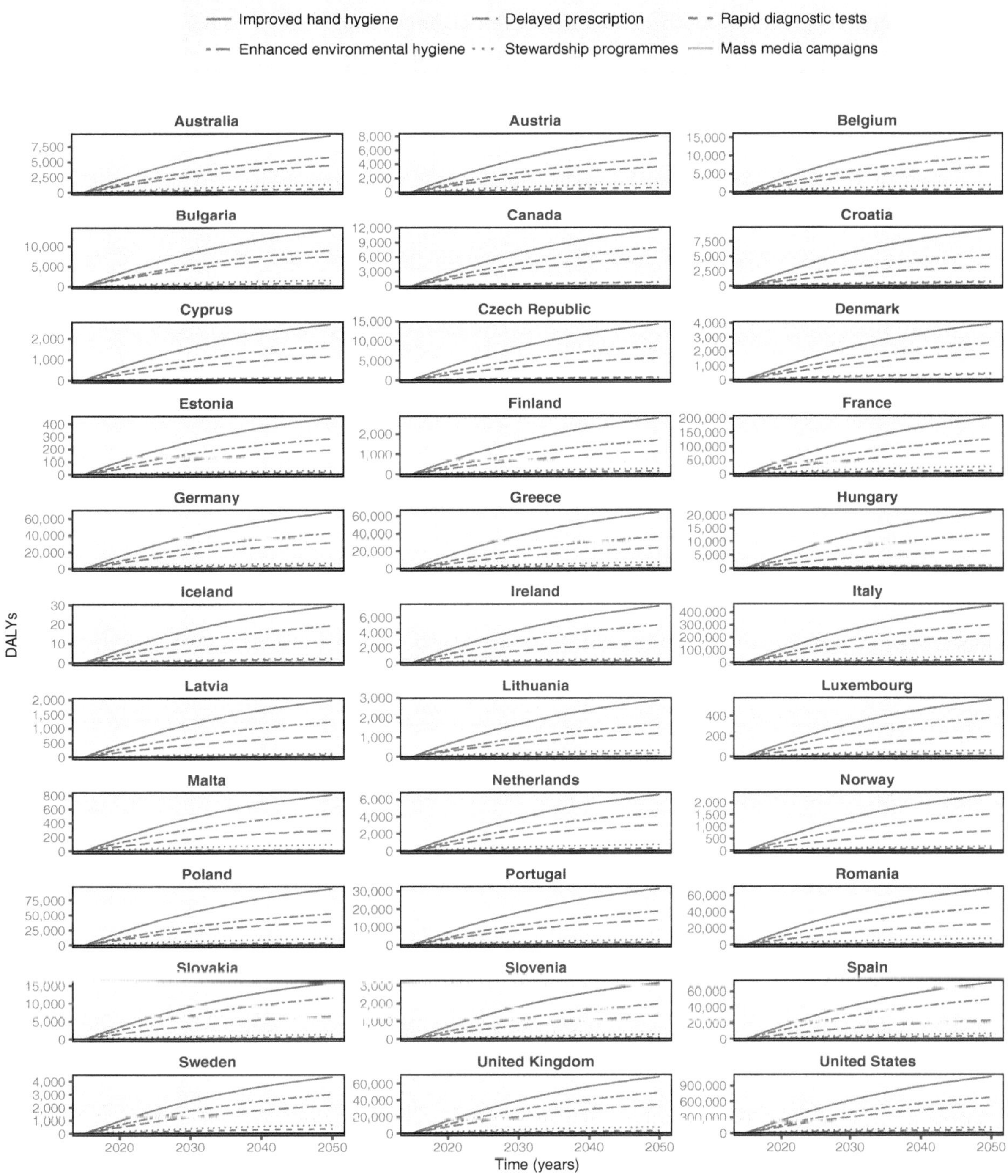

Note: Future effects are discounted at a 3% rate.
Source: OECD analysis based on the OECD SPHeP-AMR model.

StatLink http://dx.doi.org/10.1787/888933855143

6.8. Reduced burden on hospital resources

The effect of the modelled AMR control policies in terms of hospital days avoided is consistent with the results reported on health outcomes and health expenditure. The model clearly shows that the control policies, if implemented, would lead to large reductions of the number of hospital days due to AMR. However, large differences exist between countries in terms of scale of the reductions.

As for the previous model outcomes, healthcare-based policies would result in the highest number of hospital days avoided. In Italy, for example, the improved hand hygiene policy would result in around 1 000 hospital days avoided per 100 000 persons, each year. The same policy, if implemented in The Netherlands, would lead to approximately 60 hospital days avoided per 100 000 persons. These reductions would represent, for both countries, around 40% reduction in the number of hospital days due to AMR, each year. The difference in effect between the two countries translates differences in the burden of AMR, but likely also in the number of hospital admissions and average length of stay.

Logically, in absolute terms, countries with the highest burden of disease will benefit the most from the preventive effects of the control policies. However, the results also show that health systems with lower levels of AMR (supposedly as a result of more robust AMR control policies already in place) would also draw substantial benefits, in terms of health care resources, from the implementation of AMR control strategies. This applies to both hospital and community-based policies, as shown in Figure 6.5.

Figure 6.5. Number of prevented AMR hospital days, average per year, 2015-2050

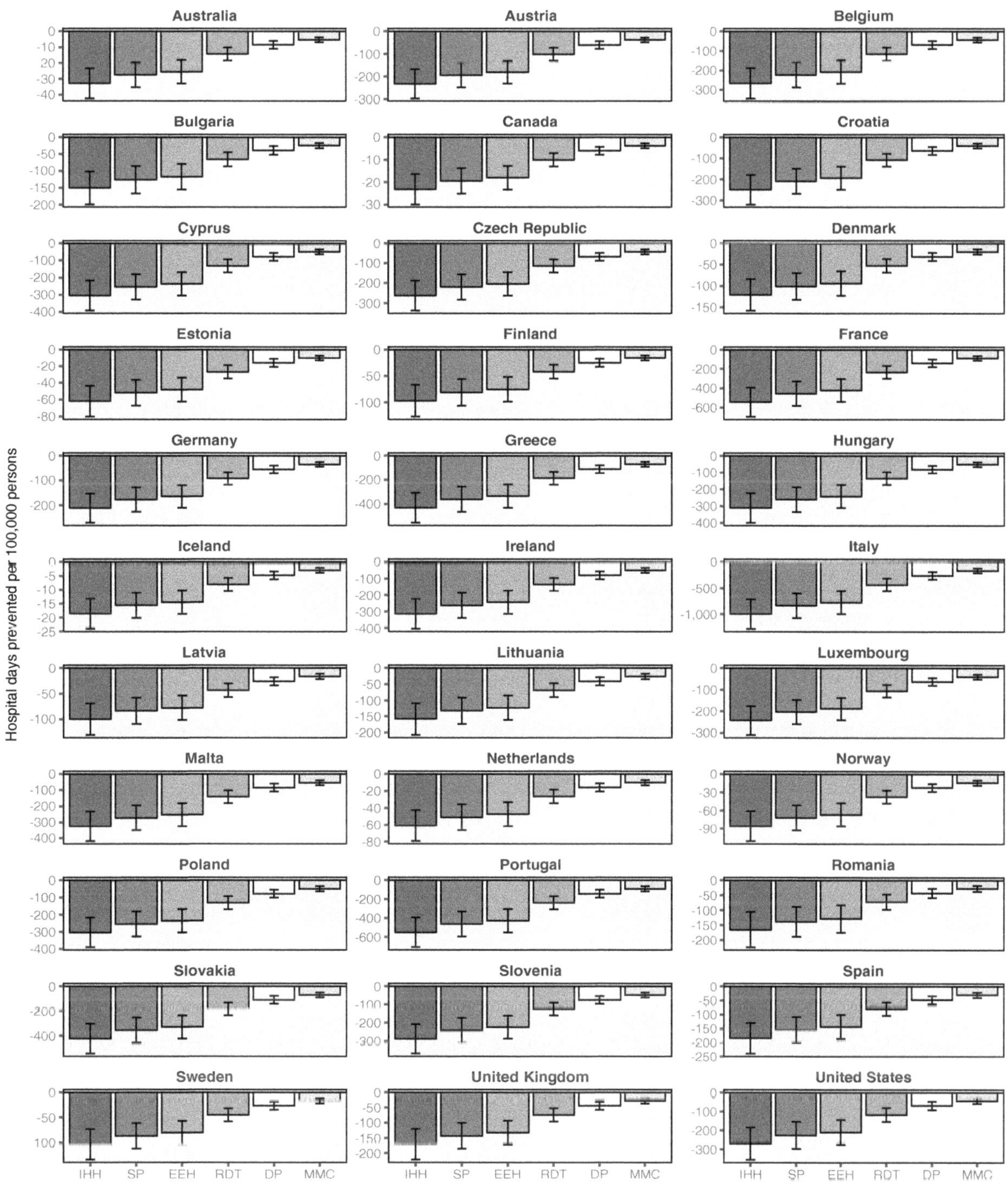

Note: IHH: improved hand hygiene, SP: stewardship programmes, EEH: enhanced environmental hygiene, RDT: rapid diagnostic tests. DP: delayed prescription, MMC: mass media campaigns.
Source: OECD analysis based on the OECD SPHeP-AMR model.

StatLink http://dx.doi.org/10.1787/888933855162

6.9. Lower health expenditure

The estimated costs of implementing the modelled AMR control policies and the potential savings over time in terms of health care expenditure are presented in Figure 6.6 and Figure 6.7. Implementation cost estimates are based on the per capita costs reported scaled up to national level by considering key drivers of expenditure including, among others, population coverage, demographic dynamic and health care system arrangements.

For all countries, enhanced environmental hygiene and stewardship programmes appear as the most expensive strategies to implement, with large variations across countries. Italy and the United States, for example, have an average annual cost for enhanced environmental hygiene policies of USD PPP 220 000-250 000 per 100 000 persons, while the implementation costs for that strategy in Australia, Canada and the most northern European countries are well below USD PPP 40 000 per 100 000 persons. The third most expensive policy is the RDT approach for community infections, which comes at an average annual cost of USD PPP 48 000 per 100 000 persons, ranging from USD PPP 1 000 to USD PPP 136 000 per 100 000 across the included countries. These high price tags are consistent with what the strategies involve in terms of staff training and recruitment as well as acquisition of special devices (e.g. no-touch cleaning devices and diagnostic technology in the cases of the enhanced environmental hygiene and the RDT policies, respectively). The three other policies tested in the model, improved hand hygiene, delayed prescription and mass media campaigns, had an average implementation cost of less than USD PPP 15 000 per 100 000 persons per year.

All the policies are expected to result in null or reduced health care expenditure. This means that the savings in health care expenditure resulting from their implementation would almost entirely and immediately offset the implementation costs associated with the different policies, including the ones involving a high initial level of government investment. The improved hand hygiene policy represents a particularly attractive investment. Its implementation cost is on average 10 times lower than the enhanced environmental hygiene policy and generates savings in health expenditure that represent, depending on the country, on average 15 times the implementation costs.

The community-based policies tested in the model – despite the somewhat higher uncertainly around their estimates and more limited effects in terms of savings over-time relative to the healthcare-based policies – would represent good investment for governments as: i) their implementation cost is gradually off-set over-time; and ii) all three policies would prevent AMR deaths and generate health benefits in the population.

Figure 6.6. Implementation cost and impact on health care expenditure of AMR control policies, average per year – 2015-2050

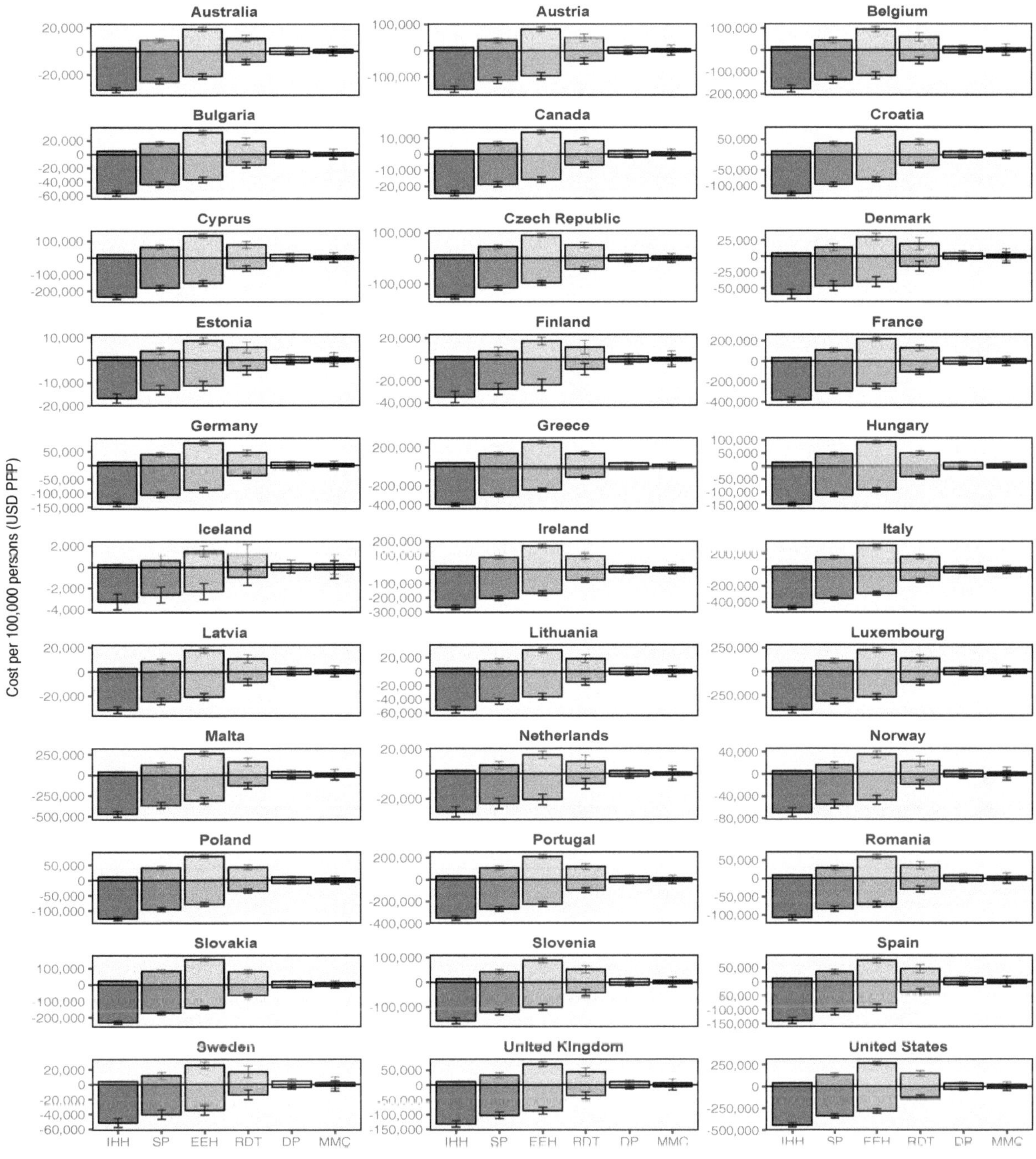

Note: IHH: improved hand hygiene, SP: stewardship programmes, EEH: enhanced environmental hygiene, RDT: rapid diagnostic tests. DP: delayed prescription, MMC: mass media campaigns.

Areas of the bars above the zero line represent the health expenditure associated with each policy. Areas below zero represent reductions in health expenditure.

Source: OECD analysis based on the OECD SPHeP-AMR model.

StatLink http://dx.doi.org/10.1787/888933855181

Figure 6.7. Savings associated with each AMR control policy over time – 2015-2050

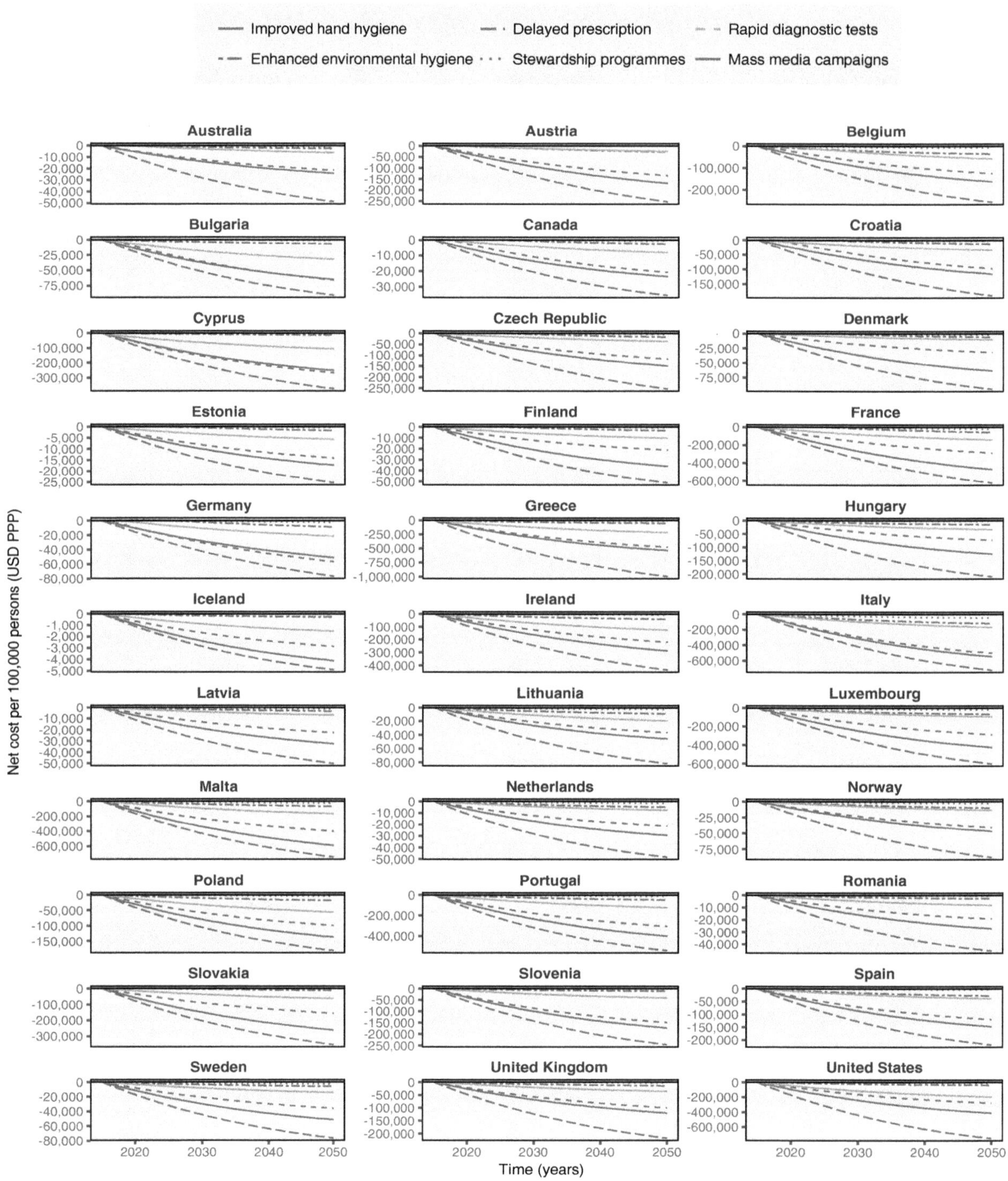

Note: Future savings are discounted at a 3% rate. The figures show the magnitude and evolution of the net savings associated with each control policy over the model's timeframe.
Source: OECD analysis based on the OECD SPHeP-AMR model.

StatLink http://dx.doi.org/10.1787/888933855200

6.10. The cost-effectiveness of AMR control

Figure 6.10 summarises the results of the country-specific cost-effectiveness analyses performed for the included AMR control policies. It shows the probability of cost-effectiveness of each strategy based on the value of its ICER (see Box 6.1). Across all countries, the implementation of the policies included in the model can be considered as “best buys” as they appear as very likely to deliver high value for money, and even cost-savings, for the health care system. The results of the OECD model are consistent with the available evidence on the cost-effectiveness of AMR control interventions (see Box 6.3). The improved hand hygiene policy would be, by far, the most efficient approach with over 90% likelihood of being cost saving. Its probability of not being cost-effective or inferior to the business-as-usual scenario is close to zero for all countries. The stewardship programme and the enhanced environmental hygiene strategies appear also as highly efficient policies with a very high probability that their implementation will result in health expenditure savings.

The implementation of community-based interventions, despite their more modest effects on health and cost outcomes described above, would deliver high returns on investment for governments. This particularly applies to the delayed prescription and the RDT policies, which are both highly likely to result in cost-savings in a majority of countries. Finally, the mass media campaigns would also represent a cost-effective investment with a very high probability of its implementation leading to cost-savings in the most populous countries.

Box 6.3. What does previous evidence on the cost-effectiveness of AMR control policies tell us?

Several studies have evaluated the cost-effectiveness of AMR control policies. All of the current estimates, however, stem from analyses focusing on "micro" interventions conducted at individual hospitals or health care units to control a specific resistant bacterium. Among the policies included in the OECD model, the stewardship programmes strategy has been evaluated the most, and studies have consistently demonstrated its cost-effectiveness. A recent report commissioned by the Dutch Ministry of Health to identify good AMR control policy practices showed that antimicrobial stewardship teams in hospitals represent a highly effective strategy to tackle AMR as they can lead to more than a 10% reduction in antimicrobial prescribing and cost-savings of over EUR 40 000 (hospital-wide), per year. Similarly, the use of RDTs to regulate antimicrobial prescribing in primary care was associated with a 40% reduction in antimicrobial prescriptions and cost-savings evaluated at EUR 7 per patient treated (Oberjé, Tanke and Jeurissen, 2016[33]).

The cost-effectiveness of improved hand hygiene programmes, at the hospital level, is well established. The WHO Guidelines on Hand Hygiene in Health Care identified several studies, conducted in a variety of countries, which have concluded that hand hygiene initiatives are highly effective in preventing transmission of health care associated infections and typically cost-saving shortly after their implementation (WHO, 2009[34]; Chen et al., 2011[35]).

The OECD model differs from previous analyses because it is the first to adopt a full health system perspective to assess the effectiveness and cost-effectiveness of AMR control policies. Overall, the findings of the model are largely consistent with the available evidence, highlighting the large potential positive impact of these policies being implemented and coordinated at the national level.

Figure 6.8. Probability of cost-effectiveness of interventions vs. business as usual

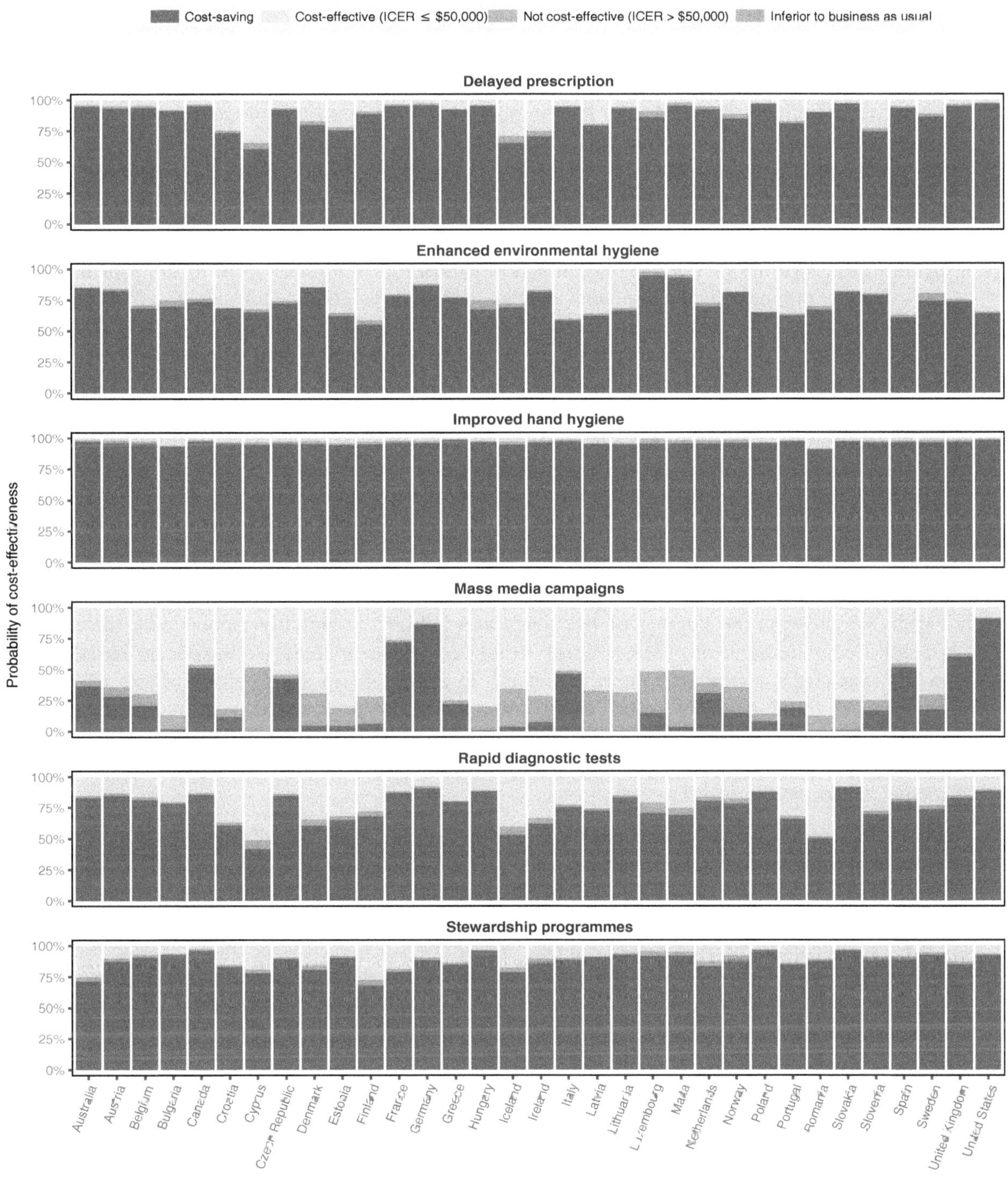

Source: OECD analysis based on the OECD SPHeP-AMR model.

StatLink http://dx.doi.org/10.1787/888933855219

6.11. More effective AMR control through combined policies

AMR is a multi-faceted public health issue which requires policy interventions in a variety of settings. The policies assessed in the cost-effectiveness analysis model address resistant infections occuring in both hospital and community settings. Even though the performance of each individual intervention is reported, the objective of the OECD model is not to identify a single or preferred AMR control policy approach. For countries that intend to effectively tackle AMR, it is important to realise that they cannot rely on a single policy to accomplish their goal. OECD analyses show that – as is often the case with prevention policies – the combined effects of multiple AMR control policies results in larger health and economic benefits.

Combining multiple AMR control policies in a broader policy package would generate overall effects (in terms disease burden and healthcare expenditure) close to the sum of the effects of the individual component policies, for all three policy packages tested in the microsimulation. The end result is broadly additive, despite an assumption of less that additive effect. This likely results from the fact that both hospital and community-based policies influence AMR from different angles, which results in a complimentary effect when they are combined. For example, improved hand hygiene reduces the risk of infection transmision from clinical staff to patients, while improved environmental hygiene reduces risk of infection through contact with contaminated objects or surfaces. Similarly, mass media campaigns create awareness in the population, while RDTs reduce the level of inappropriate use of antimicrobials. The two interventions are complementary as they impact the same cause of selection pressure – i.e. inappropriate consumption of antimicrobials – but through different vectors.

Figure 6.9 presents the number of life years and DALYs potentially gained with three possible combinations of AMR control strategies. These include a "healthcare-based policy package" combining improved hand hygiene, stewardship programmes and enhance environmental hygiene; a "community-based policy package" combining delayed prescrition, mass media campaigns and RDTs; and a broad "mixed policy package" combining stewardship programmes, enhance environmental hygiene, mass media campaigns, and RDTs.

The effect of the three policy packages are consistent with the results reported for individual interventions, in terms of scale of the impact of policies as well as the heterogeneity across countries. The healthcare-based package appears as the most effective in terms of health gains with, on average across the included countries, 118 DALYs gained and 10 life years saved per 100 000 persons, each year. Implementing the mixed package would lead to slightly lower health gains with an annual average across counties of 100 DALYs gained and 8 life years per 100 000 persons. As expected, the community-based package would have the lowest level of health benefits with around 32 DALYs gained and 3 life years per 100 000 persons.

The potential reduction in health care expenditure and savings associated with the three AMR control policy packages can be substantial for countries, as shown in Figure 6.10. The model estimates show that all three policy packages represent "best buys" as the health care expenditure associated with their implementation would be largely offset and savings would be generated. Annually, the healthcare-based package would save on average USD PPP 1.2 million per 100 000 persons. The mixed-policy and community-based policy packages, would result, respectively, in average reductions in health care expenditure of approximately USD PPP 920 000 and USD PPP 275 000 per year.

Figure 6.9. DALYs and life years saved by the policy packages – average per year 2015-2050

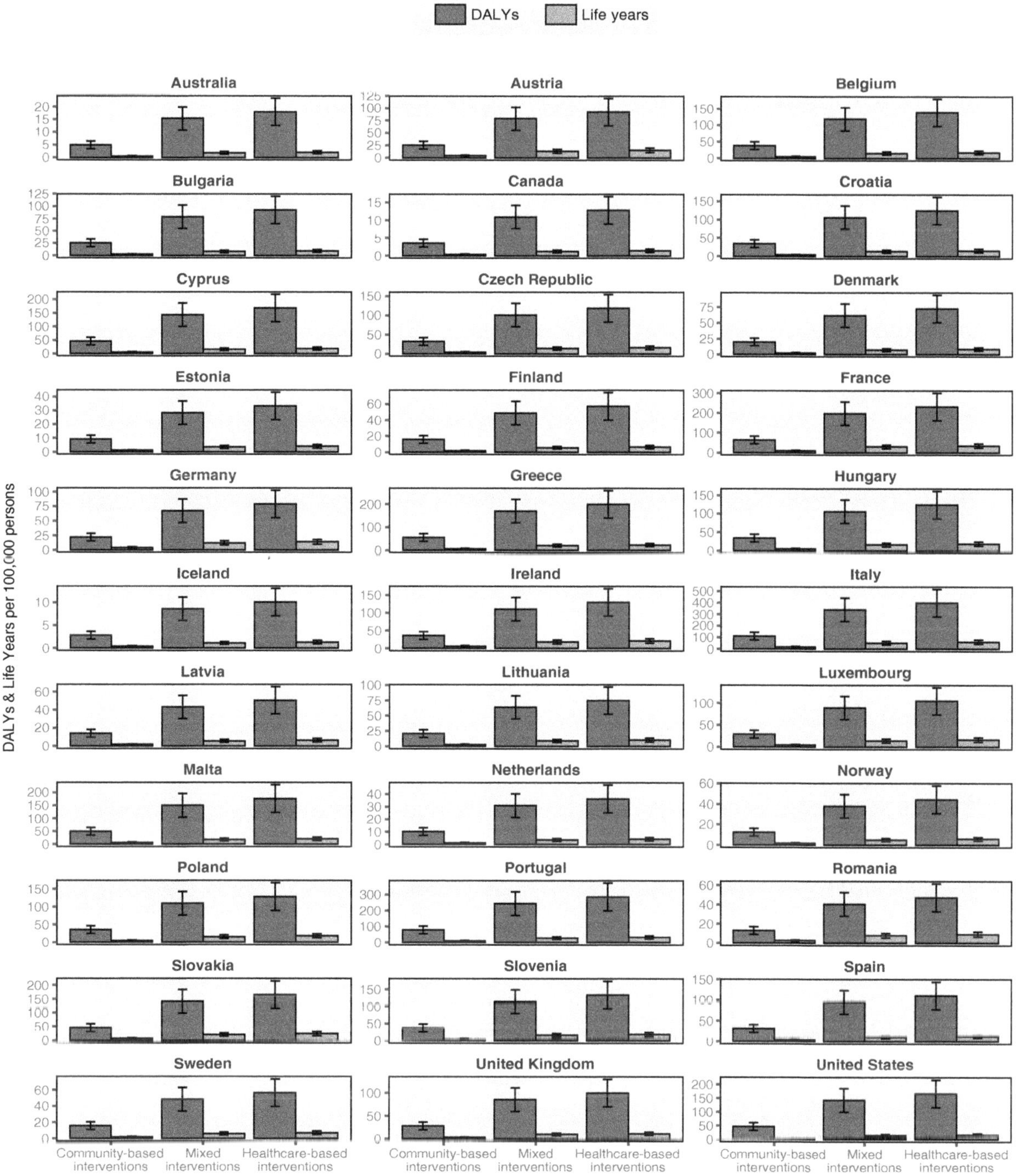

Source: OECD analysis based on the OECD SPHeP-AMR model.

StatLink http://dx.doi.org/10.1787/888933855238

Figure 6.10. Cost impact of AMR control policy packages, average per year, 2015-2050

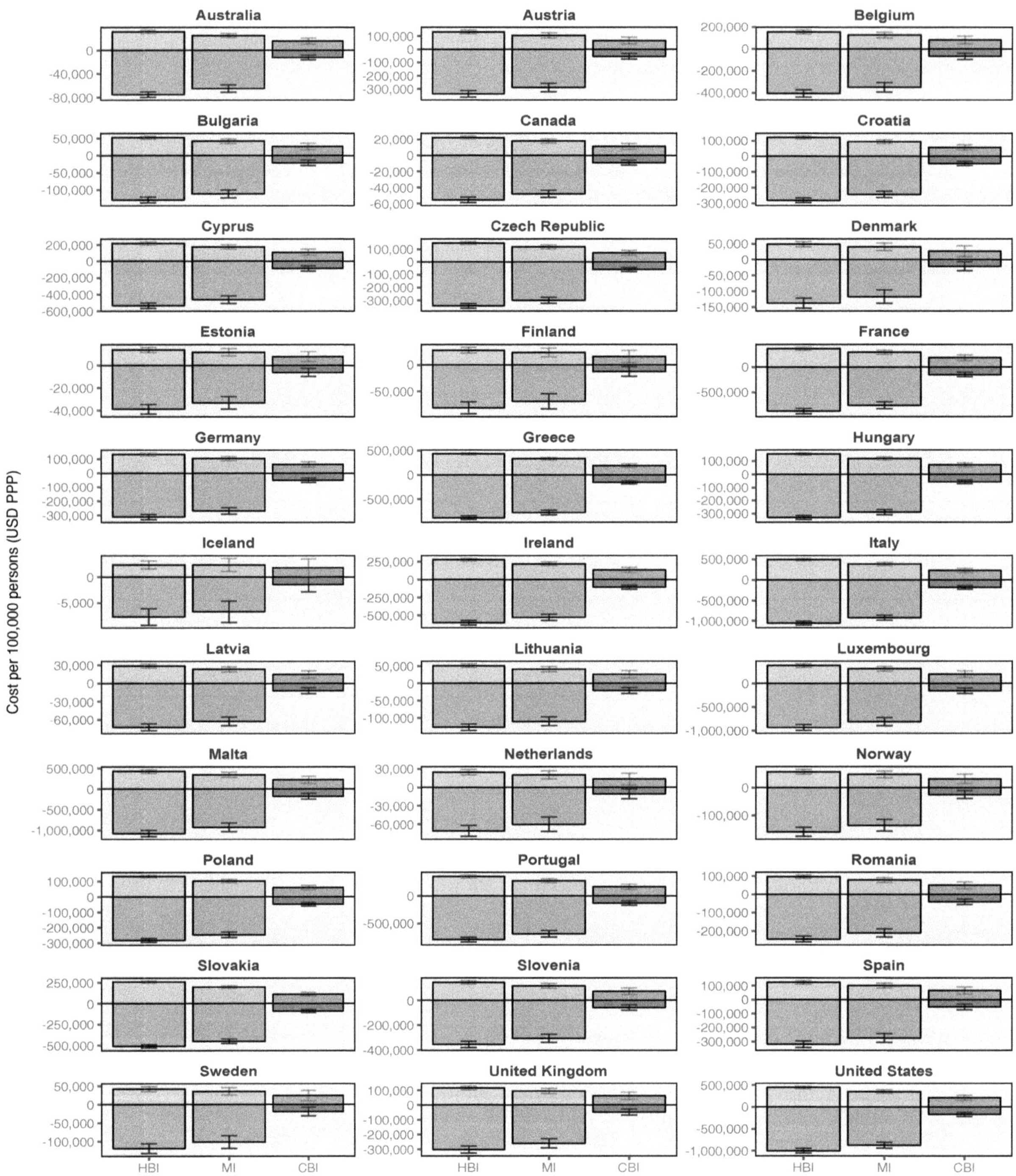

Note: HBI: healthcare-based interventions, MI: mixed interventions, CBI: community-based interventions. Areas of the bars above the zero line represent the health expenditure associated with each policy. Areas below zero represent reductions in health expenditure.

Source: OECD analysis based on the OECD SPHeP-AMR model.

StatLink http://dx.doi.org/10.1787/888933855105

6.12. Strengths and limitations of the findings

The OECD model relies on many parameters and large quantities of data, derived from a variety of sources. It also relies on several analytical decisions and assumptions made to address knowledge gaps in the epidemiology of AMR in the available costing data etc. (see Chapter 4). Therefore, as for any health-economic evaluation exercise, variations in any of these parameters will have an impact on the performance estimates of the included control policies.

Probabilistic sensitivity analysis was used to evaluate the uncertainty of the cost-effectiveness of each control policy and to generate cost-effectiveness plans showing the distribution of costs and DALYs for each evaluated AMR control policy for individual countries.

The effects of two key assumptions in the model were further tested in separate deterministic sensitivity analyses, and their effects on the probability of cost-effectiveness of the different control policies evaluated:

1. the 100% elastic relationship between consumption of antimicrobials and AMR rates, reduced to 80%
2. the 70% implementation/adherence to the control policies modelled, reduced to 50%.

Overall, the results of the sensitivity analyses and the relatively narrow uncertainty intervals around most model estimates support the validity of the findings. The reduction of the elasticity assumption and that of the level of adherence to the control policies had a similar and somewhat limited impact on the cost-effectiveness profiles of the different control policies. Under both scenarios, for most countries, the six strategies conserved high probabilities of being cost-effective. The likelihood of cost-savings was reduced considerably for all strategies, with the exception of improved hand hygiene, which would likely generate savings despite reduction in adherence or intervention effect elasticity (see Annex Figure 6.A.1 and Annex Figure 6.A.2).

The model is likely to substantially underestimate the preventive effect of the community-based interventions. This is due mainly to the limited number of community infections included in the model, which again is a result the limited data and understanding of the epidemiology of AMR in the community setting. In addition, our analysis is based on the conservative assumption that a decrease of AMR rates in community infection does not produce any decrease in AMR rates in healthcare-based infections.

An important point to highlight is the health care sector perspective adopted in the cost-effectiveness model. Such a perspective, by definition, fails to assess the indirect costs and benefits generated outside of the health care sector. The model therefore does not provide an assessment of the potential impact of AMR control on the economy as a whole. As such, it likely underestimates the beneficial effects of the control policies tested. Another major limitation of the model is its exclusive focus on human health. It is well documented that the vast majority of antimicrobials produced are destined for the livestock sector where their usage is inadequately regulated for a large number of countries. This results in selection pressure, which could lead to high levels of AMR and risk of transmission of resistant pathogens to humans, which in turn is likely to substantially affect the effectiveness and cost-effectiveness of AMR control policies.

Finally, it should be noted that the objective of the OECD cost-effectiveness model was to provide country specific data on the resources required to implement a set of AMR control policies; to generate information on feasibility, validity, reliability, and cost–effectiveness. The results reported in this chapter should be interpreted as the potential AMR reduction that could be achieved in optimal circumstances. The difficulty of implementation is recognised but beyond the scope of this modelling work

Conclusion: Tackling AMR is an excellent investment

The OECD SPHeP-AMR model is the first attempt to assess the potential impact on health outcomes, health care expenditure and cost-effectiveness of AMR control policies from the perspective of 33 different national health systems. It provides compelling evidence that the widespread implementation of the modelled policies would dramatically reduce the number of deaths due to resistant infections and generate substantial savings for health care systems. It also demonstrates that AMR is not a fatality and that it can be tackled effectively with a variety of strategies that are complementary and readily available.

References

Arroll, B., T. Kenealy and N. Kerse (2003), "Do delayed prescriptions reduce antibiotic use in respiratory tract infections? A systematic review", *British Journal of General Practice*, Vol. 53/496, pp. 871-877, https://www.ncbi.nlm.nih.gov/pubmed/14702908. [23]

Blazejewski, C. et al. (2015), "Efficiency of hydrogen peroxide in improving disinfection of ICU rooms", *Critical Care*, Vol. 19, p. 30, http://dx.doi.org/10.1186/s13054-015-0752-9. [19]

Cecchini, M., J. Langer and L. Slawomirski (2015), *Antimicrobial Resistance in G7 Countries and Beyond: Economic Issues, Policies and Options for Action*, OECD, Paris, http://www.oecd.org/els/health-systems/Antimicrobial-Resistance-in-G7-Countries-and-Beyond.pdf. [5]

Cecchini, M. and S. Lee (2017), "Low-value health care with high stakes: Promoting the rational use of antimicrobials", in *Tackling Wasteful Spending on Health*, OECD Publishing, Paris, http://dx.doi.org/10.1787/9789264266414-6-en. [7]

Cecchini, M. et al. (2010), "Tackling of unhealthy diets, physical inactivity, and obesity: health effects and cost-effectiveness", *Lancet*, Vol. 376, https://doi.org/10.1016/S0140-6736(10)61514-0. [32]

Chaplin, S. (2015), "CRP testing could reduce antibiotic prescribing", *Prescriber*, Vol. 26/18, pp. 29-30, http://dx.doi.org/10.1002/psb.1387. [29]

Chen, Y. et al. (2011), "Effectiveness and Limitations of Hand Hygiene Promotion on Decreasing Healthcare–Associated Infections", *PLoS ONE*, Vol. 6/11, p. e27163, http://dx.doi.org/10.1371/journal.pone.0027163. [35]

Davey, P. et al. (2017), "Interventions to improve antibiotic prescribing practices for hospital inpatients", in *Cochrane database of systematic reviews*, John Wiley & Sons, Ltd, http://dx.doi.org/10.1002/14651858.cd003543.pub4. [14]

Donskey, C. (2013), "Does improving surface cleaning and disinfection reduce health care-associated infections?", *American Journal of Infection Control*, Vol. 41/5 Suppl, pp. S12-9, http://dx.doi.org/10.1016/j.ajic.2012.12.010. [16]

Drees, M. et al. (2008), "Antibiotic exposure and room contamination among patients colonized with vancomycin-resistant enterococci", *Infection Control & Hospital Epidemiology*, Vol. 29/8, pp. 709-715, http://dx.doi.org/10.1086/589582. [20]

Grayson, M. et al. (2008), "Significant reductions in methicillin-resistant Staphylococcus aureus bacteraemia and clinical isolates associated with a multisite, hand hygiene culture-change program and subsequent successful statewide roll-out", *Med J Aust*, Vol. 188/11, pp. 633-640, https://www.ncbi.nlm.nih.gov/pubmed/18513171. [11]

Hanley, J. (2011), "Measuring mortality reductions in cancer screening trials", *Epidemiologic reviews*, Vol. 33/1, pp. 36-45, http://dx.doi.org/10.1093/epirev/mxq021. [31]

Hunter, R. (2015), "Cost-Effectiveness of Point-of-Care C-Reactive Protein Tests for Respiratory Tract Infection in Primary Care in England", *Advances in Therapy*, Vol. 32/1, pp. 69-85, http://dx.doi.org/10.1007/s12325-015-0180-x. [30]

Huttner, B. et al. (2010), "Characteristics and outcomes of public campaigns aimed at improving the use of antibiotics in outpatients in high-income countries", *The Lancet Infectious Diseases*, Vol. 10/1, pp. 17-31, https://doi.org/10.1016/S1473-3099(09)70305-6. [25]

Johns, B., T. Adam and D. Evans (2006), "Enhancing the comparability of costing methods: cross-country variability in the prices of non-traded inputs to health programmes", *Cost Effectiveness and Resource Allocation*, Vol. 4, p. 8, http://dx.doi.org/10.1186/1478-7547-4-8. [3]

Johns, B., R. Baltussen and R. Hutubessy (2003), "Programme costs in the economic evaluation of health interventions", *Cost Effectiveness and Resource Allocation*, Vol. 1/1, p. 1, https://www.ncbi.nlm.nih.gov/pubmed/12773220. [2]

Johnson, P. et al. (2005), "Efficacy of an alcohol/chlorhexidine hand hygiene program in a hospital with high rates of nosocomial methicillin-resistant Staphylococcus aureus (MRSA) infection", *Med J Aust*, Vol. 183/10, pp. 509-514, https://www.ncbi.nlm.nih.gov/pubmed/16296963. [12]

Kaier, K. (2011), "ECONOMIC MODELING OF THE PERSISTENCE OF ANTIMICROBIAL RESISTANCE", *Natural Resource Modeling*, Vol. 25/2, pp. 388-402, http://dx.doi.org/10.1111/j.1939-7445.2011.00114.x. [24]

Karanika, S. et al. (2016), "Systematic Review and Meta-analysis of Clinical and Economic Outcomes from the Implementation of Hospital-Based Antimicrobial Stewardship Programs", *Antimicrobial Agents and Chemotherapy*, Vol. 60/8, pp. 4840-4852, http://dx.doi.org/10.1128/AAC.00825-16. [15]

Kilpatrick, C., B. Allegranzi and D. Pittet (2011), "WHO First Global Patient Safety Challenge: Clean Care is Safer Care, Contributing to the training of health-care workers around the globe", *International Journal of Infection Control*, Vol. 7/2, http://dx.doi.org/10.3396/ijic.v7i2.011.11. [9]

Kirkland, K. et al. (2012), "Impact of a hospital-wide hand hygiene initiative on healthcare-associated infections: results of an interrupted time series", *BMJ Quality & Safety*, Vol. 21/12, pp. 1019-1026, http://dx.doi.org/10.1136/bmjqs-2012-000800. [6]

Luangasanatip, N. et al. (2015), "Comparative efficacy of interventions to promote hand hygiene in hospital: systematic review and network meta-analysis", *BMJ*, p. h3728, http://dx.doi.org/10.1136/bmj.h3728. [13]

Oberjé, E., M. Tanke and P. Jeurissen (2016), *Cost-Effectiveness of Policies to Limit Antimicrobial Resistance in Dutch Healthcare Organisations*, http://celsustalma.nl/images/Publicaties/AMR_finalreport_celsusacademie.pdf. [33]

Oppong, R. et al. (2013), "Cost-effectiveness of point-of-care C-reactive protein testing to inform antibiotic prescribing decisions", *British Journal of General Practice*, Vol. 63/612, pp. e465-e471, http://dx.doi.org/10.3399/bjgp13X669185. [28]

Otter, J. et al. (2013), "Evidence that contaminated surfaces contribute to the transmission of hospital pathogens and an overview of strategies to address contaminated surfaces in hospital settings", *American Journal of Infection Control*, Vol. 41/5 Suppl, pp. S6-11, http://dx.doi.org/10.1016/j.ajic.2012.12.004. [17]

Pittet, D. et al. (2004), "Hand Hygiene among Physicians: Performance, Beliefs, and Perceptions", *Annals of Internal Medicine*, Vol. 141/1, p. 1, http://dx.doi.org/10.7326/0003-4819-141-1-200407060-00008. [8]

Ranji, S. et al. (2008), "Interventions to reduce unnecessary antibiotic prescribing: a systematic review and quantitative analysis", *Medical Care*, Vol. 46/8, pp. 847-862, http://dx.doi.org/10.1097/MLR.0b013e318178eabd. [22]

Spurling, G. et al. (2013), "Delayed antibiotics for respiratory infections", *Cochrane database of systematic reviews* 4, p. CD004417, http://dx.doi.org/10.1002/14651858.CD004417.pub4. [21]

Stone, S. et al. (2012), "Evaluation of the national Cleanyourhands campaign to reduce Staphylococcus aureus bacteraemia and Clostridium difficile infection in hospitals in England and Wales by improved hand hygiene: four year, prospective, ecological, interrupted time series study", *BMJ*, Vol. 344/may03 2, pp. e3005-e3005, http://dx.doi.org/10.1136/bmj.e3005. [10]

Thoolen, B., D. de Ridder and G. van Lensvelt-Mulders (2012), "Patient-oriented interventions to improve antibiotic prescribing practices in respiratory tract infections: a meta-analysis", *Health Psychology Review*, Vol. 6/1, pp. 92-112, http://dx.doi.org/10.1080/17437199.2011.552061. [26]

Tonkin-Crine, S. et al. (2017), "Clinician-targeted interventions to influence antibiotic prescribing behaviour for acute respiratory infections in primary care: an overview of systematic reviews", *Cochrane Database of Systematic Reviews* 9, http://dx.doi.org/10.1002/14651858.CD012252.pub2. [27]

Weber, D., D. Anderson and W. Rutala (2013), "The role of the surface environment in healthcare-associated infections", *Current Opinion in Infectious Diseases*, Vol. 26/4, pp. 338-344, http://dx.doi.org/10.1097/QCO.0b013e3283630f04. [18]

Weinstein, M. and W. Stason (1977), "Foundations of Cost-Effectiveness Analysis for Health and Medical Practices", *New England Journal of Medicine*, Vol. 296/13, pp. 716-721, http://dx.doi.org/10.1056/NEJM197703312961304. [1]

WHO (2009), *WHO Guidelines on Hand Hygiene in Health Care First Global Patient Safety Challenge Clean Care is Safer Care*, http://apps.who.int/iris/bitstream/handle/10665/44102/9789241597906_eng.pdf;jsessionid=10F615F176A54EDDA23F6BB2F77EB29B?sequence=1 (accessed on 17 October 2018). [34]

WHO (2003), *Making Choices in Health: WHO Guide to Cost-Effectiveness Analysis*, World Health Organization, http://www.who.int/choice/publications/p_2003_generalised_cea.pdf (accessed on 4 October 2018). [4]

Annex 6.A. Sensitivity analysis of cost-effectiveness profiles

Annex Figure 6.A.1 presents the probability of cost-effectiveness of interventions relative to the business as usual scenario under the assumption of 80% elasticity between the effect of the intervention on consumption and its impact on incidence of AMR. In the main analysis, the model operates under the assumption of 100% elasticity.

Annex Figure 6.A.2 presents the probability of cost-effectiveness of interventions relative the business as usual scenario under the assumption of 50% adherence to implemented interventions. In the main analysis that assumption is of 70%.

Annex Figure 6.A.1. Probability of cost-effectiveness of interventions vs. business as usual – 80% elasticity scenario between consumption of antimicrobials and AMR rates

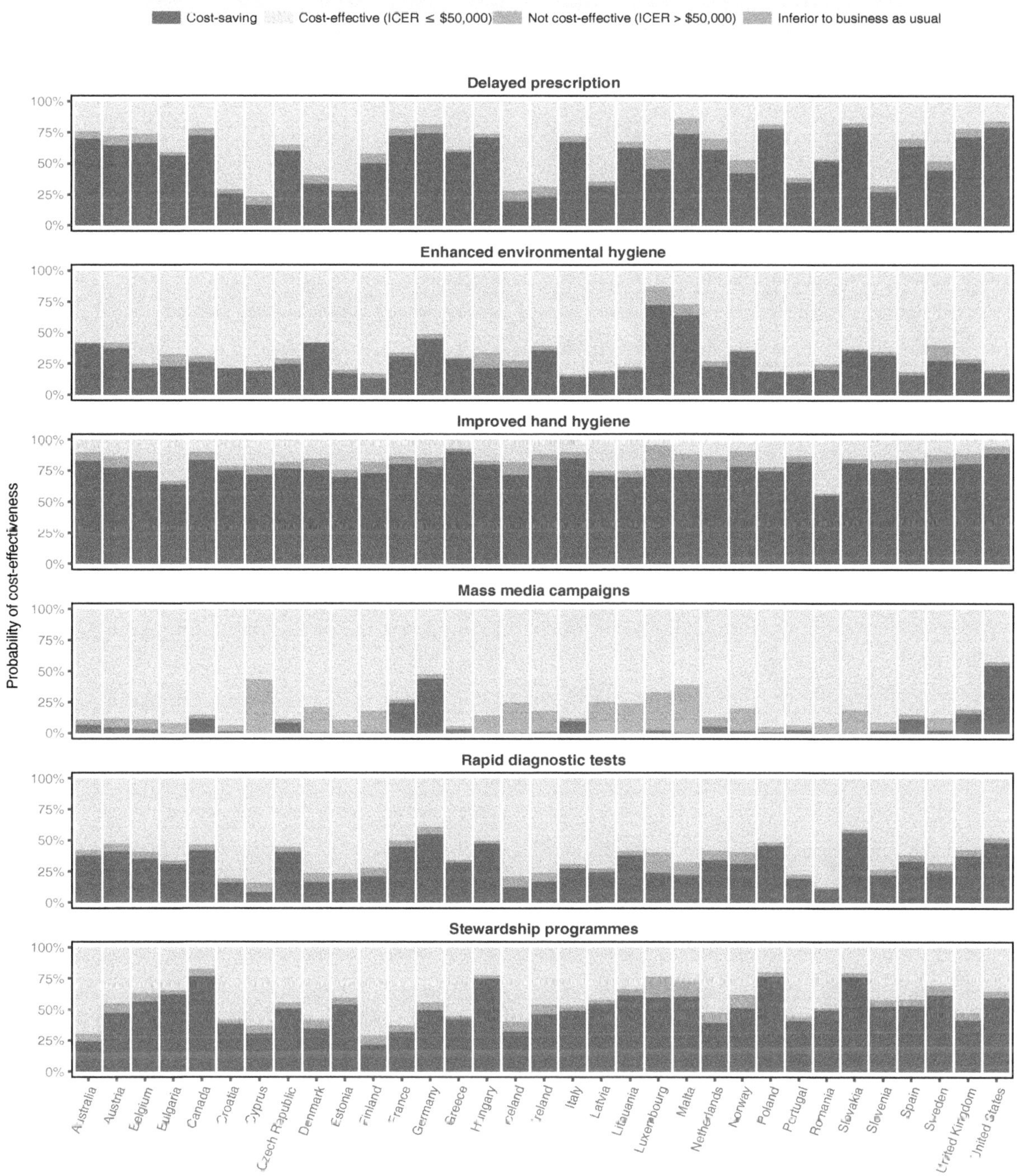

StatLink http://dx.doi.org/10.1787/888933854611

Annex Figure 6.A.2. Cost-effectiveness profile under a 50% intervention adherence scenario

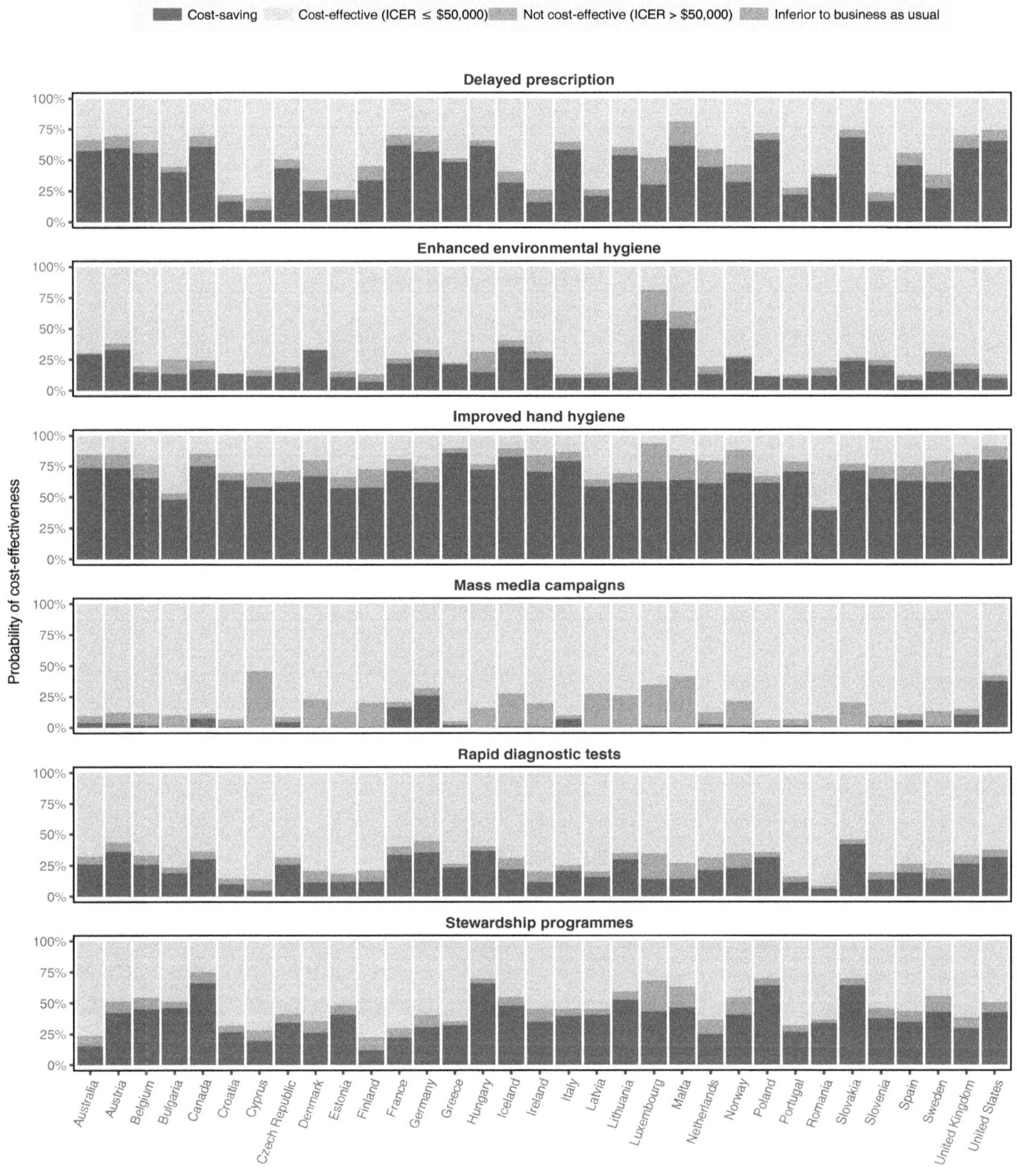

StatLink http://dx.doi.org/10.1787/888933854630

ORGANISATION FOR ECONOMIC CO-OPERATION AND DEVELOPMENT

The OECD is a unique forum where governments work together to address the economic, social and environmental challenges of globalisation. The OECD is also at the forefront of efforts to understand and to help governments respond to new developments and concerns, such as corporate governance, the information economy and the challenges of an ageing population. The Organisation provides a setting where governments can compare policy experiences, seek answers to common problems, identify good practice and work to co-ordinate domestic and international policies.

The OECD member countries are: Australia, Austria, Belgium, Canada, Chile, the Czech Republic, Denmark, Estonia, Finland, France, Germany, Greece, Hungary, Iceland, Ireland, Israel, Italy, Japan, Korea, Latvia, Lithuania, Luxembourg, Mexico, the Netherlands, New Zealand, Norway, Poland, Portugal, the Slovak Republic, Slovenia, Spain, Sweden, Switzerland, Turkey, the United Kingdom and the United States. The European Union takes part in the work of the OECD.

OECD Publishing disseminates widely the results of the Organisation's statistics gathering and research on economic, social and environmental issues, as well as the conventions, guidelines and standards agreed by its members.

OECD PUBLISHING, 2, rue André-Pascal, 75775 PARIS CEDEX 16
(81 2018 80 1 P) ISBN 978-92-64-30758-2 – 2018

www.ingramcontent.com/pod-product-compliance
Ingram Content Group UK Ltd.
Pitfield, Milton Keynes, MK11 3LW, UK
UKHW051500290926
15471UKWH00008B/1330

9 789264 307582